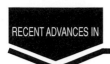

Paediatrics

Edited by

T. J. David MD PhD FRCP DCH

Professor, and Head, Department of Child Health, University of Manchester;
Honorary Consultant Paediatrician, Booth Hall Children's Hospital,
Royal Manchester Children's Hospital and St Mary's Hospital, Manchester, UK

NUMBER FIFTEEN

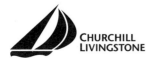

CHURCHILL
LIVINGSTONE

NEW YORK EDINBURGH LONDON MADRID MELBOURNE SAN FRANCISCO AND TOKYO 1997

CHURCHILL LIVINGSTONE
Medical Division of Pearson Professional Limited
Distributed in the United States of America by Churchill
Livingstone Inc., 650 Avenue of the Americas, New York,
N.Y. 10011, and by associated companies, branches and
representatives throughout the world.

First published 1997

ISBN 0 443 05849–0
ISSN 0 309 0140

British Library Cataloguing in Publication Data
A catalogue record for this book is available from the British
Library.

Library of Congress Cataloging in Publication Data
A catalog record for this book is available from the Library of
Congress.

Medical knowledge is constantly changing. As new information becomes available, changes in treatment, procedures,
equipment and the use of drugs become necessary. The
editors and the publishers have, as far as it is possible, taken
care to ensure that the information given in this text is accurate and up to date. However, readers are strongly advised to
confirm that the information, especially with regard to drug
usage, complies with current legislation and standards of
practice.

Typeset by B. A. & G. M. Haddock, Scotland, UK
Printed by Bell & Bain, Scotland, UK

RECENT ADVANCES IN

Paediatrics

Contents of *Recent Advances in Paediatrics 14*
Edited by T. J. David

ISBN 0 443 05308–1
ISSN 0 309 0140

You can place your order by contacting your local medical bookseller or the Sales Promotion Department, Churchill Livingstone, Robert Stevenson House, 1–3 Baxter's Place, Leith Walk, Edinburgh EH1 3AF, UK. Tel: +44 (0)131 556 2424; Fax: +44 (0)131 558 1278

Contents

Preface

The aim of *Recent Advances in Paediatrics* is to provide a review of important topics and help doctors keep abreast of developments in the subject. The book is intended for the practising clinician and the postgraduate student. The book is sold very widely in Britain, Europe, North America and Asia, and the contents and authorship are selected with this very broad readership in mind. There are 12 chapters which cover a variety of general paediatric, neonatal and community paediatric areas. As usual, the selection of topics has veered towards those of general rather than special interest.

The final chapter, an annotated literature review, is a personal selection of key articles and useful reviews published in 1995. Comment about a paper is sometimes as important as the original article, so when a paper has been followed by interesting or important correspondence this is also referred to. As with the choice of subjects for the main chapters, the selection of articles has inclined towards those of general rather than special interest. There is, however, special emphasis on community paediatrics and medicine in the tropics, as these two important areas tend to be less well covered in general paediatric journals. Trying to reduce to an acceptable size the short-list of particularly interesting articles is an especially difficult task. Each topic in the literature review section is indexed and the page number is followed by an asterisk. Therefore selected publications on (for example) vitamin A can be easily identified, as can any parts of the book that dwell on the topic.

Annual publication of this book provides the opportunity to respond to the wishes of readers, and any suggestions for topics to be included in future issues would always be welcome. Please write to me at the address below.

I am indebted to the authors for their hard work, prompt delivery of manuscripts and patience in dealing with my queries and requests. I would also like to thank my secretaries Angela Smithies, Pauline Mitchell and Val Smith, and Gill Haddock of Churchill Livingstone for all their help, and my wife and sons for all their support.

Professor T. J. David
University Department of Child Health
Booth Hall Children's Hospital
Manchester M9 7AA, UK

1997

Contributors

Linda Brown PhD RN FAAN
Associate Professor and Chair, Health Care of Women and Child-bearing Families Division, University of Pennsylvania, Pennsylvania, USA

Natasha S. Crowcroft MA MRCP MSc MFHPM
Epidemiology Section, Institute of Hygiene and Epidemiology, Brussels, Belgium

Nigel Curtis MA MRCP DTM&H
MRC Clinician Scientist, Paediatric Infectious Diseases Unit, Department of Paediatrics, Imperial College School of Medicine at St Mary's Hospital, London, UK

T. J. David MD PhD FRCP DCH
Professor and Head, Department of Child Health, University of Manchester; Honorary Consultant Paediatrician, Booth Hall Children's Hospital, Royal Manchester Children's Hospital and St Mary's Hospital, Manchester, UK

M. D. C. Donaldson MB ChB MRCP DCH
Senior Lecturer in Child Health, Royal Hospital for Sick Children, Glasgow, UK

A. D. Edwards MA FRCP
Weston Professor of Neonatal Medicine, Department of Paediatrics and Neonatal Medicine, Royal Postgraduate Medical School, Hammersmith Hospital, London, UK

D. B. Grant MD FRCP DCH
Honorary Consultant in Paediatric Endocrinology, The Great Ormond Street Hospital for Children NHS Trust, London, UK

Peter Hill MA MB BChir MRCP MRCPysch
Professor of Child and Adolescent Psychiatry, Department of Mental Health, St George's Hospital Medical School, London, UK

Louis I. Landau MD FRACP
Professor of Paediatrics, University of Western Australia, Perth, Australia

Michael Levin FRCP PhD
Professor of Paediatrics, Paediatric Infectious Diseases Unit, Department of Paediatrics, Imperial College School of Medicine at St Mary's Hospital, London, UK

Paula Meier RN DNSc FAAN
NICU Location Program Director and Director of Clinical Research, Section of
Neonatology, Rush-Presbyterian St Luke's Medical Center, Chicago, Illinois, USA

R. H. Mupanemunda BSc BM MRCP
Consultant in Neonatal Medicine, Princess of Wales Maternity Unit, Birmingham
Heartlands Hospital NHS Trust, Birmingham, UK

Michael B. O'Neill MD DCH FRCPC MHSA
Chief of Pediatrics, St Joseph's Hospital, Hamilton, Ontario, Canada

Nancy F. Olivieri MD
Division of Haematology, The Hospital for Sick Children, Toronto, Canada

Marlene Rabinovitch MD FRCPS(C) FAAC
Professor of Pediatrics, Pathology and Medicine, University of Toronto, Director of
Cardiovascular Research, The Hospital for Sick Children, Toronto, Ontario,
Canada

Mike P. Rothera FRCS
Consultant in Otolaryngology — Head and Neck Surgery, The Royal Manchester
Children's Hospital, Manchester, UK

J. A. Walker-Smith MD FRCP (Ed & Lond) FRACP
University Department of Paediatric Gastroenterology, The Royal Free Hospital,
London, UK

T. J. Woolford FRCS
Senior Registrar in Otolaryngology — Head and Neck Surgery, ENT Department,
Manchester Royal Infirmary, Manchester, UK

1

Bronchiolitis

L. I. Landau

Bronchiolitis is a syndrome recognised by the clinical features of hyper-inflation and wheeze with fine inspiratory crackles heard on auscultation of the chest. It occurs predominantly during the first year of life and during the winter months. It is usually the result of infection with the respiratory syncytial virus (RSV), although other viruses such as parainfluenza and adenovirus as well as Chlamydia can give a similar picture. Infants with cystic fibrosis, congenital heart disease or chronic neonatal lung disease (bronchopulmonary dysplasia) are particularly disadvantaged as they will develop a more severe form of bronchiolitis on exposure to these viruses. Similarly, infants in developing countries acquire a pattern of disease which may be different in relation to clinical severity, bacterial infection and response to drugs. The reasons for this difference are unknown although they may be related to the intensity of virus replication, associated bacterial colonisation, the age of infection or the nutritional and immunological status of the infant.

Wheezing lower respiratory illnesses are common during infancy. Approximately 1 in 3 infants will wheeze during the first year of life.[1] Between 5–10% of infants will be given a clinical diagnosis of bronchiolitis of whom 1 in 10 will be admitted to hospital. Those who develop wheezing illnesses are likely to be predisposed as a result of small airway calibre associated with male gender, preterm delivery, maternal cigarette smoking and a family history of asthma[3,4] as well as environmental factors associated with increased risk of viral infections such as lower socio-economical status, increased number of siblings, day care and non-breastfeeding.[2]

EPIDEMIOLOGY

RSV causes annual epidemics of respiratory disease each year during which a large proportion of the population will develop a respiratory tract infection with more than 50% of infants being infected. Almost all infants will have been infected by the virus after their second winter and many will have experienced two infections during these winters.[6]

RSV is an RNA virus first isolated from a chimpanzee in 1956 when it was called the 'chimpanzee coryza virus'. Two major subgroups of RSV, A and B, have been identified and these have been subdivided into 6 and 3 subgroups, respectively. During an epidemic, many different serotypes tend to co-circulate.[7] Strain variation is associated with differences in the F or fusion glycoprotein and G or attachment glycoprotein. The host may be re-infected by different strains or by the same strain. The reasons for re-infection by the same strain are not known but may be related to inaccurate recognition of the epitopes, impaired induction of an effective immune response or effective suppression of the immune response by the virus once re-infection has occurred through its ability to infect macrophages and lymphocytes and impair interferon production, IL-1 inhibitors and ICAM1.

RSV infection causes direct epithelial damage with inflammation involving predominantly neutrophils but also cytotoxic T cells. The role of these T cells is uncertain as some feel they are important for recovery while others argue they may contribute to the continuing problems following infection. There is associated sensitization of the cholinergic nerve fibre ends and diminished β-adrenergic function.

Based on the observation that the illness had occurred at an age when passively acquired antibody levels were generally high and that vaccination with a killed RSV vaccine had increased morbidity and mortality on exposure to the natural virus, it was proposed that the condition may result from an immune complex reaction between virus and antibodies. However, complement consumption and immune complexes have not been demonstrated and there is a tendency for high maternal antibody levels to confer some degree of protection.

Some have argued that bronchiolitis is more likely to occur in those with atopy and a family history of asthma although this observation has not been consistent. Welliver and colleagues[8] suggested that infants acquiring RSV infection produced RSV-specific IgE which was associated with more severe acute illness, histamine release in nasal secretions and persistent wheezing. However, the long term follow up of this population could not show any association between the levels of RSV-specific IgE and subsequent lower respiratory illness. There are now several good studies showing that atopy is not an important predisposing factor to an acute viral bronchiolitis.[9]

In a prospective cohort study, Young and colleagues[10] demonstrated that those who developed bronchiolitis in the first year of life had evidence of pre-existing lower respiratory symptoms and reduced airway calibre before the bronchiolitis. Those who developed symptoms diagnosed as bronchiolitis in the second year tended to be atopic and to be part of asthma spectrum (Fig. 1.1). Those with bronchiolitis are more likely to be admitted to hospital if exposed to maternal cigarette smoke during pregnancy and postnatally.

CLINICAL PRESENTATION

Acute viral bronchiolitis usually commences with a mild fever and upper respiratory symptoms such as coryza which progresses over 2–3 days to cough and tachypnoea. Wheeze may be present. On examination, the infant will

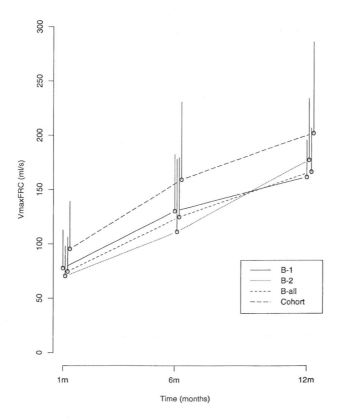

Fig. 1.1 Analysis of a prospective cohort study of patients who developed bronchiolitis in the first year of life. Abbreviations: V_{max}FRC, (mean, SD) during the first year of life; B-1, bronchiolitis during the first year; B-2, bronchiolitis during the second year; B-all, bronchiolitis during the first or second years; Cohort, children followed who did not develop bronchiolitis. Reproduced with the permission of the BMJ Publishing Group from Young et al.[10]

have hyperinflation of the chest, subcostal recession and widespread bilateral inspiratory crackles on auscultation. With progression, difficulty with feeding may develop. A chest radiograph is usually not necessary but, if obtained, will show evidence of hyperinflation and, in approximately 10% of cases, pulmonary parenchymal infiltrates or atelectasis.

The diagnosis is essentially clinical, but can be supported by identification of RSV or other respiratory viruses using immunofluorescent antibody methods. Oximetry provides a useful guide to severity and blood gases may be required in younger and smaller infants or in those with pre-existing abnormalities who are more likely to progress to respiratory failure.

Apnoea has been documented in up to 15% of infants with bronchiolitis. The mechanism responsible for apnoea is not clear but it tends to resolve within a few days. Apnoea monitors may be necessary in those demonstrating

Table 1.1 Evaluation of severity of acute bronchiolitis and likely treatment*

	Probable home management	Probable hospital management	Definite hospital management
Toxicity	Absent	Absent	Present
Physical exhaustion	No	No	Yes
Cyanosis	Absent	Absent	Present
Use of accessory muscles	Absent	Absent	Marked
Lower costal and sternal retraction	Absent	Absent	Marked
Wheeze	Mild	Present	Present
Crepititions	Occasional	Widespread	Widespread
Feeding	Well	Slowly	Poorly
Apnoea	Absent	Absent	Present
Oximetry (SaO$_2$)	> 95%	91–95%	< 91%
Psychological factors	Absent	May be present	Present

*Adapted from[34].

this phenomenon. It is more likely to develop in those born preterm and those with pre-existing lung disease. Artificial ventilation may be necessary on occasion for the apnoea.

MANAGEMENT

Monitoring for apnoea, hypoxia and exhaustion, supplemental oxygen to prevent hypoxia, appropriate provision of feeds and fluids and minimal handling are the only proven efficacious interventions in the management of infants with bronchiolitis. Criteria to use in evaluation of severity and likely treatment are shown in Table 1.1. Those who do progress to respiratory failure, usually those with pre-existing abnormalities, will require assisted ventilation. Some have reported a reduction in the need for assisted ventilation with nasal continuous positive airway pressure. Antibiotics are rarely needed as secondary bacterial infection is uncommon. However, infection with *Chlamydia* and other bacteria may be present and it is reasonable to use antibiotics in those who are particularly ill or those with atypical features. They are also used in developing countries were co-infection with bacteria appears to be a greater problem.

Failure to maintain adequate oxygenation in room air will require supplemental oxygen, usually delivered via a headbox. Occasionally, additional oxygen using nasal cannulae may be necessary.

Poor fluid intake associated with respiratory distress may require intravenous fluids. Some will use nasogastric feeding but others feel that the presence of a nasogastric tube through the nostrils blocks the airway sufficiently to cause increased work of breathing and filling the stomach may predispose to vomiting and aspiration. Inappropriate antidiuretic hormone may be present with more severe disease and justifies restricting fluids to about two-thirds maintenance in those in whom it is suspected.[11]

Studies reporting the role of bronchodilators in the management of bronchiolitis are conflicting. Most showed no benefit or minimal effect of doubtful clinical significance, although some report significant responses. If the definition is restricted to that group who commonly develop the illness between 1–4 months, then little response is documented. Those that showed benefit usually included older infants and outcome measures which were not an objective assessment of clinical status.

A number of studies have failed to show any benefit from the use of β_2-agonists.[12] Ho and colleagues[13] and Hughes and colleagues[14] have shown deterioration following nebulization of β_2-agonists. Inhalation of β_2-agonists does alter breathing patterns and may contribute to a subjective impression of improvement. Measures of airway resistance may fall due to a non-specific effect of the bronchodilator. However, measures of forced expiratory flow and oxygen saturation rarely show significant improvement. A therapeutic trial of bronchodilator may be considered in those over 6 months of age with troublesome wheeze in view of the reported response.[15,16]

Studies have failed to show any significant benefit from corticosteroid administration.[17] It was reported that a combination of β_2-agonist and steroid was more beneficial than either alone leading to a decrease in hospitalisation.[18] However, numbers were small and this observation has not been confirmed.

Ipratropium bromide was originally reported to produce improvement in respiratory mechanics but subsequent studies demonstrated no significant benefit and alteration to the course of the condition in hospital.[19] Theophylline therapy has been tried and appears of little benefit except for its respiratory stimulation in those with apneic episodes.

Adrenaline (epinephrine) was though to be more likely to be beneficial due to its vasoconstrictive and anti-oedema activity. Some have reported a greater decrease in respiratory rate and pulmonary resistance and decreased admission to hospital following nebulised epinephrine.[20] However, other studies of lung function and oxygen saturation have failed to demonstrate any benefit.[21]

Ribavirin is a virustatic agent widely used, particularly in the US, but more recent analyses have raised questions regarding its cost effectiveness. Ribavirin is administered as an aerosol produced by a small particle aerosol generator (SPAG) into a headbox for up to 18 h a day. It has been used in ventilator circuits, but there is a tendency for valves to become blocked by drug crystals. Although not incorporated into host RNA or DNA, absorption of Ribavirin by hospital personnel leading to teratogenic effects has been a concern so that exposure by pregnant women has been avoided. Side effects

include skin rashes and mild bronchospasm. Early studies suggested a clinically significant response in all but the mildest cases. However, subsequent
review of the data has shown little effect on morbidity and duration of stay.[22]
The American Academy of Pediatrics initially recommended that Ribavirin
be considered in those at high risk of severe disease which included preterm
infants, those with underlying disorders (e.g. cystic fibrosis, chronic neonatal
lung disease) and those severely ill.[23] Subsequent observations noted that
improvements in supportive therapy played a greater role in decreasing morbidity than Ribavirin. It was subsequently suggested that it be used in those
who required mechanical ventilation. However, conflicting results have again
been reported in this group and its role has yet to be determined.[24] Ribavirin
should probably be used in extremely ill infants and those who are immuno-
suppressed, although data supporting this approach are still limited.

The use of intravenous immunoglobulins has also been reported to lead to
a more rapid improvement in oxygenation and reduced length of hospitalisation, although the results are not dramatic.[25] A reduced rate of hospitalization
has been reported when given prophylactically to high risk infants.[26] The
clinical role of intravenous immunoglobulin remains uncertain. Studies are
currently being undertaken to determine the role of high titre anti-RSV antibody immunoglobulin. Monoclonal antibodies against the F glycoprotein
have been shown to be effective in animal models and this may be of value in
infants.[27]

Interferon-α was considered to have significant potential in bronchiolitis
but clinical benefit has not been demonstrated.[28]

RSV is particularly infectious and nosocomial infection is common.
Spread of infection is via large droplets or fomites. Droplets are transmitted
to hands and then to the respiratory tract. Survival of the virus on the hands
is generally short lived but, on occasions, it has been shown to be more than
24 h. Shedding of the virus in hospitalised infants continues for up to 3
weeks. Thus infants remain a potential source of nosocomial infection.
Careful attention to hand washing and cohorting of infants with RSV infection significantly reduces the incidence of nosocomial infection due to RSV.[29]

PROGNOSIS

The prognosis for most infants with acute viral bronchiolitis is excellent with
mortality rate less than 1% of those admitted to hospital. Mortality is
extremely rare in previously well children, but still does occur at a significant
rate in those with pre-existing abnormality such as congenital heart disease,
chronic neonatal lung disease or cystic fibrosis.[30]

The long term outcome and its significance remains controversial. Much
depends on the criteria for defining bronchiolitis as this has a significant
influence on the proportion of infants who develop recurrent wheezing, airway hyper-responsiveness, asthma or persisting abnormalities of lung function. Many studies are hospital based while others are community based;

some restrict their cohort to those with proven RSV infection; some limit the range to the first 12 months, while others extend this throughout infancy. All studies report increased lower respiratory symptoms in those who have had bronchiolitis compared with those who have not. Long term prospective studies of children admitted to hospital with RSV-positive bronchiolitis have shown that approximately 75% will experience wheezing in the 2 years following the initial illness, more than 50% still wheeze 3 years later and approximately 40% continue to wheeze after 5 years.[31] Some argue that those more likely to wheeze were children born to parents with a history of atopy, however others found that atopy in the family was not a significant risk factor for bronchiolitis.[31] Personal atopy was more prevalent in those symptomatic after bronchiolitis.

Murray et al.[31] found an increased incidence of bronchial hyper-responsiveness to chemical mediator after bronchiolitis, confirming previous studies suggesting 60–80% of infants will demonstrate bronchial hyper-responsiveness. However, they found that few of the patients with bronchial hyper-responsiveness had troublesome symptoms and that bronchial hyper-responsiveness did not correlate with wheezing.

McConnochie and Roghmann[32] evaluated children 7–8 years after bronchiolitis managed in a community based paediatric practice. Upper respiratory allergy, bronchiolitis and passive smoke exposure were significantly related to subsequent wheezing but bronchiolitis accounted for only 1% of the risk for subsequent wheezing.

Welliver and colleagues collected nasal secretions from infants with documented RSV infection and found that those with bronchiolitis and pneumonia who also wheezed had higher titres of RSV-specific IgE antibody in their nasal secretions. This group also had greater concentrations of histamine in their nasal secretions and lower arterial oxygen saturations. In the next 2 years, over 70% of those will high IgE antibody titres experienced wheezing compared with 20% of those with undetectable titres. However, 7–8 years later, abnormalities of respiratory function and airway reactivity were related to atopy and passive cigarette smoke exposure and not RSV-specific IgE response.[8]

Young et al.[10] found that infants who developed bronchiolitis in the first year of life had evidence of pre-existing small airways suggesting that those who develop bronchiolitis have pre-existing abnormalities of airway calibre which is likely to cause recurrent wheezing through the early years of life, but not necessarily persisting into later childhood. Certainly, some of these will have asthma and will continue to have recurrent wheeze throughout life.

CONCLUSIONS

With an increased understanding of the natural history of bronchiolitis, we are able to better aim to reduce the incidence and morbidity associated with this common condition. Reducing maternal smoking will decrease the risk for severe bronchiolitis. For 30 years, attempts have been made to introduce a vaccine to prevent significant RSV lower respiratory illness. Trials in the 1960s with inactivated virus found excess morbidity and mortality in immunised children subsequently exposed to wild virus.[33] The explanation for this problem remains elusive, although the complex humoral response to infection appears important. The vaccines clearly failed to generate adequate antibody levels to the important glycoproteins. Attempts to produce live attenuated vaccines to be administered topically to the respiratory tract have not been particularly successful due to failure to replicate or reversion to pathogenic strains. Newer preparations are currently being tested. Recently, attempts to produce subunit vaccines appear to have been more successful and are under trial at present.

KEY POINTS FOR CLINICAL PRACTICE

1. Wheezing lower respiratory illnesses in infancy are common. They occur in approximately 30% of infants and 25% of these will present a picture of acute viral bronchiolitis. Two-thirds will have recurrent wheezing in infancy but cease to have wheezing illnesses after the first year or two.

2. Specific predisposing conditions, such as cystic fibrosis, congenital cardiac abnormalities, chronic neonatal lung disease or milk inhalation may predispose to more severe bronchiolitis.

3. The term bronchiolitis should be reserved for those infants with wheeze, hyperinflation and fine inspiratory crackles in the first year of life. Those with this picture in subsequent years are more likely to be part of the asthma spectrum.

4. Environmental tobacco smoke is a major risk factor for hospitalization with acute viral bronchiolitis. Maternal smoking should be discouraged from early pregnancy.

5. The only effective treatment for acute viral bronchiolitis with respiratory distress is supplemental oxygen with maintenance of adequate hydration.

6. No medications are currently available which significantly affect the natural history of the majority of infants with acute viral bronchiolitis.

7. Nosocomial infection is important and hand washing and cohorting important for reduction of the spread of infection in hospitals.

8. It is likely that an effective vaccine will be developed to prevent RSV bronchiolitis in the future.

REFERENCES

1. Martinez FD, Morgan WJ, Wright AL, Holberg CJ, Taussig LM. Diminished lung function as a predisposing factor for wheezing respiratory illness in infants. N Engl J Med 1988; 319: 112–117
2. Wright A, Holberg C, Martinez F, Morgan WJ, Taussig LM. Breast feeding and lower respiratory tract illness in the first year of life. BMJ 1989; 299: 946–949
3. Ware JH, Dockerty D, Spiro A, Speizer FE, Ferris BG. Passive smoking, gas cooking and respiratory health of children living in six cities. Am Rev Respir Dis 1984; 129: 366–374
4. Tepper R, Morgan W, Cota K, Wright A, Taussig LM. Physiologic growth and development of the lung during the first year. Am Rev Respir Dis 1986; 134: 513–519.
5. Young S, Le Souëf PN, Geelhoed G, Stick SM, Turner KJ, Landau LI. The influence of a family history of asthma and parental smoking on the level of airway responsiveness in infants soon after birth. N Engl J Med 1991; 324: 1168–1173
6. Glazen WP, Taber LN, Frank AL, Kasel JA. Risk of primary infection and reinfection with respiratory syncytial virus. Am J Dis Child 1986; 140: 543–546
7. Anderson LJ, Hendry RM, Pierik LT et al. Multicentre study of strains of respiratory syncytial virus. J Inf Dis 1991; 163: 687–692
8. Welliver RC, Duffy L. The relationship of RSV specific immunoglobulin E antibody responses in infancy, recurrent wheezing and pulmonary function at age 7–8 years. Pediatr Pulmonol 1993; 15: 19–27
9. Carlsen KH, Larsen S, Bjerve O, Leegaard J. Acute bronchiolitis: predisposing factors and characterisation of infants at risk. Pediatr Pulmonol 1987; 3: 153–160
10. Young S, O'Keeffe PT, Arnott J, Landau LI. Infant lung function, airway responsiveness, atopic status and respiratory symptoms before and after bronchiolitis. Arch Dis Child 1995; 72: 16–24
11. Van Steensel-Moll NA, Hazelet JA, Van der Voort E et al. Excessive secretion of antidiuretic hormone in infections with respiratory syncytial virus. Arch Dis Child 1990; 65: 1237–1239
12 Wang EEL, Milner R, Allen U et al. Bronchodilators for treatment of mild bronchiolitis: a factorial randomised trial. Arch Dis Child 1992; 67: 289–293
13. Ho L, Collis G, Landau LI, Le Souëf PN. Effect of salbutamol on respiratory mechanics in bronchiolitis. Pediatr Res 1987; 22: 83–86
14. Hughes PM, Le Souëf PN, Landau LI. Effect of salbutamol on respiratory mechanics in bronchiolitis. Pediatr Res 1987; 22: 83–86
15. Schuh S, Canny G, Reisman JJ et al. Nebulised albuterol in acute bronchiolitis. J Pediatr 1990; 117: 663–667
16. Gadomski AM, Lichtenstein R, Horton L et al. Efficacy of albuterol in wheezing infants. Pediatrics 1994; 93: 907–912
17. Springer C, Bar Yishay E, Vwayyed K et al. Corticosteroids do not affect the clinical or physiological status of infants with bronchiolitis. Pediatr Pulmonol 1990; 9: 181–185
18. Tal R, Bavilski C, Yohai O et al. Dexamethasone and salbutamol in the treatment of acute wheezing in infants. Pediatrics 1983; 71: 13–18
19. Henry RL, Milner AD, Stokes EM. Ineffectiveness of ipratropium bromide in acute bronchiolitis. Arch Dis Child 1983; 58: 925–926
20. Menon K, Sutcliffe T, Klassen TP. A randomised trial comparing the efficacy of epinephrine with salbutamol in the treatment of acute bronchiolitis. J Pediatr 1995; 126: 1004–1007
21. Henderson AJW, Arnott J, Young S et al. The effect of inhaled adrenaline on lung function of recurrently wheezy infants less than 18 months old. Pediatr Pulmonol 1995; 20: 9–15
22. Isaacs D, Moxon ER, Harvey D et al. Ribavirin in respiratory syncytial virus infection. A double blind placebo controlled trial is needed. Arch Dis Child 1988; 63: 986–990
23. American Academy of Pediatrics Committee on Infections Disease. Ribavirin therapy of respiratory syncytial virus. Pediatrics 1987; 79: 475–478
24. Krafte-Jacobs B, Holbrook PR. Ribavirin in severe respiratory syncytial virus infection. Crit Care Med 1994; 22: 541–543
25. Hemming VE, Rodriguez W, Kim HW et al. Intravenous immunoglobulin treatment of respiratory syncytial virus infections in infants and young children. Antimicrob Agents Chemother 1987; 31: 1882–1886
26. Groothius JR, Simoes EAF, Levin MJ et al. Prophylactic administration of respiratory

syncytial virus immune globulin to high risk infants and young children. N Engl J Med 1993; 329: 1524–1530

27. Levin MJ. Treatment and prevention options for respiratory syncytial virus infections. J Pediatr 1994; 124: 522–527
28. Chipps BE, Sullivan WF, Portnoy JM. Alpha 2A interferon for treatment of bronchiolitis caused by respiratory syncytial virus. Pediatr Inf Dis J 1993; 12: 653–658
29. Isaacs D, Dickson H, O'Callaghan C et al. Handwashing and cohorting in prevention of hospital acquired infections with respiratory syncytial virus. Arch Dis Child 1991; 66: 227–231
30. Wang EEL, Lau BJ, Stephens D et al. Pediatric Investigators Collaborative Network on Infections in Canada (PICNIC) prospective study of risk factors and outcomes in patients hospitalized with respiratory syncytial viral lower respiratory tract infection. J Pediatr 1995; 126: 212–219
31. Murray M, Webb MSC, O'Callaghan C. Respiratory status and allergy after bronchiolitis. Arch Dis Child 1992; 67: 482–487
32. McConnochie K, Roghmann K. Bronchiolitis as a possible cause of wheezing in childhood; new evidence. Pediatrics 1984; 74: 1–10
33. Kim HW, Canchola JE, Brandt CD et al. Respiratory syncytial virus disease in infants despite prior administration of antigenic inactivated virus. Am J Epidemiol 1969; 89: 422–434
34. Dawson K, Kennedy D, Asher I et al. Consensus view: the management of acute bronchiolitis. J Pediatr Child Health 1993; 29: 335–337

Triangles	Copies
⭕ 2	$2\frac{1}{2}$.
✚ 3	$3\frac{1}{2}$
◻ 4	$4\frac{1}{2}$.
△ ($4\frac{3}{4}$.	$5\frac{1}{4}$)
◇	

	M	FM/A.	S+L.	S rse he
8/52	S head control	fixingr following	smiling	responsiv
9/12	sitting ~~crawling~~ getting around	palmar gasp hold 2 cubes	2 syllable babble	finger feed stranger anx
18/12	walking	pincer grasp 3 bricks scribbling	few words	spoon. cup. imaginative play with mom symbolic play
3	walking up r down stairs	drawing ~~square~~ circle. cross. bridge -	sentences whats happened	play with other dress - help.
4	Running Jumping	imitates square bridges with blocks	details prepositions	

2

Identification and management of large airway disease in the first year of life

M. P. Rothera   T. J. Woolford

In the first year of life, small changes in the diameter of the larynx and trachea can cause a considerable increase in airflow resistance. By the time stridor becomes apparent, a significant proportion of the airway lumen has already been lost and even minor changes can precipitate respiratory obstruction.

There is a wide spectrum of pathology which can embarrass the airway of a neonate. Stridor is the presenting feature. The character, severity and timing all provide important information but associated symptoms of coughing, choking, feeding difficulties and apnoea all contribute to the diagnosis. Assessing the severity of the obstruction is not always easy but has an important influence on the time scale for investigation and treatment.

PATHOPHYSIOLOGY

The infant larynx is approximately one-third of its adult size and is significantly higher in relation to the hyoid and tongue base than in the older child. This may help separate feeding and respiration during suckling, but tongue enlargement and posterior tongue position secondary to micrognathia can result in oropharyngeal obstruction. Some of the most difficult airways to protect at birth are found in children with the Pierre Robin or the Treacher Collins syndrome.

The infant epiglottis is softer and relatively more bulky than the adult. Prolapse occurs if there is a pronounced omega configuration with prominent aryepiglottic folds. Laryngomalacia is possibly the commonest cause of noisy breathing in neonates. However, it is important to recognise that all inspiratory stridor is not due this condition. Other causes of laryngeal obstruction, such as webs, cysts or vocal cord palsies, can produce similar stridor and must be considered.

The laryngeal airway is the narrowest portion of the upper respiratory tract. In adults, the glottis has the smallest cross sectional area, but in neonates the subglottis, with a diameter of 4.5 mm, is the limiting factor. The subglottis is also an unforgiving area of the paediatric airway, being surrounded by the cricoid, the only non distensible complete ring of cartilage in the larynx and trachea. This region is lined by epithelia with a lax sub-mucosa which readily becomes oedematous. If the pressure on the mucosa from an endotracheal

11

Table 2.1 Large airway disease classified according to anatomical divisions

Nasal obstruction	Dislocation of the nasal septum Turbinate hypertrophy Congenital nasal masses Choanal atresia and stenosis
Facial skeletal abnormalities	Micrognathia (Pierre Robin and Treacher Collins syndromes) Apert's syndrome Crouzon's syndrome
Oropharyngeal obstruction	Adeno tonsillar hypertrophy Macroglossia Retropharyngeal abscess Haemangioma of the tongue Cystic hygroma Vallecular cysts
Laryngeal obstruction	Laryngomalacia Acute epiglottitis and croup Post intubation oedema and granulations Subglottic stenosis Unilateral/bilateral vocal cord palsy Supraglottic cysts Juvenile papillomata Laryngeal webs Subglottic haemangioma Laryngo-oesophageal clefts
Tracheal obstruction	Foreign bodies Tracheomalacia Bacterial tracheitis Vascular compression Tracheal stenosis Cardiac enlargement Mediastinal masses
Bronchial obstruction	Bronchomalacia

tube exceeds the perfusion pressure of 40 mmHg, progressive damage occurs. Initially simple oedema develops, followed by mucosal ulceration, perichondritis and eventually scar tissue formation resulting in an acquired subglottic stenosis.

The 19th Century French physician Poiseuille stated that the resistance to flow of a substance of a given density through a tube of a given length was inversely proportional to the 4th power of the radius, i.e. every time the radius is halved, the resistance to flow increases 16 times. Fortunately, the body has been designed with a large degree of biological reserve, and even infants have a much larger airway than is required for normal respiration. Stridor at rest only occurs when 75% of the airway has been lost, but the degree of narrowing needed to convert mild stridor to severe obstruction is minimal. In a neonate, 1 mm of circumferential mucosal swelling reduces the cross sectional area of the subglottis by 60%. Even a minor increase in swelling may therefore precipitate dramatic changes in obstruction.

Oxygen consumption and carbon dioxide production, relative to body weight, may be 2–3 times greater in a baby than in an older child. Infants have a low functional residual capacity and consequently less respiratory reserve. Airway obstruction rapidly leads to hypoxia and hypercarbia. Small children rely predominantly on diaphragmatic breathing rather than inter-costal activity and, as the diaphragm has few type 1 slow twitch muscle fibres, they are prone to fatigue.

Laryngeal neuropathology causing vocal cord paralysis, altered sensation or incoordination of swallowing and respiration may result in aspiration lead-ing to recurrent respiratory tract infections. Most cases are clinically evident, but mild sub-clinical aspiration requires careful evaluation if long term pul-monary damage is to be avoided.

The physiology of the thorax dictates that any obstruction or collapse of the intrathoracic trachea will be accentuated in expiration. Stridor is classi-cally biphasic, but not invariably so. The dynamics of the trachea, a close anatomical relationship with mediastinal vessels and the potential for col-lapse if tracheal rings are weakened, causes a nebulous group of intermittent respiratory symptoms. Coughing, choking, intermittent stridor, occasional cyanosis and failure to thrive are seen, often accompanied by recurrent lower respiratory tract infections. A high level of clinical suspicion is required to ini-tiate the correct investigations if the diagnosis of a vascular compression syn-drome is to be recognised.

SPECTRUM OF PATHOLOGY

From a clinical perspective, a classification based on the anatomical divisions is helpful (see Table 2.1).

PRESENTATION

History

Infants with upper respiratory or tracheal obstruction nearly all present with some degree of noisy breathing, turbulent air flow causing vibrations of the narrowed segment. The age at which the stridor is first noted and the natural history varies with the underlying pathology. Bilateral vocal cord palsies pre-sent with stridor at birth whereas a subglottic haemangioma might present with progressively worsening stridor over several weeks. Some clues to the site of obstruction can be gained from the character and timing of this noise. Nasal obstruction causes a stertorious sound, oropharyngeal obstruction has a snoring quality. Laryngomalacia often sounds rather dramatic, the stridor being disproportionate to the other symptoms and signs of respiratory tract obstruction. Subglottic stenosis typically has a constant level of stridor with predictable changes accompanying increases in activity. Tracheal stridor may have an expiratory component and can vary in intensity, often being quiet at rest but with episodes of more severe obstruction when the child is crying or feeding. The rate of onset, progression and presence of precipitating factors are all important.

Whilst croup has its characteristic cough, intermittent simple recurrent coughing should raise the possibility of aspiration which occurs with neurological problems, tracheo-oesophageal clefts and tracheomalacia. Infective causes of stridor are reasonably straightforward to diagnose, but a retropharyngeal abscess can be surprisingly silent and nearly always occurs within the first year of life.

Cyanosis, which is a late and unreliable indicator of hypoxia, is rare in children with upper respiratory tract obstructions. However tracheomalacia and vascular compression syndromes can cause transient episodes of cyanosis, even progressing to life threatening obstructive apnoea and should be investigated accordingly. There is an associated risk of congenital heart disease with many developmental causes of airway obstruction and episodes of cyanosis should initiate a cardiological opinion. A history of prolonged intubation (with possible subglottic stenosis) and the presence of any symptoms of reflux all contribute to the process of pattern recognition.

Examination

On many occasions there is a history of stridor but no detectable noise when the infant is brought to clinic. Auscultation of the neck as well as the chest should be performed and examination during feeding or crying is helpful to unmask a latent stridor. A cooled silver tongue depressor held below the nostrils to demonstrate a misting pattern is a simple technique for assessing nasal airflow or excluding choanal atresia. Tracheal tug in the suprasternal notch during inspiration is an early sign of obstruction. More severe restriction leads to intercostal and subcostal recession and eventually to sternal recession. In supraglottic and oropharyngeal obstruction an opisthotonic posture is often adopted. Fever, drooling and toxicity suggests a serious infective cause.

Assessing the degree of respiratory effort can be difficult. As Wilson[1] pointed out, probably the greatest error made in the diagnosis of respiratory distress in children is not in the cause but in the assessment of the degree of compromise. The severity of the airway obstruction and the need for intervention are judged on clinical signs, but pulse oximetry and transcutaneous carbon dioxide levels provide important additional objective information. It is important to realise that the infant who seems to be improving with reduced respiratory effort and improving stridor may just be exhausted and slipping into respiratory failure.

Investigations

Laryngobronchoscopy

A small number of patients may require very specific investigations to establish a diagnosis, but for the majority of cases presenting in the first year of life there is no substitute for direct examination of the respiratory tract. Storz™ laryngoscopes and rigid ventilating bronchoscopes allow a detailed examination of all areas whilst protecting the airway. The addition of Hopkins™ rod telescopes improves illumination and visualisation. The nose, post nasal space, mouth, larynx, large airways, pharynx and, on occasion, the oesophagus should all be examined to obtain a complete static and dynamic assessment of the airway. Fibreoptic endoscopy can be used to supplement the examination, analysis the movements of the vocal cords and assist in the intubation of difficult airways but does not give the same degree of protection or quality of image.

No endoscopic airway assessment is complete without a formal examination of the trachea and main bronchi in order to diagnose primary and secondary tracheomalacia. In addition to examining the trachea during assisted ventilation, observations should take place during onset of spontaneous breathing when the normal negative intra-thoracic pressure may unmask tracheal collapse. Video recording and instant prints are now easily obtained during the procedure and provide accurate documentation.

The temptation to have 'a quick look' with a fibreoptic endoscope on the SCBU should generally be resisted. If endoscopy is indicated, examination in theatre with an experienced paediatric anaesthetist is safer and allows a complete sequential and unhurried evaluation of the entire upper respiratory tract. No airway procedure is without risk and, in infants, even minimal trauma can produce significant mucosal swelling. To adequately perform a paediatric laryngobronchoscopy a range of Storz™ bronchoscopes from 2.5–4.0 are required, along with a 2.5 mm Hopkins™ telescope. The exact size of any stenotic segment can be measured by passing a Portex™ endotracheal tube, noting whether it passes easily or feels a little tight. The ventilation pressure required to just produce a leak around the tube is also noted. The complication rate of this endoscopic examination is 2–3%[2] and in high risk patients the possibility of postoperative intubation or even a tracheostomy must be discussed with the parents before the procedure.

Imaging

AP and lateral X-rays of the soft tissue of the upper airway can help delineate narrowing of the trachea but a normal film does not exclude pathology and X-rays are rarely requested. Plain radiographs of the chest are useful in cases of a suspected foreign body, tracheal compression or mediastinal masses. Specific changes have been described in cases of retropharyngeal abscess (Fig. 2.1) and epiglottitis,[3,4] but in croup the diagnostic value of plain films

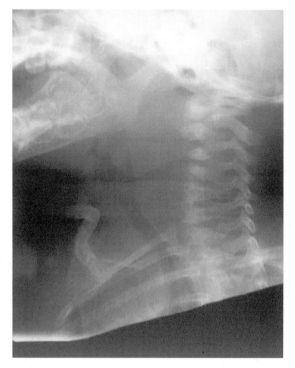

Fig. 2.1 Lateral soft tissue neck X-ray showing retropharyngeal abscess.

has been questioned.[5] It must be stressed that the X-ray department is a dangerous place for any child with airway (or potential airway) obstruction and, in cases of suspected epiglottitis, X-rays should not be performed.

CT is used to define the anatomical details of choanal atresia but has the disadvantage of a high radiation dose. MR imaging has become the investigation of choice for identifying vascular compression of the trachea and mediastinal masses.[6] Angiography is left to the discretion of the radiologist or cardiothoracic surgeon. Echocardiography and a barium swallow are still useful adjuncts in the early investigation of vascular anomalies.

TREATMENT

General principles

Although the main objective of many treatments is to avoid the need for ventilatory support, in a minority of cases intubation will be required. The laryngologist becomes involved if there are difficulties with intubation or when attempts at extubation have failed. In recent years there have been a number of specific advances which have influenced the management of both of these dilemmas.

Intubation

Rigid laryngoscope

Storz™ instruments should now be regarded as essential equipment in any unit likely to manage paediatric airway problems. Fibreoptic illumination combined with specific design features makes laryngoscopy possible even in cases of severe micrognathia. In these cases, an extreme lateral route may be used rather than the normal paramedian approach.

Fibreoptic laryngoscopes

In severe cases, a 3.8 mm intubating fibreoptic endoscope can be passed via a laryngeal mask airway (LMA) to assess the larynx. A guide wire is then introduced through the larynx under direct vision followed by a ureteric catheter over the guide wire. Carbon dioxide monitoring from the catheter confirms correct positioning. The LMA is then removed and a 3.0 endotracheal tube advanced over the catheter affecting intubation in a controlled fashion. In older children the scope can be introduced directly into the trachea acting as a guide for the endotracheal tube. Fibreoptic laryngoscopes with external diameters as small as 2.2 mm are available but without a suction or instrumentation channel – they are useful for checking the position of endotracheal tubes.

The difficult extubation

Another common problem encountered is the infant who develops signs of respiratory obstruction soon after extubation. Often a couple of attempts have been made to remove the tube before the ENT surgeons are contacted. Unless there was a previous narrowing of the trachea, the most probable cause of failure of extubation will be mucosal oedema of the subglottis.

One in a thousand children will have a subglottic diameter well below normal and intubation with a standard sized tube will traumatise the mucosa which will swell when the tube is withdrawn. Reintubation, excessive movement of the tube, infections of the upper and lower respiratory tract and gastro-oesophageal reflux all increase the risk of sub-glottic damage.[7]

In cases of failed attempts at extubation, the first line of management should be an examination under general anaesthetic. A number of studies have reported the effective use of steroids and nebulised adrenaline in the treatment of post extubation oedema.[8–10] A specific protocol has been used for the last 5 years in our department. This involves micro-surgical removal of any florid polypoid fringe from the vocal cords and reintubation with a correctly sized nasal ET tube smeared with Tri Adcortyl ointment (which contains triamcinolone acetonide 0.1%, gramicidin 0.025%, neomycin 0.25% and nystatin 100,000 units/g). Systemic antibiotics are commenced and dexamethasone (1 mg/kg per day) is also started 48 h prior to the next attempt at extubation. Immediately after the tube has been removed, nebulised 1 in 1000 adrenaline is given, repeated as required over the next 24 h. In most of cases, this treatment will control mucosal swelling which would otherwise precipitate reintubation. Once the aggravating effect of the endotracheal tube has been removed, the oedema generally resolves spontaneously. Failure to extubate at this stage suggests more severe damage with a potential sub-glottic stenosis. Further management is discussed under this topic below.

SPECIFIC CONDITIONS AND THEIR TREATMENT

It would seem appropriate to discuss the management and recent changes in treatment of these conditions in the order in which they most frequently present.

Laryngomalacia

This is the commonest cause of congenital stridor and the presentation of this condition is well known to paediatricians. Characteristic inspiratory stridor becomes evident within a few days or weeks after birth and is most noticeable when the child is active or excited. The stridor settles at night, or when the child is placed in the prone position. Stridor in the absence of any other signs of respiratory obstruction is common but tracheal tug and sternal recession may occur. Occasionally the condition is so severe that the child fails to thrive due to a combination of increased energy expenditure and compromised feeding. In these cases micro-surgical or laser laryngoplasty has proved effective[11] and obviates the need for a tracheostomy.

The anatomical features that predispose to laryngomalacia have been discussed above. Direct laryngoscopy with spontaneous breathing confirms the diagnosis. In most cases the natural history is one of resolution over 18 months to 3 years. Any deviation from the standard presentation should certainly initiate a request for a direct examination, and we have a low clinical threshold for proceeding to endoscopic examination in children referred with even slightly atypical histories. This generally confirms the diagnosis of laryngomalacia – reassuring to parents and physician alike. However, it is important to appreciate that other causes of stridor may mimic laryngomalacia, and some 15% of children referred to our unit with a provisional diagnosis of laryngomalacia are found to have other airway pathology. Failure to make a correct diagnosis can have serious consequences.

Subglottic stenosis

The reason paediatric laryngologists are so keen to prevent this condition is that once a stenosis is established, it is likely to involve a tracheostomy for at least 1 year and possibly reconstructive laryngotracheal surgery. The former has major implications for the child and family, the results of the latter with regard to both voice and respiration are unpredictable.

There is little that can be done about the relatively rare cases of congenital sub-glottic stenosis except to recognise them and try not to make the situation worse with prolonged intubation. A full term infant with a subglottis less than 4 mm in diameter is defined as having sub-glottic stenosis. A more practical definition is that the same child should be able to be intubated with a 3.0 Portex™ tube and still have a leak at pressures below 30 mm of water. In premature babies, a diameter of less than 3 mm is used as a criteria for diagnosis, although this will obviously depend upon the child's weight.

Acquired sub-glottic stenosis has had a fluctuating incidence over the years. Advances in neonatology enable increasingly premature babies to survive, many of whom require prolonged ventilation. Although no specific aetiology has been identified, several factors have been suggested. The use of inappropriately large endotracheal tubes, sub-optimal tube fixation with transmitted movements from the ventilator, upper and lower respiratory tract infections and the presence of uncorrected reflux all contribute to this problem.[12]

The earliest pathological changes in the subglottis occur if the pressure from the endotracheal tube exceeds the transmucosal blood pressure of 40 mm of mercury. Initial swelling is followed by ulceration and eventually granulation tissue formation. Healing, thought in the past to be prevented by the presence of a tube, does in fact take place by a process of fibrosis and re-epithelialisation. Stenosis occurs if the damage extends to the perichondrium due to circumferential scarring.[13] Early involvement of a laryngologist, particularly after failed extubation, helps identify the nature of the sub-glottic pathology and may allow treatment to commence which could prevent a more severe stenosis.

Subglottic stenosis presents either with failed attempts at extubation or with stridor which may get worse with respiratory tract infections. The severity of the stenosis can be inferred from the history and examination, but correct diagnosis requires rigid endoscopy with sizing of the narrowed segment using endotracheal tubes. The staging system from the Children's Hospital in Cincinnati is clinically useful.

Grade 1 stenosis   narrowing of up to 70% of the lumen.

Grade 2 stenosis   narrowing between 70–90% of the lumen.

Grade 3 stenosis   narrowing greater than 90% of the lumen.

Grade 4 stenosis   total obstruction.

In the early stages of subglottic damage where the general clinical situation allows extubation of the child, the protocol described earlier is useful. If extubation fails or the damage is more severe there are two other options before a tracheostomy is considered.

TREATMENT TO PREVENT OR LIMIT SUBGLOTTIC STENOSIS

Anterior cricoid split

This operation, which releases the complete ring of cricoid cartilage anteriorly, may allow intubation to continue with the same size endotracheal tube. Transmucosal pressures are reduced thereby facilitating healing and re-epithelialisation. It is important to rule out all other possible causes for obstruction, such as a vocal cord palsy, laryngomalacia or tracheomalacia. Cotton, who developed the technique, outlines several criteria concerning the general health of the child which should be met before surgery is performed.[14]

Reintubation

Formal reintubation for incipient neonatal subglottic stenosis was first suggested by Graham[15] in 1994. He performed a prospective study of babies who failed extubation and would have been candidates for an anterior cricoid split. They were carefully examined and then reintubated with a nasal endotracheal tube of a size that fitted comfortably but with no leak. The children were then sedated and nursed intensively for 2 weeks. Six of the 10 infants were successfully extubated. The hypothesis, which initially seems contradictory, is that reintubation controls the acute inflammatory swelling, stabilises the submucosa, encourages re-epithelialisation thereby limiting cicatrization. These promising results have been supported by Hoeve[16] who reports success in 22 of 23 cases using a similar technique.

Tracheostomy

If these procedures fail, the accepted treatment has been to perform an elective tracheostomy. Many paediatricians and parents are understandably reluctant to consider this alternative. However, if a tracheostomy is performed before significant perichondrial damage occurs, the subglottis is 'rested', thereby allowing normal healing with minimal scar tissue formation. The tracheostomy can subsequently be removed, usually within a few months. Even if one has to wait substantially longer to allow for laryngeal growth, there is a good chance that the sub-glottic narrowing will be limited and the child will not be totally tracheostomy dependent.

The care of a child with a tracheostomy is challenging,[17] but most of these children can eventually be managed at home. Adequate care relies upon intensive training of the parents and the support of a nurse specialist working between the hospital, family and community medical services.[18] In the UK, a parents association, Aid for Children with Tracheostomies (ACT) provides additional support and advice.

TREATMENT OF ESTABLISHED SUBGLOTTIC STENOSIS

Once a stenosis has become established there are a number of options. Some relatively mild cases can be treated expectantly, provided the parents and general practitioners have clear guideline on when to contact the hospital should the stridor get worse. More severe grade 1 stenosis can usually be managed with a tracheostomy which protects the airway until the stenosis is corrected by natural laryngeal growth. However, this is not without risk, and even in a carefully supervised environment a tracheostomy has a small but significant mortality (0–6%).[19] Laser treatment is another option. Vaporisation of granulation tissue, thin webs and partial stenosis using multiple treatments with low power to limit the zone of tissue damage can be effective.

Laryngotracheal reconstruction

Laryngotracheal reconstruction is now the established technique for more severe stenosis, though in general, surgery is not performed on a child less than 10 kg. Details of the various techniques are described by Cotton[20] but in essence the surgery involves expansion of the cricoid and related trachea, augmentation with rib cartilage and stenting of the lumen with a teflon tube. With this technique it is possible to extubate 70% of patients after a single reconstruction, but 30% need revision surgery before the tracheostomy tube can finally be removed. Laryngeal growth after this type of surgery seems to be satisfactory in most long term studies, and children who are successfully extubated rarely encounter problems of increasing obstruction as they get older, although their exercise tolerance may always be limited. Voice quality is much less predictable and expert speech therapy is often required.

Single stage reconstruction

One recent development in laryngotracheal reconstruction is early single stage surgery.[21] Instead of performing a tracheostomy the cricoid ring is split, cartilage grafts are inserted to open the subglottic region and the area is stented with an endotracheal tube. The child is then extubated 7–10 days postoperatively. The advantage of this technique is that a tracheostomy is not required, however, only selected cases are suitable and a paediatric intensive care unit capable of very careful supervision of the endotracheal tube is an absolute prerequisite.

Balloon dilatation

Simple dilatation of a stenosis with conventional bougies has a reputation for making the situation worse. Recent reports of balloon dilatation have been encouraging.[22,23] We have had a number of cases of post-intubation sub-glottic and tracheal stenosis with gradual onset of stridor over a 1–2 week period following extubation. A soft granular stenosis has been identified and balloon dilatation using a cardiac valvotomy catheter inflated to 6 atmospheres has provided sufficient improvement to avoid a tracheostomy. The airway is dilated without the shearing forces to the mucosa of conventional bouginage which was thought to be responsible for subsequent re-stenosis.

Croup, epiglottitis and acute tracheitis

The symptoms of croup are well known to all practitioners who care for children. There are two excellent recent reviews of inflammatory disease of the airway by Wilson[1] and Cressman and Myer.[24] A number of recent advances have influenced diagnosis and treatment. Most children with croup do not require hospitalisation but in the small number (1–2%) who do, very careful clinical evaluation is needed to differentiate more serious causes and to decide when intervention is required.

Croup, or more correctly acute laryngotracheobronchitis, has a peak incidence between the age of 1–2 years but is not uncommon below the age of 12 months, particularly in boys. The diagnosis is usually clear but needs to be differentiated from acute epiglottitis and bacterial tracheitis.

Whilst there has been a marked decline in cases of acute epiglottitis since the introduction of Hib conjugate vaccine,[25] bacterial tracheitis seems to be making a re-emergence. *Staphylococcus aureus* is the commonest isolate but *Haemophilus influenzae, Streptococcus pneumoniae* and the β haemolytic streptococcus have been reported. Eckel et al.[26] conducted a study to try and identify patients with bacterial tracheitis on clinical grounds. Stridor and respiratory distress were always present but cough, hoarseness and fever were inconsistent. None of the children had drooling, a feature specific to acute epiglottitis. They recommended endoscopy to confirm the diagnosis in patients presenting with an initial diagnosis of viral croup that does not respond to conventional treatment. Removal of any thick tracheal or subglottic secretions can be accomplished at the same time.

Successful treatment of critical croup with nebulised 1 in 1000 adrenaline (5 ml repeated every 2 h) has been reported by Meakin.[27] There is also clear evidence, from controlled trials, of benefit from nebulised budesonide in children with acute croup.[28,29,29a]

Vocal cord palsies and laryngo–oesophageal clefts

Vocal cord paralysis accounts for 10% of all congenital laryngeal lesions.[30] A unilateral vocal cord palsy should be considered when there is a weak, breathy cry with occasional aspiration causing choking and possibly recurrent chest infections. Stridor is seldom a prominent feature and, as with children found to have minor laryngo-oesophageal clefts, the signs and symptoms can be subtle. Diagnosis is made by laryngoscopy and both of these conditions can be missed if the mobility of the vocal cords or the inter-arytenoid region of the larynx are not specifically assessed. Most unilateral vocal cord palsies are idiopathic and the majority of cases improve spontaneously. Other than careful clinical examination no specific investigations or treatment are needed.

In patients where the protective function of the larynx has been compromised by neurological or structural pathology the risks of sub-clinical aspiration must be considered. A grossly incompetent larynx is clinically obvious but minor degrees of aspiration, particularly associated with nocturnal reflux, are more difficult to detect and can lead to permanent structural changes in the lungs. Contrast studies in these cases are often normal but an isotope labelled milk scan with imaging of the lungs after 24 h is a sensitive method of detection.[31] If significant aspiration is demonstrated a number of remedial actions are possible.[32] Gastro-oesophageal reflux is also increasingly being recognised as an important contributory factor in many different causes of large airway obstruction.[33]

Bilateral vocal cord palsies are rare but can produce marked stridor and even cyanosis. Presentation is usually at birth but the onset can be delayed. The cry may be normal but aspiration is usually clinically evident unless the lesion occurs below the level of the superior laryngeal nerves. An incomplete bilateral palsy can be mistaken for croup or asthma. Central nervous system anomalies are the commonest cause of bilateral vocal cord palsies of which the Arnold Chiari malformation is the best known example. In this condition, the vagus is damaged by traction to the nerve rootlets or possibly by abnormal nuclear development.[34] Early neurosurgical decompression provides the best chance of recovering some vocal cord movement. Hydrocephalus needs to be excluded, and neonatal myasthenia gravis, congenital hypotonia and Charcot Marie-Tooth disease must all be considered.

A tracheostomy may be clearly indicated to safeguard the airway but the decision to intervene may take several weeks in less severe cases. Recent reports advocate a more conservative approach.[35] Although understandably perceived as a major step by the parents, a tracheostomy is one of the few reversible forms of intervention available. All other surgery to the larynx should be delayed for at least 1 year to allow for spontaneous recovery.

Laryngeal webs

Laryngeal webs of various degrees and thickness are a relatively common congenital anomaly within the larynx. The glottic narrowing can be dramatic with only a 2 mm opening remaining. If the child can be safely transferred to an ENT unit, definitive vapourisation of the web with the laser is the treatment of choice. However, if in extremis, most webs can be disrupted with an endotracheal tube and always with a 2.5 Storz™ bronchoscope followed by intubation.

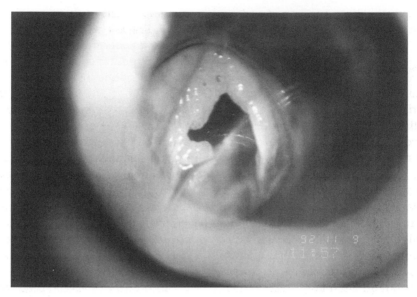

Fig. 2.2 Juvenile papillomatosis of the larynx.

Papillomata

Various other pathologies can occur in the larynx during the first year of life causing airway obstruction. Some, such as papillomata, have a deceptive history and the infant is often treated for recurrent croup before alternative diagnoses are considered and diagnostic laryngoscopy performed.[36] Although rare, cases of laryngeal papillomata below the age of 1 year have been reported (Fig. 2.2). Microsurgical and laser removal are still the mainstay of treatment.

Haemangioma

A cutaneous haemangioma should always raise the possibility of a similar sub-glottic lesion. These may be present at birth or gradually over the first few months. Symptoms are exacerbated by upper respiratory tract infections and the condition can mimic croup. There is usually a dramatic response to nebulised adrenaline, which may reinforce the misdiagnosis.

Supraglottic cysts

A supraglottic cyst is one of the commonest conditions associated with delayed referral. These lesions arise either in the vallecula or the supraglottis, usually as a mucus retention cyst. The cysts can assume quite large proportions before airway obstruction becomes a feature. Feeding problems and a tendency to extend the head and neck to improve breathing are consistent hallmarks. Treatment by simple excision is rewarding and effective.

Choanal atresia

Young babies tend to be obligate, or at least preferential, nasal breathers and restriction of the nasal airway will cause various degrees of distress depending on the severity of the obstruction. Bilateral choanal atresia is rapidly diagnosed at birth. Absence of a mist pattern, failure to pass a naso-gastric tube and respiratory obstruction without an oropharyngeal airway are all indicative. Treatment requires the immediate establishment of an oro-pharyngeal airway. A feeding bottle teat with the end cut off is enough to safeguard the airway until a proper oro-pharyngeal tube is available. In unilateral cases or where there is stenosis rather than complete atresia, regular treatment with a nasal decongestant may be sufficient. Surgery to correct the atresia is now predominantly performed via a transnasal route, the bony plate being drilled out under microscopic control.[37] Some centres continue to use long term stents but an alternative approach is early correction of the atresia, followed by regular examination with dilatation and lasering of granulation tissue. As with other congenital anomalies, it is important to search for other anomalies (e.g. the CHARGE syndrome or the VATER syndrome).

Micrognathia

Micrognathia, either as an isolated first arch anomaly, or associated with the Pierre Robin or the Treacher Collins syndrome, can present particular problems. The tongue base and hyoid are both suspended from the mandible and the retrognathia causes the tongue to prolapse posteriorly and the supraglottis to fall against the posterior pharyngeal wall. In severe cases breathing can be obstructed at birth. Intubation may be very difficult or even impossible but ventilation can usually be maintained with a nasopharyngeal airway until help can be summoned. If intubation was traumatic, both for the infant and doctor, strong consideration should be given to a tracheostomy. With mandibular growth, extubation is nearly always possible but should be delayed until any associated cleft palate has been repaired.

Foreign bodies

Paediatric laryngologists have a low threshold for performing a laryngobronchoscopy on children with a history suggestive of an inhaled foreign body. Those lodged in the larynx present dramatically or fatally but if the foreign body passes into a bronchus there is frequently a significant delay in referral, and the adage about a sudden onset of asthma after a choking attack is still uncomfortably true. Telescopic Hopkins™ guided forceps used via a ventilating bronchoscope have made examination and extraction a much more relaxed procedure. Most problems are caused by late presentation, particularly if peanuts have been inhaled.

Tracheomalacia

Respiratory obstruction due to collapse or compression of the trachea can be the most difficult cases to diagnose. The symptoms may fluctuate in severity, often with minimal signs of embarrassment until the child becomes distressed by a crying or coughing spell. This may then precipitate cyanosis or even a cardio-respiratory arrest. Less severe cases can be mistaken for breath holding attacks or may mimic cyanotic heart disease. Rarely, the presentation may be with recurrent chest infections due to sub-clinical aspiration.[38]

Primary tracheomalacia is a congenital weakness of the cartilaginous rings causing an isolated segment of the trachea to collapse on expiration. Secondary tracheomalacia occurs at the same level as a tracheo-oesophageal fistula. After surgical repair, there is a tendency for the trachealis muscle to balloon forwards which compounds the problem of collapsing tracheal rings. A high rate of improvement after aortopexy has been reported.[39] Very minor

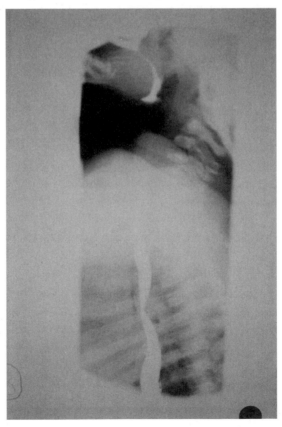

Fig. 2.3 Barium swallow showing posterior indentation from R aortic arch.

tracheo-oesophageal fistulae are notoriously difficult to diagnose and should be considered in any child who has repeated episodes of chest infection and intermittent stridor.

Vascular syndromes

Vascular compression of the trachea is most commonly caused by a right aortic arch with a restricting left sided ligamentum. Less commonly, the compression is due to a double aortic arch, anomalous right subclavian or aberrant innominate artery. These vascular syndromes result in a nebulous group of upper respiratory tract symptoms,[40] though a complete ring is usually associated with more severe symptoms which tend deteriorate with time. Feeding difficulties and apnoeic episodes are common, but any infant presenting with stridor should be assessed to exclude a vascular cause. Diagnosis may be suggested by tracheal narrowing or an indistinct aortic arch on plain X-ray and a barium swallow is still a useful screening test (Fig. 2.3). Diagnosis is, however, dependent upon direct examination of the trachea with spontaneous ventilation to show the degree and position of compression. MR is then the investigation of choice followed by angiography in cases where surgery is being considered.

KEY POINTS FOR CLINICAL PRACTICE

1. Significant upper airway pathology may present with a number of symptoms; stridor may be minimal or even absent. Conditions such as tracheomalacia, vascular anomalies and laryngeal clefts may present with feeding difficulties, cough, recurrent chest infections and cyanotic episodes.

2. Although laryngomalacia is the commonest cause of stridor, the diagnosis cannot be made from the history and examination alone. Other causes of stridor may mimic this condition or may co-exist.

3. Direct examination of the airway is indicated in all children with a history of chronic stridor to enable a definitive diagnosis to be reached. This endoscopy must be complete and incorporate a dynamic examination of the airway during spontaneous breathing.

4. The safest technique for paediatric laryngobronchoscopy is for the procedure to be undertaken by skilled personnel in an operating theatre. There is no place for the 'quick look'.

5. X-rays are rarely useful in cases of acute inflammatory airway obstruction. The X-ray department is unsafe for children with airway obstruction (or possible airway obstruction), and cases of suspected epiglottitis should not be sent for an X-ray.

6. In cases where extubation has been unsuccessful on more than one occasion, direct examination of the larynx and trachea is indicated to establish the cause. Subsequent management may then enable successful extubation and reduce the likelihood of subglottic stenosis formation.

7. There is frequently a delay in referral of children who have aspirated a foreign body. Any persistent airway symptoms developing after a choking episode should raise the suspicion of aspiration and warrant prompt referral.

8. Recurrent lower respiratory tract infections may be caused by sub-clinical aspiration. Careful evaluation, including an isotope milk scan, are needed to establish the diagnosis.

9. Gastro-oesophageal reflux is a common complicating factor in many cases of airway obstruction and may require treatment in addition to the alleviation of the obstruction.

REFERENCES

1. Wilson FW. Inflammatory diseases of the airway. In: Myer 3rd CM, Cotton RT, Shott SR, eds. The pediatric airway: an interdisciplinary approach. Philadelphia: Lippincott, 1995; 67–99
2. Hoeve LJ, Rombout J, Meursing AE. Complications of rigid laryngo-bronchoscopy in children. Int J Pediatr Otorhinolaryngol 1993; 26: 47–56
3. Mahboubi S, Kramer SS. The pediatric airway. J Thorac Imaging 1995; 10: 156–170
4. Strife JL, Emery KH. Imaging of airway obstruction in infants and children. In: Myer 3rd CM, Cotton RT, Shott SR, eds. The pediatric airway: an interdisciplinary approach. Philadelphia: Lippincott, 1995; 45–66
5. Dawson KP, Steinberg A, Capaldi N. The lateral radiograph of neck in laryngo-tracheo-bronchitis (croup). J Qual Clin Pract 1994; 14: 39–43
6. Simoneaux SF, Bank ER, Webber JB et al. MR imaging of the pediatric airway. Radiographics 1995; 15: 287–299
7. Gould SJ, Graham JM. Long-term pathological sequaelae of neonatal endoteacheal intubation. Clin Otolaryngol 1989; 103: 622–625
8. Couser RJ , Ferrara TB, Falde B et al. Effectiveness of dexamethasone in preventing extubation failure in preterm infants at increased risk for airway edema. J Pediatr 1992; 1214: 591–596
9. Nutman J, Brooks LJ, Deakins KM et al. Racemic versus l-epinephrine aerosolin the treatment of postextubation laryngeal edema: results from a prospective, randomized, double-blind study. Crit Care Med 1994; 22: 1591–1594
10. Hoeve LJ, Verwood CD. The management of difficult extubation in pre-term infants. Int J Pediatr Otorhinolaryngol 1995; 32 Suppl: S97–S99
11. Roger G, Denoyelle F, Triglia JM et al. Severe laryngomalacia: surgical indications and results in 115 patients. Laryngoscope 1995; 105: 1111–1117
12. Dankle SK, Shuller DE, McClead RE. Risk factors for neonatal acquired subglottic stenosis. Ann Otol Rhinol Laryngol 1995; 97: 439–443
13. Quiney RE, Gould SJ. Subglottic stenosis: a clinicopathological study. Clin Otolaryngol 1985; 10: 315–327
14. Silver AM, Myer 3rd CM, Cotton RT. Anterior cricoid split. Update 1991. Am J Otolaryngol 1991; 12: 343–346
15. Graham JM. Formal reintubation for incipient neonatal subglottic stenosis. J Laryngol

Otol 1994; 108: 474–478
16. Hoeve LJ, Eskici O, Verwood CDA. Therapeutic reintubation for post-intubation laryngotracheal injury in preterm infants. Int J Pediatr Otorhinolaryngol 1995; 31: 7–13
17. Simma B, Spehler D, Burger R et al. Tracheostomy in children. Eur J Pediatr 1994; 153: 291–296
18. Campbel JB, Morgan DW, Pearman K. Experience with the home-care of tracheotomised paediatric patients. Arch Otolaryngol 1989; 246: 345–348
19. Gianoli GJ, Miller RH, Guarisco JL. Tracheostomy in the first year of life. Ann Otol Rhinol Laryngol 1990; 99: 896–901
20. Willging JP, Cotton RT. Subglottic stenosis in the pediatric patient. In: Myer 3rd CM, Cotton RT, Shott SR, eds. The pediatric airway : an interdisciplinary approach. Philadelphia: Lippincott, 1995; 111–132
21. Cotton RT, Myer CM, O'Connor DM et al. Pediatric laryngotracheal reconstruction with cartilage grafts and endotracheal tube stenting: the single-stage approach. Laryngoscope 1995; 105: 818–821
22. Hebra A, Powell DD, Smith CD. Balloon tracheoplasty in children: results of a 15 year experience. J Pediatr Surg 1991; 26: 957–961
23. Otherson Jr HB. Subglottic tracheal stenosis. Semin Thorac Cardiovasc Surg 1994; 6: 200–204
24. Cressman WR, Myer 3rd CM. Diagnosis and management of croup and epiglottitis. Pediatr Clin North Am 1994; 41: 265–276
25. Takala AK, Peltola H, Eskola J. Disappearance of epiglottitis during large scale vaccination with *Haemophilus influenzae* type B conjugate vaccine among children in Finland. Laryngoscope 1994; 104: 731–735
26. Eckel HE, Widemann B, Damm M et al. Airway endoscopy in the diagnosis and treatment of bacterial tracheitis in children. Int J Pediatr Otorhinolaryngol 1993; 27: 147–157
27. Remington S, Meakin G. Nebulised adrenaline 1.1000 in the treatment of croup. Anaesthesia 1986; 41: 923–926
28. Husby S, Agertoft SM, Mortensen S et al. Treatment of croup with nebulised steroid (budesonide): a double blind, placebo controlled study. Arch Dis Child 1993; 68: 352–355
29. Klassen TP, Feldman ME, Watters LK et al. Nebulized budesonide for children with mild-to-moderate croup. N Engl J Med 1994; 331: 285–289
29a. Skolnik NS. Treatment of croup: a critical review. Am J Dis Child 1989; 143: 1045–1049
30. Holinger LD, Holinger PC, Holinger PH. Etiology of bilateral abductor vocal cord paralysis: a review of 389 cases. Ann Otol Rhinol Laryngol 1976; 85: 428–436
31. McVeagh P, Howman-Giles R, Kemp A. Pulmonary aspiration studied by radionuclide milk scanning and barium swallow roentgenography. Am J Dis Child 1987; 141: 917
32. Benjamin BN, Gray SD, Bailey CM. Neonatal vocal cord paralysis. Head Neck 1993; 15: 169–172
33. Rudolph CD. Gastroesophageal reflux and airway disorders. In: Myer 3rd CM, Cotton RT, Shott SR, eds. The pediatric airway: an interdisciplinary approach. Philadelphia: Lippincott, 1995; 327–357
34. Oren J, Kelley DH, Todres ID et al. Respiratory complications in patients with myelodysplasia and Anold-Chiari malformation. Am J Dis Child 1886; 140: 221–224
35. Murty GE, Shinkwin C, Gibbin KP. Bilateral vocal fold paralysis in infants: tracheostomy or not? J Laryngol Otol 1994; 108: 329–331
36. Derkay CS, Darrow DH. Recurrent respiratory papillomatosis. Curr Opin Otolaryngol Head Neck Surg 1994; 2: 449–503
37. Morgan DW, Bailey CM. Current management of choanal atresia. Int J Pediatr Otorhinolaryngol 1990; 19: 1–13
38. Mair EA, Parsons DS. Pediatric tracheobronchomalacia and major airway collapse. Ann Otol Rhinol Laryngol 1992; 101: 300–309
39. Corbally MT, Spitz L, Kiely E et al. Aortopexy for tracheomalacia in oesophageal anomalies. Eur J Pediatr Surg 1993; 3: 264–266
40. Andrews TM, Myer 3rd CM, Bailey WW, Vester SR. Intrathoracic lesions involving the tracheobronchial tree. In: Myer 3rd CM, Cotton RT, Shott SR, eds. The pediatric airway: an interdisciplinary approach. Philadelphia: Lippincott, 1995; 223–245

3

Superantigen diseases

N. Curtis   M. Levin

Since the first description of superantigens in 1989, there has been a proliferation of interest in these proteins and their interaction with the immune system;
in 1995 more than 200 papers on superantigens were published compared
with only 29 in 1990.

Superantigens are produced by some viruses and *Mycoplasma* species but
to date only superantigens from bacteria have been conclusively shown to
cause disease in humans. Superantigens are defined by the unique way in
which they interact with the immune system. The discovery of this mechanism of action has dramatically enhanced the understanding of the pathogenesis of a number of diseases and offers exciting opportunities for the design of
novel and improved treatments as well as new immunisation strategies.

The first diseases recognised to be superantigen mediated were those
caused by the exotoxins produced by *Staphylococcus aureus* and *Streptococcus
pyrogenes*. These include staphylococcal toxic shock syndrome and scalded
skin syndrome, and streptococcal toxic shock-like syndrome, scarlet fever and
erysipelas. Recently, new staphylococcal and streptococcal superantigen toxins have been described. In addition, there is evidence to suggest that toxins
produced by a number of other bacteria are able to act as superantigens
(Table 3.1). However, the role of these new superantigen toxins in causing
disease in humans has not yet been fully defined. Conversely, there is evidence to implicate superantigen toxins in a wide range of diseases in which a
specific superantigen has not yet been identified, including some autoimmune
diseases (Table 3.2).

This chapter discusses the immunological properties of superantigens and
the mechanisms by which their interaction with the host immune system may
cause disease. It focuses on a number of bacterial diseases for which there is
good evidence of superantigen involvement. Diseases for which there has
been a recent surge in interest in their possible association with a superantigen
are also discussed. Finally, it examines some of the factors which may predispose to, or are associated with, superantigen disease.

SUPERANTIGEN IMMUNOLOGY

One of the exciting developments in the understanding of bacterial diseases

Table 3.1 Bacterial superantigens[a]

Toxin	Names	Size (kDa)	Vβ affinity
Staphylococcal			
TSST	Toxic shock syndrome toxin (Staphylococcal enterotoxin F, SEF)	22.0	2
SEA	Staphylococcal enterotoxin A	27.8	1.1, 5, 6's, 7.3, 7.4, 9.1
SEB	B	28.3	3, 12, 14, 15, 17, 20
SEC1	C1	26.0	3, 6.4, 6.9, 12, 15
SEC2	C2	26.0	12, 13.2, 14, 15, 17, 20
SEC3	C3	28.9	3, 5, 12, 13.2
SED	D	27.3	5, 12
SEE	E	29.6	5.1, 6's, 8, 18
SEG	G	27.1	
SEH[8]	H	25.0	
ExT A[b]	Epidermolytic toxin A Exfoliative toxin A Exfoliatin, Epidermolysin	27.0	2
ExT B	Epidermolytic toxin B	27.3	2
Streptococcal			
SPE A	Streptococcal pyrogenic exotoxin A Erythrogenic toxin A Scarlet fever toxin	25.8	2[c], 12, 14, 15[c]
SPE B[d]	Streptococcal pyrogenic exotoxin B Streptococcal proteinase, Streptopain Precursor form of cysteine protease Interleukin-1β activator	27.6	
SPE C	Streptococcal pyrogenic exotoxin C	24.4	1, 2, 5.1, 10
M protein fragments[e]	pep M5 pep M6 pep M18 pep M19 pep M24 pep M2	27.0	2, 4, 8 1, 2, 4, 8 1, 2, 4, 5.2 4, 5.2, 8 1, 4, 5.2, 8 2
SSA	Streptococcal superantigen[12]	28.0	1, 3, (5.2),15
SPE F	Streptococcal pyrogenic exotoxin F[13] Mitogenic factor (MF)	25.4	2, 4, 8, 15, 19
SPE X	Uncharacterised novel toxin (see[3])		8
Unknown	Uncharacterised novel toxin(s) (see[14])		1, 5.1, 12
SPM	*Streptococcus pyogenes* mitogen	28.0	includes 21
Other			
YPM	*Yersinia pseudotuberculosis* mitogen	21.0	3, 9, 13.1, 13.2
YEM	*Yersinia enterocolitica* mitogen		
PAE-A	*Pseudomonas aeruginosa* exotoxin A	66.6	8
CPET	*Clostridium perfringens* enterotoxin	31.3	6.9, 22
Gp B SPE	Group B streptococcus pyrogenic exotoxin	12.0	
Gp G SPE	Group G streptococcus pyrogenic exotoxin		
F-2	*Streptococcus mitis* 108 fraction F-2	> 60	2, 5.2

[a] From[2,3,5,15,28].   [b] The superantigen properties of the epidermolytic toxins is disputed[3].   [c] These Vβ affinities are disputed[3].   [d] The literature differs on whether SPE B acts as a superantigen. It is now generally accepted that SPE B is *not* a superantigen and that the superantigen properties previously attributed to it were due to contamination with other SPEs[3]. SPE B has been found to be identical to cysteine protease and is an important virulence factor in its own right (reviewed in[15]).   [e] Recent evidence suggests that the superantigen activity associated with pep M5 is caused by contamination with SPE C and SPE F (reviewed in[15]).

Table 3.2 Diseases for which a superantigen mediated process has been postulated

Toxic shock	Staphylococcal toxic shock syndrome[7—9,35]
	Streptococcal toxic shock-like syndrome[10,12—14]
Scarlet fever	
Skin diseases	Atopic dermatitis[28]
	Guttate psoriasis[28—30]
	Scalded skin syndrome
	Erysipelas
Kawasaki disease[21—24,26,27]	
Other	Autoimmune disease[6] including
	Rheumatoid arthritis
	Rheumatic fever
	Multiple sclerosis
	Thyroiditis
	Sarcoidosis
	Systemic sclerosis
	Inflammatory myopathies
	Sjorgren's syndrome
	Endogenous posterior uveitis
	Systemic lupus erythematosis
	Myaesthenia gravis
	Sudden infant death syndrome[31—33]
	Insulin dependent diabetes
	Crohn's disease
	Tuberculosis

Note that the role of a superantigen in many of the diseases in this list (especially those under the heading 'Other') remains speculative. Further studies are needed to confirm the association in these cases.

has been the recognition of the unique immunological properties of a number of bacterial toxins, called superantigens.[1-5] Bacterial superantigens are globular proteins which are generally of between 20 and 30 kDa in size. There is considerable similarity in the amino acid sequence among superantigens, but it is the tertiary structure of these molecules that is responsible for their superantigen properties.

How does T cell stimulation by superantigens differ from stimulation by conventional antigens?

Superantigens stimulate T cells by directly binding Class II molecules on antigen presenting cells to the T cell receptor. This unique mechanism differs to conventional antigen stimulation in a number of key ways (Fig. 3.1).

Lack of antigen processing

Conventional antigens are ingested by antigen presenting cells and broken down into peptide fragments for presentation on the antigen presenting cell surface in the groove of major histocompatability complex (MHC) Class II

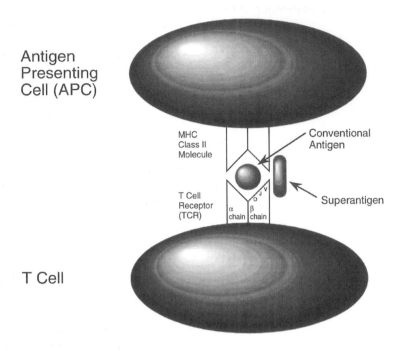

Fig. 3.1 Composite diagram contrasting T cell stimulation by a conventional antigen and a superantigen.

molecules. Superantigens do not undergo antigen processing but interact directly with the Class II molecule.

Lack of MHC restriction

Conventional antigen fragments are presented on the antigen presenting cell surface in conjunction with an MHC Class II molecule. T cell recognition of this MHC-antigen complex is, therefore, 'MHC restricted'. Whilst super-antigen stimulation requires MHC Class II expression ('MHC dependent') it is not restricted.

T cell receptor Vβ specificity and intense immune activation

T cell recognition of conventional antigen is highly specific involving all domains of both chains of the T cell receptor. Only a small proportion of T cells (perhaps 1 in 10^6) will possess a receptor that recognises a given MHC-antigen complex and thus be stimulated. In contrast, superantigen binding to T cells is restricted only by the variable region of the β chain of the T cell receptor, the 'Vβ region'. Each T cell belongs to one of only 25 different Vβ families, based on the sequence of their Vβ domain. Each superantigen has a specificity for one or a limited set of Vβ families and can stimulate all T cells bearing those Vβ regions, irrespective of the antigen specificity of the T cell receptor (Table 3.1). By this mechanism, superantigens are able to stimulate a large proportion (up to 1 in 5) of all T cells.

The particular set of Vβ families that many of the known superantigens will stimulate has been established. For example, staphylococcal toxic shock syndrome toxin only stimulates T cells bearing Vβ2; streptococcal pyrogenic exotoxin A only stimulates T cells expressing Vβ2, 12, 14 or 15 (Table 3.1). This specificity is not predictable from the superantigen's amino acid sequence as it is dependent on the three dimensional structure of the super-antigen. The specific amino acids critical for interaction with both the MHC molecule and the T cell receptor have been defined for some superantigens (reviewed in[5]).

What are the consequences of superantigen stimulation?

The major consequence of superantigen stimulation is T cell activation and proliferation of Vβ restricted clones of T cells specific to that superantigen, in turn leading to cytokine release (Fig. 3.2). However, there are other alterna-tive outcomes possible depending on co-stimulatory signals from the antigen presenting cell and the cytokine environment of the T cell. Stimulated T cells may undergo apoptosis (programmed cell death) leading to clonal deletion or become anergised leading to non-responsiveness (Fig. 3.3).

How do superantigens cause disease?

The exact mechanism by which superantigens cause disease remains unclear. Superantigen stimulation of T cells leads to the release of cytokines both from

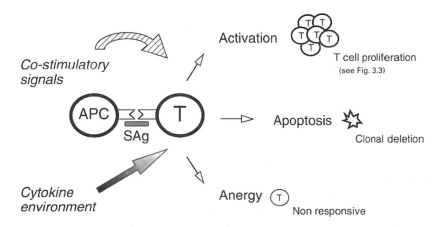

Fig. 3.2 The possible consequences following superantigen stimulation of a T cell.

T cells and other cells of the immune system. These cytokines include tumour necrosis factor-α, interleukin-1, interleukin-2 and interferon-γ (Fig. 3.3). The intense cytokine release brought about by superantigens, especially the release of tumour necrosis factor-α, is believed to be particularly important in the pathogenesis of the capillary leak underlying toxic shock. The cascade of cytokine release and immune activation is similar to lipopolysaccharide induced septic shock in Gram negative bacteraemia, but there are clear differences in the pattern, cell requirements and kinetics of cytokine release. Whilst the mechanisms of superantigen and lipopolysaccharide induced shock are distinct, another important pathological mechanism may be the ability of superantigens to enhance endotoxic shock. Moreover, there is additional evidence that superantigens can alter capillary permeability by a direct effect on the endothelium.

Superantigens have a number of other effects on the immune system which may contribute to their role in disease. It is suggested that, by their capacity to bind T cells and MHC Class II expressing cells, superantigens cause a polyclonal B cell activation leading to hypergammaglobulinaemia and antibody production. They may also activate natural killer cells.

How might superantigens be involved in autoimmune disease?

Autoimmune disease sometimes follows bacterial infection, e.g. rheumatic fever after group A streptococcal disease. There are a number of theoretical

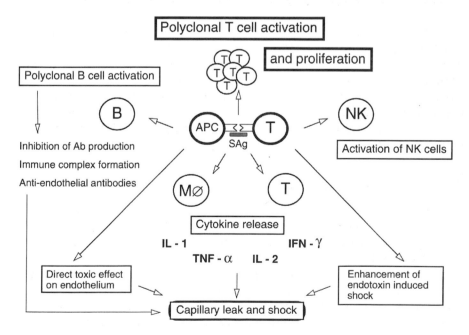

Fig. 3.3 Immunological effects of superantigens.

mechanisms by which superantigens could cause autoimmune disease.[5,6] First, the non specific activation of large numbers of T cells may allow self reactive clones, which are normally anergised or present in low numbers, to expand. Second, superantigen mediated polyclonal B cell activation could lead to autoantibody production. Last, the altered cytokine pattern caused by superantigens may lead to abnormal presentation of self proteins leading to the formation of autoantibodies.

A number of autoimmune diseases, including rheumatoid arthritis and insulin dependent diabetes, have been proposed to be superantigen mediated. Although there is some evidence to support these hypotheses, the role of superantigens in autoimmune disease remains speculative (Table 3.2).[6]

SUPERANTIGENS IN HUMAN DISEASE

Background

What is the evidence that superantigens have a role in human disease?

Superantigens have been proposed as the cause of a wide range of human diseases. Whilst there is no direct proof for the role of superantigens in the pathogenesis of many of these, there is indirect evidence from epidemiological, microbiological and immunological studies. The strength of this evidence varies considerably. The isolation of toxin-producing organisms from patients with the disease, together with evidence of a serological response to the toxin, is usually taken as good evidence for the role of the toxin in the pathogenesis of the disease. However, the best evidence that a superantigen is associated with a disease comes from studies of the T cell Vβ repertoire in patients. These have shown that staphylococcal toxic shock syndrome and streptococcal toxic shock-like syndrome are mediated by superantigens (discussed below). In contrast, for many other diseases in which a superantigen has been proposed, there is only indirect evidence and the role of superantigens remains uncertain. Further studies are needed to confirm the association in these cases.

Do superantigen mediated diseases have similar clinical features?

The diseases caused by staphylococcal and streptococcal toxins were the first to be recognised as being superantigen mediated. There is considerable overlap in the clinical features of these diseases: for example scarlet fever and toxic shock syndrome are both febrile illnesses with an erythematous desquamating rash and strawberry tongue; conjunctivitis is an additional feature common to both staphylococcal toxic shock syndrome and streptococcal toxic shock-like syndrome. The fact that Kawasaki disease shares many of these clinical features has led to the suggestion that it is another example of a superantigen mediated disease.

Table 3.3 Diagnostic criteria for staphylococcal toxic shock syndrome

Staphylococcal toxic shock syndrome is probable when 3 or more major criteria are met in the presence of desquamation or more than 5 are met in its absence.

- **Fever** > 38.9°C
- **Rash** diffuse erythematous,
    with desquamation 1–2 weeks after onset of illness
- **Hypotension or shock**
- **Involvement of 3 or more of the following organ systems:**

Mucous membranes	vaginal, conjunctival or oropharyngeal hyperaemia
Gastrointestinal	vomiting, profuse diarrhoea
Muscular	severe myalgia or ↑ CPK
Renal	↑ urea/creatinine or pyuria in absence of UTI
Hepatic	abnormal liver function tests indicative of hepatitis
Haematological	platelets < 100
Central nervous system	disorientation or alteration in consciousness without focal signs

- **Exclusion of Rocky Mountain spotted fever, leptospirosis and measles**

What other diseases might be caused by superantigens?

More recently, it has been suggested that a superantigen is involved in the pathogenesis of a number of other diseases of unknown aetiology that have dissimilar clinical presentations. Examples include Crohn's disease, TB and insulin dependent diabetes (Table 3.2). In most cases this is based on the finding of a skewed T cell Vβ repertoire in patients with the disease (see below). The strength of evidence supporting these claims varies considerably. The actual superantigen or the organism producing it is unknown in most instances. Until further confirmatory evidence is published such claims should be viewed with caution.

This section focuses on those diseases of interest to paediatricians for which there is good evidence of superantigen involvement. Diseases for which there has been a recent surge in interest in their possible association with a superantigen are also discussed.

Staphylococcal toxic shock syndrome

Although staphylococcal toxic shock syndrome received most attention following an epidemic in 1980, associated with the use of hyper absorbable tampons by menstruating women, it was first described in children.[7] Staphylococcal toxic shock syndrome is a severe multisystem disease characterised by hypotension, fever, a diffuse erythematous skin rash that desquamates in convalescence and multi-organ failure secondary to capillary leak and shock (Table 3.3). In the majority of childhood cases, the focus of staphylococcal infection is a cutaneous or subcutaneous infection, which may in itself be quite trivial.

What is the cause of staphylococcal toxic shock syndrome?

90% of isolates from patients with menstrual staphylococcal toxic shock syndrome and 63% of isolates from non-menstrual cases produce toxic shock syndrome toxin compared with 30% of non-toxic shock syndrome strains. Other toxins, notably staphylococcal enterotoxins B and C are also implicated, more commonly in non-menstrual cases, including paediatric patients. The toxin responsible is not identified in up to one-third of non-menstrual cases and may be due to as yet uncharacterised superantigen toxins. One such candidate toxin has recently been described. Staphylococcal enterotoxin H[8] was isolated from a patient with non-menstrual staphylococcal toxic shock syndrome and has been shown to fulfil the criteria for a superantigen.

Do staphylococcal toxins act as superantigens in staphylococcal toxic shock syndrome?

The isolation of toxin-producing strains of bacteria from patients together with serological studies correlating the lack of neutralising antibody with susceptibility is good evidence for the role of a staphylococcal toxins in the pathogenesis of the disease. However, it does not necessarily follow that the disease is caused by the toxins acting as superantigens. This is illustrated by staphylococcal food poisoning. The symptoms of nausea, vomiting, abdominal pains, diarrhoea, headache and myalgia are caused by ingesting preformed staphylococcal enterotoxins. Their mechanism of action in this illness is unclear but is not thought to be due to a superantigen effect because mutant enterotoxins which have no effect on T cells remain enterotoxic in experimental animals. It is proposed that enterotoxins cause the symptoms of food poisoning by inducing the release of as yet unidentified neuropeptides from intestinal cells and/or histamine from mast cells in the gut.

What is the evidence for a superantigen mediated process in staphylococcal toxic shock syndrome?

Proof that a disease is superantigen mediated can only be obtained from immunological studies of patients. The hallmark of a superantigen mediated disease is a skewed pattern of Vβ expression in the population of T cells from patients with the disease. This is caused by the preferential stimulation and proliferation of T cells belonging to Vβ families specific to the superantigen. The specific pattern ('Vβ repertoire') should reflect the in vitro Vβ specificity (or 'signature') of the causative superantigen. Staphylococcal toxic shock syndrome was the first disease in which an altered T cell Vβ repertoire was detected in patients. A disproportionately high number of T cells bearing Vβ2 were found in 7 out of 12 patients with staphylococcal toxic shock syndrome.[9] This correlated with the in vitro Vβ specificity of toxic shock syndrome toxin which stimulates T cells bearing Vβ2.

Table 3.4 Diagnostic criteria for streptococcal toxic shock-like syndrome

◆ **Isolation of group A streptococci**	
From a normally sterile site (definite case)	
From a non-sterile site (probable case)	
◆ **Hypotension or shock**	
◆ **2 or more of the following:**	
Fever	> 38.5°C
Rash	diffuse erythematous macular, with subsequent desquamation
Vomiting and diarrhoea	
Hepatic dysfunction	abnormal liver function tests
Renal impairment	↑ creatinine
Adult respiratory distress syndrome	
Coagulopathy	platelets < 100 or disseminated intravascular coagulation
Soft tissue necrosis	including necrotising fasciitis/myositis or gangrene
◆ **Exclusion of other aetiology for illness**	

Invasive group A streptococcal infection and streptococcal toxic shock-like syndrome

Streptococcal toxic shock-like syndrome was first described in 1987.[10] It has been described in adults and children[11] and can affect otherwise healthy individuals. The disease is similar to staphylococcal toxic shock syndrome with fever, hypotension and multisystem organ failure (Table 3.4). Desquamation in convalescence is seen less commonly in streptococcal toxic shock-like syndrome. In contrast to staphylococcal toxic shock syndrome, which can be associated with even a trivial abrasion, streptococcal toxic shock-like syndrome is usually associated with severe focal infection, extensive soft tissue infection and septicaemia. It may be associated with necrotising fasciitis. The case fatality rate is 5 times higher for streptococcal toxic shock-like syndrome than staphylococcal toxic shock syndrome. However, staphylococcal toxic shock syndrome and streptococcal toxic shock-like syndrome may be indistinguishable in the early stages.

What is the cause of streptococcal toxic shock-like syndrome?

Group A streptococci are isolated from the blood in over 50% of streptococcal toxic shock-like syndrome cases. Streptococcal pyrogenic exotoxin A producing strains are most common: in one study 74% of isolates were M type 1 or 3 and 85% of these strains possessed the gene encoding streptococcal pyrogenic exotoxin A compared with 15% of a sample of general isolates. Streptococcal pyrogenic exotoxins B and C have also been implicated in this syndrome, especially in Europe. Two new streptococcal superantigen toxins, with unique patterns of T cell Vβ stimulation, have recently been isolated from patients with streptococcal toxic shock-like syndrome. Streptococcal superantigen[12] is structurally more similar to some of the staphylococcal enterotoxins than the streptococcal pyrogenic exotoxins. It is thought that the streptococcal superantigen gene has only recently been acquired by group A streptococci. Streptococcal pyrogenic exotoxin F[13] (previously called mitogenic factor) does not show any nucleotide homology with the known superantigens. There is also evidence that further as yet uncharacterised superantigens may be involved in streptococcal toxic shock-like syndrome.[14]

Are superantigens responsible for the resurgence of invasive group A streptococcal infections?

During the 1980s there was a resurgence of severe invasive group A streptococcal infections worldwide both in adults and children. A change in the epidemiology of group A streptococci with the emergence of more virulent strains, in particular those producing streptococcal pyrogenic exotoxins, is thought to be an important contributing factor (reviewed in[15]).

Kawasaki disease

Kawasaki disease is a systemic febrile vasculitis characterised by fever, a polymorphous rash, conjunctivitis, mucositis, cervical lymphadenopathy and swelling of the hands and feet (Table 3.5).[16,17] The major complication of Kawasaki disease is coronary artery involvement, predominantly dilatation and aneurysm formation, which occurs in 20–30% of untreated patients. Death from myocardial infarction, aneurysm rupture and dysrhythmias can occur in the acute phase of the illness. The case fatality rate in the UK in 1990 was 3.7%.[18] It is also recognised that there is considerable long term morbidity as a result of scar formation, intimal thickening and accelerated atherosclerosis. These complications have been associated with sudden deaths in adolescence. With the decline in rheumatic heart disease, Kawasaki disease is now the commonest cause of acquired heart disease in developed countries. It has been shown that intravenous immunoglobulin (a single dose of 2 g/kg over 10 h) given within 10 days of the start of the illness dramatically lessens the risk of developing coronary artery aneurysms. Treatment with intravenous immunoglobulin after this time has not been subjected to a formal trial. It may be beneficial if there is evidence of on going inflammation (e.g. fever, acute phase reactants). Aspirin is also given, initially for its anti-inflammatory properties and later for its action on platelets.[19]

What is the cause of Kawasaki disease?

Kawasaki disease affects children predominantly between the age of 6 months and 4 years, implicating a lack of protective antibody in the development of the disease. Epidemics, clusters and seasonal peaks of the disease have been described, and its wave-like spread has been tracked across Japan.

Table 3.5 Diagnostic criteria for Kawasaki disease

Note that there are cases of Kawasaki disease which do not strictly fulfil these criteria.[42] Such patients with 'atypical' or 'incomplete' Kawasaki disease may still suffer cardiac complications and their recognition and treatment is therefore important.

A. **Fever** persisting for 5 days or more

B. Presence of **four** of the following five conditions
  (1) Bilateral bulbar conjunctival injection (non-purulent)
  (2) Changes in the mucous membranes and upper respiratory tract, such as injected pharynx, reddened or dry cracked lips, strawberry tongue
  (3) Changes in the hands and feet, including erythema of the palms and soles, indurative oedema, desquamation (in convalesence) of the skin
  (4) Polymorphous rash
  (5) Cervical lymphadenopathy

C. Exclusion of: staphylococcal and streptococcal infection, measles, leptospirosis, rickettsial disease, Steven's Johnson syndrome, drug reaction and juvenile rheumatoid arthritis

In the presence of coronary artery aneurysms (A) plus three of the five criteria in (B) are sufficient.

Other features which may occur in Kawasaki disease

Cardiac	(see text)
Joints	Arthralgia, arthritis
Neurological	Extreme irritability, aseptic meningitis, VII nerve palsy, subdural effusion
Gastrointestinal	Abdominal pain, diarrhoea, vomiting, hydrops of the gallbladder, mild hepatitis, abdominal distension, acute abdomen from ischaemic bowel, paralytic ileus, splenomegaly
Ocular	Uveitis
Renal	Sterile pyuria, proteinuria
Respiratory	Pneumonitis, pleural effusions, sterile otitis media
Skin	Erythema and induration at site of BCG scar

Laboratory findings may include:

Neutrophilia	Hypoalbuminaemia
Raised ESR	Thrombocytosis (Note: usually a late feature and
Raised CRP	therefore **not** useful for early diagnosis)
Anaemia	Raised serum IgE
Raised serum transaminases	

The cause of Kawasaki disease remains unknown but these epidemiological features strongly suggest that it is caused by an infectious agent to which everyone is exposed and to which most acquire immunity in childhood. A wide variety of different organisms have been proposed as the cause of Kawasaki disease but none have been proven. There are striking clinical and immunological similarities between Kawasaki disease and the staphylococcal and streptococcal toxic shock syndromes and scarlet fever. This has raised the possibility that Kawasaki disease is another superantigen mediated disease.[20]

What is the evidence for a superantigen mediated process in Kawasaki disease?

The T cell Vβ repertoire in patients with Kawasaki disease has been investigated. Two studies have shown an increased proportion of Vβ2 bearing T cells in Kawasaki disease patients when compared with controls.[21,22] The detection of increased Vβ expression is critically dependent on the timing of the investigation with respect to the onset of disease.[9,22] It may not be possible to detect a rise in patients studied early in the disease and this may explain the failure of some other studies to find a Vβ restricted T cell repertoire in Kawasaki disease.[23]

What is the superantigen in Kawasaki disease?

It has been suggested that toxic shock syndrome toxin, secreted from a new clone of *S. aureus* which has distinct phenotypic properties (including growth as white rather than gold colonies on agar), is the cause of Kawasaki disease.[24] However, this remains controversial.[25] Strains of *S. aureus* producing a variety of other superantigen toxins have also been isolated from patients with Kawasaki disease.[26] However, direct evidence against a central role for the known staphylococcal toxins in Kawasaki disease has been provided by serological studies which demonstrate pre-existing specific anti-toxin IgG in Kawasaki disease patients in the acute stage of the illness, a lack of IgM antibody and the absence of seroconversion to any known toxin during the course of the illness. The finding of strains of bacteria which produce superantigen activity that can not be explained by any of the known toxins has raised the interesting possibility that a previously unrecognised superantigen toxin is involved in the disease.[26,27]

Skin diseases

Atopic dermatitis

S. aureus can be isolated from more than 90% of patients with atopic dermatitis and it has been shown that more than half of these isolates have the capacity to secrete identifiable superantigen toxins.[28] In addition, antistaphylococcal antibiotics can augment the effectiveness of topical corticosteroids in the treatment of chronic atopic dermatitis.[28] These observations raise the possibility that staphylococcal toxins play a role in the pathogenesis of this disorder.

A number of mechanisms whereby superantigen toxins could be involved in the pathogenesis of atopic dermatitis have been proposed,[28] but the immunological criteria for a superantigen mediated disease have by no means been conclusively demonstrated. Superantigens secreted at the skin surface could penetrate the inflamed skin and, by binding with epidermal macrophages or Langerhans cells, stimulate the release of pro-inflammatory cytokines. Alternatively, superantigens may act as allergens stimulating the production of anti-staphylococcal superantigen toxin IgE. IgE-mediated histamine release could then trigger the itch-scratch cycle that exacerbates atopic dermatitis.

Psoriasis

T cell activation predominates in the histopathology of psoriasis and drugs that inhibit T cell activation and cytokine release, such as corticosteroids, anti CD4 monoclonal antibodies and cyclosporin A, are effective in treating the condition. Psoriatic plaques represent areas of ongoing cellular immune response with cytokine release. The agents driving this process are not known but it has been suggested that bacterial infection may be one factor: 50% of patients with psoriasis carry *S. aureus* on their skin. In addition, streptococcal throat infection is known to be an important precipitating factor in guttate psoriasis and systemic antibiotics are effective in this type of psoriasis.

It has recently been shown that keratinocytes can act as accessory cells for superantigen stimulation. It has been speculated that staphylococcal or streptococcal superantigen toxins could, therefore, activate keratinocytes as well as infiltrating T cells and monocytes. This could lead to cytokine release, keratinocyte proliferation, endothelial cell activation and other features of psoriasis.[29] Evidence to support this hypothesis has recently been provided by the demonstration that skin biopsies from patients with guttate psoriasis have a selective increase in Vβ2 bearing T cells.[30] Furthermore, all streptococcal isolates from the patients in this study produced streptococcal pyrogenic exotoxin C, whose Vβ specificity includes Vβ2. Further studies to confirm the aetiological role of streptococcal toxins in psoriasis are awaited.

Sudden infant death syndrome

One theory for the cause of sudden infant death syndrome involves bacterial toxins.[31] It proposes that sudden death is due to toxins produced by nasopharyngeal bacterial overgrowth that occurs after a viral upper respiratory tract infection. There is some laboratory evidence to support this hypothesis: there is increased carriage of staphylococci, streptococci and enterobacteria in the nasopharyngeal bacterial flora of sudden infant death syndrome cases when compared with controls.

It has also been shown, in a chick embryo bioassay, that toxins from sudden infant death syndrome cases are more likely to have a lethal effect and that certain combinations of toxins from the same infant are synergistic. Furthermore, nicotine in very low concentrations has been shown to potentiate the effects of these toxins and could, therefore, explain why parental smoking increases the risk of sudden infant death syndrome.[32]

A role for superantigen toxins in this theory has been proposed. Staphylococcal enterotoxins have been demonstrated immunohistologically in the kidney of sudden infant death syndrome cases.[33] In addition, endotoxaemia has also been implicated in sudden infant death syndrome; the ability of superantigen toxins to enhance the effect of endotoxin has been suggested as a further mechanism by which superantigens may be involved in this syndrome. In common with many theories that have been proposed for the cause of cot death, the association with superantigens remains to be proven.

WHAT DETERMINES SUSCEPTIBILITY TO SUPERANTIGEN MEDIATED DISEASE?

What is the importance of host immunity?

A large proportion of commensal skin and mucous membrane flora (staphylococci and streptococci in particular) in healthy individuals are superantigen toxin producers. There is an increase in the prevalence of antibodies to these toxins with age implying asymptomatic acquisition of immunity is common.

The importance of antibodies in protecting against superantigen mediated disease is illustrated by the fact that patients with staphylococcal toxic shock syndrome have been shown to lack anti-toxin antibodies at presentation. Patients with pre-existing antibodies are unlikely to develop staphylococcal toxic shock syndrome even if colonised by toxin-producing strains. Similarly, the lack of neutralising antibodies to streptococcal pyrogenic exotoxin F has been correlated with severe infection.[34]

The development of disease, therefore, represents infection with a toxin producing strain in an individual who does not have protective antibodies to the toxin. However, the age related prevalence of antibodies to superantigen toxins does not correlate well with the incidence of clinical disease. Additional factors must therefore be important.

What other factors predispose to superantigen mediated disease?

Association with tampon use

The association of hyperabsorbable tampons with staphylococcal toxic shock syndrome is well documented.[35] It is believed that the use of these particular tampons alters micro environmental conditions in such a way as to favour toxin production. Of particular importance is the ability of these tampons to bind magnesium ions which has been shown to increase toxin production.

Varicella

The association of invasive group A streptococcal infection and staphylococcal disease with varicella (chicken pox) has received increasing recognition.[15,36—38] Varicella has been associated with up to 47% of patients in published series of cases with invasive group A streptococcal disease.[37] Secondary bacterial infection by group A streptococci or *S. aureus* is the most common complication of varicella in immunocompetent children. Reported complications include cellulitis, myositis, necrotising fasciitis, pneumonia, epiglottitis and streptococcal toxic shock-like syndrome. The reason for the association of invasive bacterial infection in varicella may simply be the decreased integrity of the skin and mucous membranes as a result of varicella lesions or the co-incident peak seasonal activity of the two infectious diseases. An alternative (but unproven) explanation is that varicella impairs host immune responses either directly or by means of secreted proteins (virokines).

Detecting bacterial superinfection in patients with varicella may be difficult. However, temperature above 38.9°C, 3 days or more after the onset of chicken pox lesions is unusual in uncomplicated varicella. The possibility of secondary bacterial infection should, therefore, be considered in any child with varicella who has persistent or recurrent fever after the third day of the illness, or when additional signs, such as localised swelling, pain or erythema appear. Early antibiotic administration and surgical drainage of infective foci may be life-saving in patients with septicaemia or toxic shock syndrome.

Nonsteroidal anti-inflammatory drugs

There have been numerous reports suggesting an association between the use of nonsteroidal anti-inflammatory drugs and the progression to invasive group A streptococcal infections.[15,36] It is proposed that the underlying basis for this link is the ability of nonsteroidal anti-inflammatory drugs to inhibit neutrophil function, augment cytokine (particularly tumour necrosis factor-α) production and attenuate cardinal signs of inflammation.[39] It is, therefore, recommended that these drugs are not used as anti-pyretics where the cause of fever is not known.

TREATMENT OF SUPERANTIGEN MEDIATED DISEASES

The treatment of staphylococcal toxic shock syndrome and streptococcal toxic shock-like syndrome outlined below illustrates the principles of management that can be applied from an understanding of the mechanism of action of superantigen toxins.

Identification and treatment of focus of infection

An essential component of the initial management of both staphylococcal toxic shock syndrome and streptococcal toxic shock-like syndrome is the urgent identification and treatment of any focus of infection. This may involve surgical exploration and removal by drainage, lavage or debridement. Fasciotomies may be necessary in the case of streptococcal toxic shock-like syndrome with necrotising fasciitis.

Antibiotics

Elimination of the infecting bacteria using anti-staphylococcal or anti-streptococcal antibiotics is also part of the initial management of toxic shock. In cases of toxic shock in which the causative bacteria is not yet known, antibiotics directed against both organisms should be started. Flucloxacillin remains the antibiotic of choice for the first line treatment of staphylococcal disease. Penicillin has historically been used for streptococcal disease. However, clindamycin may be preferable to penicillin in the treatment of severe invasive group A streptococcal infection (reviewed in[15]). Penicillin is less efficacious where there are large numbers of organisms present (the 'Eagle effect'). Large inocula reach stationary phase rapidly and penicillin is less active against slowly growing organisms. In addition, some penicillin binding proteins are not expressed by streptococci during stationary phase. Clindamycin does not suffer these disadvantages. Moreover, clindamycin may also have immunomodulatory properties in addition to its antimicrobial activity. It has recently been shown to block toxin and protease production as well as inhibit streptococcal M protein (an important group A streptococcus virulence factor) synthesis. It also has the ability to modulate host cytokine synthesis in vitro.[40]

Treatment of shock and multi-organ failure

Aggressive support of the circulation with fluid replacement and inotropes may be necessary together with support of multi-organ failure.

Adjunctive therapy

Superantigens trigger a complex cascade of immunological events and it is this rather than the superantigen or the bacteria itself that is responsible for the clinical features of disease. Therefore, anti-bacterial treatment alone is unlikely to be effective once this process has started. Therapy aimed at modulating toxin production or the immune response may be useful.

Steroids

Among their many actions, steroids inhibit toxin-induced T cell activation and cytokine production. Steroids have been associated with improvement when given early in the course of staphylococcal toxic shock syndrome but have not been subjected to a controlled trial. Their use should probably, therefore, be restricted to patients unresponsive to fluid resuscitation.

Intravenous immunoglobulin

Intravenous immunoglobulin has multiple immunomodulatory properties. In particular it contains specific antibodies that inhibit the activation of T cells by superantigens and has the ability to down regulate cytokine production (reviewed in[15]). Intravenous immunoglobulin has been successfully used in staphylococcal toxic shock syndrome and streptococcal toxic shock-like syndrome but there have been no formal prospective trials.

THE FUTURE

Novel superantigens and superantigen-mediated diseases

With the continuing flurry of research into superantigens, it is likely that more superantigens will be isolated and characterised. The list of different organisms capable of producing superantigens may grow; and the range of disease for which a role for superantigens is postulated will increase. Although it has been suggested that a superantigen mechanism may play an important part in the pathogenesis of AIDS,[4,41] definitive proof of a viral superantigen causing disease in humans is awaited. Further immunological studies of patients are needed to elucidate the role of superantigens in many of the bacterial and autoimmune diseases in which this role remains speculative.

New therapeutic strategies

The appreciation of the immunological mechanisms by which superantigens cause disease permits the development of new agents that more specifically target the immune response to superantigens. Agents that impede T cell activation such as cyclosporin and interferon, or that inhibit cytokine release, such as pentoxifylline and thalidomide, have been shown to be effective in vitro but have not been assessed in human trials. Anti Vβ monoclonal antibodies and anti Vβ specific cytotoxic T cells may be useful to eliminate specific subsets of Vβ bearing T cells if these are confirmed as important in the pathogenesis of autoimmune disease. Other bacterial virulence factors that interact with superantigens may also be important in disease pathogenesis (reviewed in[15]). These may be additional targets for future therapy.

Vaccines against superantigen diseases

Immunisation to prevent superantigen mediated diseases in susceptible individuals or even on a population basis may be possible. Attempts have been made to construct mutant toxins that have no T cell activity or toxicity but which are still immunogenic. Such toxins could safely be used in vaccines to induce the development of protective antibodies. Studies in vitro and in animals using mutant superantigen toxins have been encouraging, but trials in humans are still a distant prospect.

Superantigens as therapy

It has been shown that superantigens can activate and direct T cells to eradicate class II expressing cells. This is called superantigen dependent cellular cytotoxicity. Attempts are being made to exploit this unique property as a therapeutic strategy in treating autoimmune disease and in killing class II expressing tumour cells (reviewed in[5]). Another strategy for the use of superantigens as anti-tumour agents (superantigen directed T cell killing) involves the conjugating of a superantigen to a monoclonal antibody specific for a tumour antigen. By this technique, the superantigen can be used to initiate T cell dependent killing specifically targeted at tumour cells.

KEY POINTS FOR CLINICAL PRACTICE

1. A number of diseases are mediated by bacterial toxins acting as superantigens. Many of the clinical features of these diseases can be explained by the interaction of the bacterial superantigen with the host immune system.

2. Superantigens stimulate T cells by a unique mechanism and thereby cause a profound and widespread activation of the immune system characterised by T cell activation/proliferation and cytokine release.

3. The list of diseases that are postulated as being superantigen mediated is growing rapidly. Confirmation of the role of a superantigen in a disease requires rigorous immunological studies in patients.

4. The management of severe invasive staphylococcal and streptococcal disease requires the removal of any focus of infection, elimination of the infecting bacteria using antibiotics and aggressive support of the circulation and multi-organ failure. Additional treatment with agents that reduce the inflammatory response may be beneficial.

5. Clindamycin may be preferable to penicillin in the treatment of severe invasive group A streptococcal infection because it does not suffer from the 'Eagle effect' and may also have beneficial immunomodulatory properties.

6. Agents that modulate the immune response (e.g. steroids or intravenous immunoglobulin) and/or toxin production (e.g. clindamycin) may offer therapeutic benefits but have not been subjected to formal evaluation.

7. Staphylococcal and streptococcal superinfection are the commonest complications of varicella. Strains producing superantigen toxins can lead rapidly to invasive disease. Early recognition and treatment can be life-saving.

8. There is a suggestion that nonsteroidal anti-inflammatory drugs may predispose to invasive streptococcal disease and should therefore be avoided as anti-pyretics where the cause of fever is unknown.

9. Understanding the mechanism by which superantigens mediate disease may be exploited to formulate novel strategies for vaccines and to design new and improved therapies which target the immune response more specifically to superantigens.

REFERENCES

1. Marrack P, Kappler J. The staphylococcal enterotoxins and their relatives. Science 1990; 248: 705–711
2. Kotzin BL, Leung DY, Kappler J, Marrack P. Superantigens and their potential role in human disease. Adv Immunol 1993; 54: 99–166
3. Fleischer B. Superantigens. Apmis 1994; 102: 3–12
4. Schafer R, Sheil JM. Superantigens and their role in infectious disease. Adv Pediatr Infect Dis 1995; 10: 369–390
5. Kotb M. Bacterial pyrogenic exotoxins as superantigens. Clin Microbiol Rev 1995; 8: 411–426
6. Davis MM, Buxbaum J. T-cell receptor use in human autoimmune disease. Ann NY Acad Sci 1995; 756: 1–464.
7. Todd J, Fishaut M. Toxic-shock syndrome associated with phage-group-I staphylococci. Lancet 1978; 2: 1116–1118
8. Ren K, Bannan JD, Pancholi V et al. Characterization and biological properties of a new staphylococcal exotoxin. J Exp Med 1994; 180: 1675–1683
9. Choi Y, Lafferty JA, Clements JR et al. Selective expansion of T cells expressing V beta 2 in toxic shock syndrome. J Exp Med 1990; 172: 981–984
10. Cone LA, Woodard DR, Schlievert PM, Tomory GS. Clinical and bacteriologic observations of a toxic shock-like syndrome due to *Streptococcus pyogenes*. N Engl J Med 1987; 317: 146–149
11. Torres MC, Mehta D, Butt A, Levin M. Streptococcus associated toxic shock. Arch Dis Child 1992; 67: 126–130
12. Mollick JA, Miller GG, Musser JM, Cook RG, Grossman D, Rich RR. A novel superantigen isolated from pathogenic strains of *Streptococcus pyogenes* with aminoterminal homology to staphylococcal enterotoxins B and C. J Clin Invest 1993; 92: 710–719
13. Norrby TA, Newton D, Kotb M, Holm SE, Norgren M. Superantigenic properties of the group A streptococcal exotoxin SpeF (MF). Infect Immun 1994; 62: 5227–5233
14. Watanabe OR, Low DE, McGeer A et al. Selective depletion of V beta-bearing T cells in patients with severe invasive group A streptococcal infections and streptococcal toxic shock syndrome. Ontario Streptococcal Study Project. J Infect Dis 1995; 171: 74–84
15. Curtis N. Invasive group A streptococcal infection. Curr Opin Infect Dis 1996; 9: 191–202
16. Nadel S, Levin M. Kawasaki disease. In: David TJ, ed. Recent Advances in Paediatrics vol 11. Edinburgh: Churchill Livingstone, 1993; 103–116
17. Kato H, Akagi T, Sugimura T et al. Kawasaki disease. Coron Artery Dis 1995; 6: 194–206
18. Dhillon R, Newton L, Rudd PT, Hall SM. Management of Kawasaki disease in the British Isles. Arch Dis Child 1993; 69: 631–636
19. Newburger JW. Treatment of Kawasaki disease. Lancet 1996; 347: 1128
20. Levin M, Tizard EJ, Dillon MJ. Kawasaki disease: recent advances. Arch Dis Child 1991; 66: 1369–1372
21. Abe J, Kotzin BL, Jujo K et al. Selective expansion of T cells expressing T-cell receptor variable regions V beta 2 and V beta 8 in Kawasaki disease. Proc Natl Acad Sci USA 1992; 89: 4066–4070
22. Curtis N, Zheng R, Lamb JR, Levin M. Evidence for a superantigen mediated process in Kawasaki disease. Arch Dis Child 1995; 72: 308–311
23. De Inocencio J, Hirsh R. Evidence for a superantigen mediated process in Kawasaki disease. Arch Dis Child 1995; 73: 275–276
24. Leung DY, Meissner HC, Fulton DR, Murray DL, Kotzin BL, Schlievert PM. Toxic shock syndrome toxin-secreting *Staphylococcus aureus* in Kawasaki syndrome. Lancet 1993; 342: 1385–1388
25. Terai M, Miwa K, Williams T et al. The absence of evidence of staphylococcal toxin

involvement in the pathogenesis of Kawasaki disease. J Infect Dis 1995; 172: 558–561

26. Curtis N, Chan B, Levin M. Toxic shock syndrome toxin-secreting *Staphylococcus aureus* in Kawasaki syndrome. Lancet 1994; 343: 299

27. Curtis N, Chan B, Levin M. Is Kawasaki disease caused by a novel superantigen toxin? In: Kato H, ed. Kawasaki disease. Amsterdam: Elsevier, 1995; 133–138

28. Leung DY, Travers JB, Norris DA. The role of superantigens in skin disease. J Invest Dermatol 1995; 105 (Suppl. 1): S37–S42

29. Valdimarsson H, Baker BS, Jonsdottir I, Powles A, Fry L. Psoriasis: a T-cell-mediated autoimmune disease induced by streptococcal superantigens? Immunol Today 1995; 16: 145–149

30. Leung DYM, Travers JB, Giorno R et al. Evidence for a streptococcal superantigen-driven process in acute guttate psoriasis. J Clin Invest 1995; 96: 2106–2112

31. Blackwell CC, Saadi AT, Raza MW, Weir DM, Busuttil A. The potential role of bacterial toxins in sudden infant death syndrome (SIDS). Int J Legal Med 1993; 105: 333–338

32. Sayers NM, Drucker DB, Telford DR, Morris JA. Effects of nicotine on bacterial toxins associated with cot death. Arch Dis Child 1995; 73: 549–551

33. Malam JE, Carrick GF, Telford DR, Morris JA. Staphylococcal toxins and sudden infant death syndrome. J Clin Pathol 1992; 45: 716–721

34. Norrby TA, Pauksens K, Holm SE, Norgren M. Relation between low capacity of human sera to inhibit streptococcal mitogens and serious manifestation of disease. J Infect Dis 1994; 170: 585–591

35. Kass EH, Parsonnet J. On the pathogenesis of toxic shock syndrome. Rev Infect Dis 1987; 9 (Suppl. 5): S482–S489

36. Brogan TV, Nizet V, Waldhausen JH, Rubens CE, Clarke WR. Group A streptococcal necrotizing fasciitis complicating primary varicella: a series of fourteen patients. Pediatr Infect Dis J 1995; 14: 588–594

37. Peterson CL, Vugia DJ, Meyers HB et al. Risk factors for invasive group A streptococcal infections in children with varicella: a case-control study. Pediatr Infect Dis J 1996; 15: 151–156

38. Pollard AJ, Isaacs A, Lyall EGH et al. Life-threatening bacterial infection associated with varicella. BMJ 1996; 313: 283–285

39. Stevens DL. Could nonsteroidal antiinflammatory drugs (NSAIDs) enhance the progression of bacterial infections to toxic shock syndrome? Clin Infect Dis 1995; 21: 977–980

40. Stevens DL, Bryant AE, Hackett SP. Antibiotic effects on bacterial viability, toxin production, and host response. Clin Infect Dis 1995; 20 (Suppl. 2): S154–S157

41. Dobrescu D, Ursea B, Pope M, Asch AS, Posnett DN. Enhanced HIV-1 replication in V beta 12 T cells due to human cytomegalovirus in monocytes: evidence for a putative herpesvirus superantigen. Cell 1995; 82: 753–763

42. Fukushige J, Takahashi N, Ueda Y, Ueda K. Incidence and clinical features of incomplete Kawasaki disease. Acta Paediatr 1994; 83: 1057–1060

4

Thalassaemia

N. F. Olivieri

The thalassaemias are hereditary anaemias which occur as a result of mutations that affect the synthesis of hemoglobin. Decreases in the synthesis of either the alpha or beta chains of hemoglobin produce the distinct clinical phenotypes of alpha and beta thalassaemia. Alpha thalassaemia, resulting for the most part from deletion mutations within the duplicated alpha genes on chromosome 16, is common in populations from China, Indochina, Malaysia, and Africa. The beta thalassaemias, for which over 130 mutations within the beta globin gene on chromosome 11 have been described, are concentrated in populations of the Mediterranean, Africa, the Middle East, India and Pakistan, and China.[1] The most clinically important thalassaemia syndrome, homozygous beta thalassaemia, will be discussed in this chapter; the primary focus of discussion will be transfusion-dependent beta thalassaemia, or thalassaemia major. The reader is referred to an excellent review of alpha thalassaemia for discussion of these disorders.[2]

MOLECULAR ASPECTS OF BETA THALASSAEMIA

The beta thalassaemias are a heterogeneous group of autosomal recessive disorders characterized by deficient or absent beta-globin chain synthesis. Reduced beta chain production results in imbalanced synthesis of globin chains and in varying degrees of ineffective erythropoiesis, with production of small and poorly hemoglobinized red cells.[1] Globin chain imbalance, the major determinant of the severity of beta thalassaemia, is influenced by three main factors: (i) the presence of a mild beta thalassaemia defect, associated with a high residual production of beta globin chains; (ii) co-inheritance of alpha thalassaemia which reduces globin chain imbalance; and (iii) the presence of genetic factors associated with increased gamma chain production, also thereby reducing globin chain imbalance. The molecular heterogeneity of the beta thalassaemias explains the wide spectrum of clinical syndromes, with severity varying between common transfusion-dependent thalassaemia major to mild non-transfusion-dependent thalassaemia 'intermedia'.[3]

The large majority of the beta thalassaemia defects are single nucleotide mutations affecting one of the molecular processes involved in beta globin gene expression, including transcription, RNA processing, and translation.

In each ethnic population, a limited number of mutations (usually not more than 5–8) account for 90% of the molecular defects.[3]

CLINICAL MANAGEMENT OF BETA THALASSAEMIA

Red cell transfusions

Regular red cell transfusions eliminate the complications of anaemia and ineffective erythropoiesis, permit normal growth and development throughout childhood, and extend survival in thalassaemia major.[1] The decision to initiate a programme of regular red cell transfusions is based on the severity of anaemia, decline in growth velocity, splenomegaly, and the presence and severity of bone marrow expansion. The institution of a transfusion programme is often based upon the observation of a peripheral hemoglobin concentration of less than 7 g/dl at monthly intervals over 3 consecutive months, a finding usually associated with poor growth, splenic enlargement, and/or marrow expansion. Determination of the molecular basis of homozygous beta thalassaemia is rarely of value in predicting a requirement for regular transfusions. Prior to the first transfusion, the iron and folate status of each patient should be assessed, hepatitis B vaccine series should be initiated, and a complete red cell phenotype should be obtained, so that subsequent alloimmunization may be detected.

The transfusion regimen itself appears critical for the control of body iron loading. Adoption of a regimen to maintain pre-transfusion hemoglobin concentrations not exceeding 9.5 g/dl has been shown to result in a reduced transfusion requirement and improved control of body iron burden, compared to a regimen (termed 'supertransfusion') in which baseline hemoglobins exceed 11 g/dl.[4] The individualization of a transfusion regimen for each patient is necessary. Pre-transfusion hemoglobins, volume administered, weight and spleen size should recorded at each visit to permit evaluation of the need for splenectomy.

Type of red cell concentrates

Clinical studies of the use of neocytes, or young red blood cells, have confirmed that prolonged in vivo survival of these concentrates reduce the red cell mass required to maintain appropriate baseline hemoglobin concentrations. A recent analysis reported that a 15% extension of transfusion interval during administration of neocyte concentrates, which would be expected to minimally reduce the requirement for iron chelation therapy, was achieved through increased exposure to donated units and a 5-fold increase in preparation costs over those of standard concentrates.[5] Hence, the use of neocytes should have a small impact on the long-term management of most chronically transfused patients.

Splenectomy

In the past, most patients with homozygous beta thalassaemia developed significant hypersplenism and an increase in yearly red cell requirements during the first decade of life. While hypersplenism may sometimes be avoided by early and regular transfusion, many thalassaemia patients will nevertheless ultimately require splenectomy. Splenectomy should reduce red cell requirements by 30% in a patient whose transfusion index (calculated by addition of the total of packed cells administered over 1 year, divided by the mid-year weight in kg) exceeds 200 ml/kg/year.[6] Because of the risk of post-splenectomy infection, splenectomy should generally be delayed until the age of 5 years. Prior to splenectomy, immunization with 23-valent pneumococcal vaccine and *Haemophilus influenzae* type B vaccine (if not administered previously) is recommended; after splenectomy, compliance with longterm prophylactic penicillin (250–300 mg twice daily) should be monitored.

COMPLICATIONS OF RED CELL TRANSFUSION

Viral hepatitis

Liver disease is reported as a common cause of death in patients with thalassaemia over the age of 15 years. Iron-induced hepatic damage is influenced by a second complication of transfusions, infection with hepatitis C virus, the most frequent cause of hepatitis in thalassemic children. The high incidence of liver failure and hepatocellular carcinoma in patients who have acquired the virus through transfusions support the use of antiviral therapy for patients with thalassaemia. The results of recent trials of interferon-alpha in hepatitis-C-infected patients with thalassaemia suggest that the clinical and pathologic responses to this agent may be inversely related to body iron burden.[7]

Yersinia infection

Yersinia sepsis is encountered much more frequently in patients with thalassaemia and iron overload than in the normal host. This infection should also be suspected in patients with iron overload who present with an acute diarrheal illness and high fever. Even in the absence of a positive blood culture for *Yersinia* in this clinical setting, therapy with intravenous gentamicin and oral trimethoprim-sulphamethoxazole should be promptly instituted, and continued for 7 days.

Iron overload

Iron overload is the most important consequence of life-saving transfusions in thalassaemia.[6] The toxicity of iron has been thoroughly reviewed previously;[8] the clinical complications of iron overload and the impact of iron chelating therapy will be reviewed here.

CLINICAL COMPLICATIONS OF IRON OVERLOAD

In the absence of chelating therapy, myocardial disease remains the most severe, life-limiting complication of transfusional iron overload. Irregularly transfused, unchelated children usually developed left ventricular hypertrophy and conduction disturbances by late childhood and ventricular arrhythmias and refractory congestive failure by the mid-teens.[6] Within the liver, the main repository of transfused iron, parenchymal iron accumulation, accelerated by viral infection, may rapidly progress to portal fibrosis in a significant percentage of patients.[6] The most common endocrine abnormalities observed in modern cohorts of patients with thalassaemia include hypogonadotropic hypogonadism, growth hormone deficiency, and diabetes mellitus. Although rates of prepubertal linear growth are normal in patients maintained on regular transfusion programs,[9] poor pubertal growth has been observed even in well-transfused patients. Poor growth has been attributed to iron-induced selective central hypogonadism, impaired growth hormone responses to growth hormone-releasing hormone, hyposecretion of adrenal androgen, delay in pubertal development itself, zinc deficiency, and desferrioxamine therapy. Diabetes mellitus in thalassaemia has been attributed both to impaired insulin secretion secondary to chronic pancreatic iron overload, and to insulin resistance as a result of iron deposition within liver or skeletal muscle.[10]

IRON CHELATING THERAPY

The only iron chelating agent presently available for clinical use is desferrioxamine B, a trihydroxamic acid produced by *Streptomyces pilosus*.[6] Desferrioxamine is poorly absorbed orally and rapidly metabolized in plasma, conferring on the drug its principal drawback: the requirement for prolonged parenteral infusions to achieve efficacy.[6]

The impact of desferrioxamine therapy

Only in the present decade did patients who started desferrioxamine in early childhood reach an age at which cardiac disease free survival could be assessed with certainty. Two recent trials have demonstrated that long-term desferrioxamine is associated with cardiac disease free survival in thalassaemia major.[11,12] One analysis reported that an increased incidence of cardiac disease and death was observed in patients who had begun desferrioxamine at a more advanced age, and who had used less desferrioxamine in relation to transfusional iron load, than had another cohort who had maintained low body iron burdens over 4–12 years of therapy.[11] The cohort in whom most complications were observed had maintained concentrations of hepatic iron exceeding 15 mg (normal approximately 1 mg) iron per g liver tissue, dry weight over the period of treatment. In a second study, patients who maintained low body iron burden as estimated by serum ferritin concentration had an estimated cardiac disease free survival of 91% after 15 years of desferrioxamine, while the cardiac disease free survival in patients in whom most serum ferritin concentrations had exceeded a value of 2500 mg/l was less than 20%.[12] Both these trials established that the magnitude of the body iron burden is the principal determinant of clinical outcome in thalassaemia major.

Reports of reduction of liver iron, improvement in laboratory abnormalities of liver function, and arrest of hepatic fibrosis support the beneficial effects of subcutaneous desferrioxamine on iron loading in the liver.[6]

Finally, the effectiveness of desferrioxamine in the preservation of gonadal function in thalassaemia was reported in a cohort of patients treated with desferrioxamine since the age of 7 years: 90% of these patients achieved normal growth and pubertal status. In contrast, in a group of patients who had administered a relatively lower total dose of desferrioxamine since a relatively later age, only 38% reached normal puberty.[13] While a striking increase in fertility in thalassaemia has been reported over the last decade, secondary amenorrhea may eventually develop in thalassemic girls with previous evidence of normal pituitary function.[14] Reduction in the risk of diabetes mellitus and glucose intolerance has been reported in patients who maintained low body iron burdens, compared to a group who had begun chelation therapy later in life and who had used less desferrioxamine less intensively.[11]

MANAGEMENT OF CHELATION THERAPY

Several practical problems are associated with chelation therapy. These include the accurate assessment of body iron burden, the appropriate age of initiation of desferrioxamine, the maintenance of balance between drug effectiveness and toxicity, and the difficulties of compliance with desferrioxamine.

Assessment of body iron burden and the effectiveness of chelating therapy

24 h DFO-induced urinary iron excretion

Because the relative amounts of iron excreted into stool and urine vary with the dose of desferrioxamine, body iron burden, and erythroid activity,[15] there exists a poor correlation between urinary iron excretion induced by desferrioxamine and hepatic iron concentration, the reference method of body iron quantitation.

Serum or plasma estimates of body iron burden

Although the measurement of plasma ferritin is the most commonly used indirect estimate of body iron stores,[15] interpretation of serum or plasma ferritin may be complicated by several conditions that are common in thalassaemia major and that alter concentrations independently of changes in body iron burden. These include ascorbate deficiency, fever, acute infection, chronic inflammation, acute and chronic hepatic damage, hemolysis and ineffective erythropoiesis. Careful studies have observed that only about 57% of the variation in plasma ferritin is accounted for by changes in hepatic iron concentration.[16] Thus, reliance on this parameter alone can lead to inaccurate assessment of body iron burden in individual patients.

Imaging of tissue iron

Computed tomography[17] and magnetic resonance imaging[18] have been used to evaluate tissue iron stores in patients with iron overload. Studies using different magnetic resonance imaging techniques have confirmed biopsy-demonstrated reductions in hepatic iron in chelated patients,[19] but correlation with biopsy-determined hepatic iron concentrations have varied with different methods of magnetic resonance imaging. This modality is not been validated as a method of providing measurements of liver iron quantitatively equivalent to that determined at biopsy. At present, magnetic resonance represents the only modality with the potential to estimate iron stores within the heart and anterior pituitary gland.

Assessment of organ function

Cardiac function. Electro- or resting echo-cardiograms are not sufficiently sensitive in the detection of iron-induced cardiac dysfunction.[20] By contrast, multi-gated exercise cardiac radionuclide angiography or low-dose dobutamine stimulation may be useful in the diagnosis of early iron-induced cardiac disease.[20] Diastolic dysfunction in asymptomatic individuals has been suggested to have prognostic significance for the development of symptomatic iron-induced cardiac disease in some, but not all, studies.

Anterior pituitary reserve. Measurement of peak serum luteinizing hormone following a bolus of gonadotropin releasing hormone is useful in the evaluation of pituitary reserve.[13] Because secondary amenorrhea may develop in thalassemic girls with previous evidence of normal pituitary function,[14] a history of menstrual pattern should be obtained regularly. Bone densities may be abnormally low in hypogonadal thalassaemia patients; because of this risk, full replacement doses of estrogen or testosterone should be prescribed to hypogonadal patients.

Direct assessment of body iron

Measurement of hepatic iron concentration is the most quantitative, specific, and sensitive means of assessing body iron stores in patients with thalassaemia major.[15] Liver biopsy provides information regarding both the pattern of iron accumulation and the histology of the liver. Superconducting magnetic susceptometry (SQUID) of hepatic iron stores offers a non-invasive method for quantitation of hepatic iron;[21] this instrument has been validated as a method of providing measurements of liver iron quantitatively equivalent to those determined at biopsy.[21]

Initiation of iron chelation therapy

Uncertainties exist as to the optimal age at which patients with thalassaemia major, transfused since infancy, should begin therapy with desferrioxamine. Because of the imprecision of indirect measurements, initiation of therapy should be based upon the severity of body iron loading, as determined by hepatic iron concentration obtained after about a year of regular transfusions; liver biopsy under ultrasound guidance has been shown to be safe in very young children.[22] One recommended endpoint of therapy is maintenance of hepatic storage iron concentration between approximately 3–7 mg (normal, 1 mg) per g dry weight liver tissue, in the range associated with long-term survival in heterozygotes for hereditary hemochromatosis.[23] If liver biopsy is not available, therapy with subcutaneous desferrioxamine, not exceeding 25 mg desferrioxamine per kg body weight/24 h in young children, should be initiated after 1 year of regular transfusions.

Balance between effectiveness and toxicity of desferrioxamine

Many toxicities associated with desferrioxamine therapy have been observed during administration of excess desferrioxamine in the presence of a relatively modest body iron burden, and include ocular, auditory, and sensorimotor neurotoxicity, renal abnormalities, and pulmonary toxicity.[24] An important desferrioxamine-induced toxicity in young children with modest body iron burdens is abnormalities of linear growth, associated with cartilaginous dysplasia of the long bones and spine.[25,26] Declines in height percentile should not be expected in a well-transfused, chelated patient, and any fall-off in growth should be investigated promptly with review of growth velocities, and metaphyseal and thoraco-lumbar-sacral spine radiographs. If evidence of widening or irregularity of the unossified metaphyseal matrix, decreased spinal height, vertebral flattening, anterior elongation or disk calcification are observed, direct assessment of body iron load should be obtained immediately, and dose reduction or discontinuation of desferrioxamine should be considered, especially in patients with hepatic iron concentrations less than 7 mg per g dry weight liver tissue.

Most desferrioxamine-induced toxicities can be avoided by regular direct assessment of body iron burden, with maintenance of hepatic iron concentration between 3–7 mg per g dry weight liver tissue. If hepatic iron is not regularly assessed, a 'toxicity' index[27] defined as the mean daily dose of desferrioxamine (in mg/kg) divided by the serum ferritin concentration in mg/l should be calculated every 6 months and should not exceed 0.025. Desferrioxamine doses should never exceed 50 mg/kg body weight/24 h, even in heavily iron loaded patients treated with intravenous regimens.

Alternatives to subcutaneous desferrioxamine infusions

Intravenous desferrioxamine

Regimens of intravenous ambulatory desferrioxamine administered through implantable venous access ports reduce local pain and irritation of subcutaneous infusions, and are associated with rapid reduction of body iron burden. Protocols of continuous intravenous ambulatory desferrioxamine in which the infusion site is changed weekly by medical personnel require infusion site care and a weekly clinic visit, but remove the need for nightly self-administration and improve patient compliance.[28]

Bone marrow transplantation

The cure of homozygous beta thalassaemia with allogeneic bone marrow transplantation, first reported over a decade ago, now offers an alternative to standard clinical management with blood transfusions and iron chelation therapy. Bone marrow transplantation is now an accepted treatment for thalassaemia; at present, disease-free survival in this disorder cannot be provided by any other therapy. Despite the cure of many patients with beta thalassaemia with marrow transplantation optimal procedures for the selection of patients, the timing of transplantation, and the preparative regimen have not yet been determined.

The most extensive experience with bone marrow transplantation in thalassaemia has been reported by Lucarelli and his colleagues in Pesaro, Italy. These investigators have identified three characteristics as significantly associated with survival and event-free survival following allogeneic bone marrow transplantation for homozygous beta thalassaemia:[29] (i) the degree of hepatomegaly; (ii) the presence of portal fibrosis on liver biopsy; and (iii) the effectiveness of therapy with desferrioxamine prior to allogeneic bone marrow transplantation. In patients in whom none of these three factors were present prior to allogeneic bone marrow transplantation (identified as Class 1 patients), event-free survival exceeded 90%. By contrast, in patients with all three of these factors (Class 3 patients), event-free survival was only 70%. These factors may be related to the severity of iron overload at the time of transplantation.

Many patients with thalassaemia major are inevitably confronted with the choice between standard therapy and bone marrow transplantation. On the one hand, the excellent results from Pesaro suggest that bone marrow transplantation should be offered to any patient with a compatible donor. On the other hand, several other factors render the choice between these therapeutic approaches difficult for knowledgeable clinicians and families. One factor includes the increased expectation of survival with standard therapy: the estimated 15 year cardiac disease free survival of transfused patients regularly compliant with desferrioxamine is 91%, comparable to that with achieved with bone marrow transplantation in Class 1 patients. Second, event-free survival following marrow transplantation for thalassaemia in North America is much lower than that reported from Pesaro. Lastly, the late complications of marrow transplantation for thalassaemia are not fully known. In support of marrow transplantation as a treatment option, this procedure renders patients not merely cardiac disease free, but also thalassaemia free. Moreover, the long-term cost of transfusion and chelation therapy greatly exceeds the cost of bone marrow transplantation.

Iron chelation following bone marrow transplantation

Successful allogeneic bone marrow transplantation does not eliminate the necessity for iron chelating therapy in all patients; hepatic iron overload persists in older patients who do not receive post-transplant desferrioxamine therapy. Both phlebotomy and short-term desferrioxamine are safe and effective in the reduction of tissue iron in the 'ex-thalassemic'[30] and should be initiated 1 year following successful marrow transplantation if the hepatic iron concentration exceeds 7 mg/g dry weight liver tissue at that time.

ORALLY ACTIVE IRON CHELATING AGENTS

The expense and inconvenience of desferrioxamine has mandated a search for an orally active iron chelator. The orally active agent most extensively evaluated to date is 1,2-dimethyl-3-hydroxypyridin-4-one (deferiprone; L1), patented in 1982 as an alternative to desferrioxamine for the treatment of chronic iron overload. In transfused patients with thalassaemia major, 75 mg of deferiprone per kg body weight induces urinary iron excretion approximately equivalent to that achieved with 30–40 mg of desferrioxamine per kg,[31] sufficient to induce net negative iron balance in many patients with thalassaemia major. Although the short term efficacy of deferiprone is unquestionably inferior to that of desferrioxamine, the long-term effectiveness of deferiprone may be sufficient to induce net negative iron balance in some, although not all, patients.

Effectiveness of deferiprone

While early studies reported no sustained decrease in serum ferritin concentration over 1–15 months of deferiprone therapy, subsequent trials reported statistically significant reductions in mean serum ferritin concentration in patients with thalassaemia major, with the most substantial declines observed in those whose pre-study ferritin concentrations exceeded 5000 mg/l, and in whom treatment had been administered for at least 18 months.[32] Direct reduction in body iron burden as determined by the hepatic iron concentration during deferiprone treatment was recently demonstrated in both thalassaemia 'intermedia'[19] and thalassaemia major.[33] Deferiprone was able to reduce and maintain, over 3 years of therapy, hepatic iron at concentrations associated with prolonged survival free of the clinical complications of iron overload in patients with thalassaemia major,[33] using criteria derived from a prospective trial in desferrioxamine-treated patients.[11] Although deferiprone has now been administered for several years to many iron loaded patients, the evaluation of its effect on cardiac iron in vivo is still complicated by our lack of ability to quantitate cardiac iron overload. Conclusions regarding the impact of deferiprone on cardiac disease-free survival in thalassaemia major must await at least a decade of observation, as was required with therapy with desferrioxamine.[11,12]

Toxicity of deferiprone – animal studies

In animal studies of deferiprone, anaemia, leucopenia and thrombocytopenia, adrenal hypertrophy, gonadal and thymic atrophy, bone marrow atrophy and pancytopenia, growth retardation, and embryotoxicity have been reported.[34] Most of these adverse effects have not been observed in patients treated with deferiprone.

Toxicity of deferiprone – human trials

Arthropathy

The most common adverse effect associated with deferiprone treatment (occurring in up to 38% of patients in some series) has been arthropathy.[35] Generalized joint pain, swelling and muscle stiffness have usually resolved after dose reduction or discontinuation of therapy. Arthroscopy, aspiration and biopsy have revealed a sterile transudate without inflammatory cells, lining cell proliferation and extensive iron deposition, with no evidence of an inflammatory or allergic reaction.[35] The etiology of deferiprone-associated arthropathy remains elusive.

Agranulocytosis and neutropenia

The most serious adverse effect associated with the administration of deferiprone is severe neutropenia or agranulocytosis, reported to date in 13 patients, of whom 10 have thalassaemia major.[32] Agranulocytosis has been observed as early as 6 weeks, and up to 21 months, after the initiation of deferiprone. Recovery periods after drug withdrawal have varied between 1–17 weeks, with complete recovery in all patients; no deaths have been reported as a result of this adverse effect. The mechanism of deferiprone-induced neutropenia is unknown. There is no evidence for increased in vitro sensitivity of myeloid precursors to deferiprone, nor of antibody-mediated white cell destruction, in patients in whom this toxicity has developed. This adverse effect associated with deferiprone may limit the widespread application of the drug. A large trial of deferiprone ongoing in Italy and the US is expected to provide an estimate of the incidence of this adverse effect.

Other adverse effects

Although one case report suggested deferiprone-induced systemic lupus erythematosus as a cause of death in a patient in India,[36] prospective studies in patients treated with deferiprone for over 3 years have suggested no adverse effect of deferiprone on immunologic function.[33] Nausea and transient liver enzyme abnormalities have also been reported;[37] dermatologic changes associated with declines in serum zinc concentration in patients receiving deferiprone have resolved with oral zinc supplementation.[37]

The licensing of deferiprone

The data from available animal toxicity studies and clinical trials of deferiprone were recently reviewed by representatives of the US Food and Drug Administration, at which time it was judged that a prospective, randomized trial to compare therapy with deferiprone with desferrioxamine, and a second prospective study to estimate the incidence of serious adverse effects of deferiprone in a larger cohort of patients, would be required for the licensing of deferiprone in the US. In 1995, deferiprone was licensed for sale in India.

Summary

While data from several trials have provided direct and supportive evidence for the short-term efficacy of deferiprone, the toxicity of this agent mandates a careful evaluation of the balance between risk and benefit of deferiprone in patients with thalassaemia, in most of whom desferrioxamine is a safe and efficacious treatment.

EXPERIMENTAL THERAPIES

Augmentation of fetal hemoglobin

Humans and other primates undergo a switch from fetal hemoglobin ($\alpha_2\gamma_2$), hemoglobin F, the main hemoglobin during gestation, to adult hemoglobin ($\alpha_2\beta_2$), hemoglobin A, at or around the time of birth. As a result of the switch to beta globin gene synthesis, hemoglobin A comprises approximately 97% of the total hemoglobin and fetal hemoglobin less than 1% in normal individuals after the first year of life.[1] In the vast majority of individuals with thalassaemia major, the upstream gamma globin genes are intact and fully functional, and if these genes could be reactivated, functional hemoglobin synthesis could be maintained during adult life, eliminating the phenotype of the disease entirely.

During the last decade, studies in vitro and in animal models have demonstrated that several cell cycle specific agents including 5-azacytidine, cytarabine, vinblastine, and hydroxyurea, as well as non-chemotherapeutic agents, including hematopoietic growth factors and short-chain fatty acids, stimulate gamma globin synthesis and fetal hemoglobin production through a variety of proposed mechanisms.[38] Clinical trials aimed at augmentation of fetal hemoglobin synthesis in thalassaemia have included short and long term administration of 5-azacytidine, hydroxyurea, recombinant human erythropoietin and butyric acid compounds, as well as combinations of these agents. The successes and failures associated with these therapies in patients with homozygous beta thalassaemia in vivo have been reviewed recently and will be summarized here.

5-azacytidine therapy in beta thalassaemia

In the first application of therapy to augment fetal hemoglobin in vivo, Ley and colleagues reported the results of administration of 5-azacytidine in a patient with homozygous beta thalassaemia in 1982.[39] Subsequently, the results of treatment with 5-azacytidine have been reported in a total of 6 patients with beta thalassaemia.[38] Increases in total hemoglobin exceeding 2 g/dl have been observed during 5 treatment courses of intravenous 5-azacytidine. The data suggest that the intravenous route of administration is associated with consistent laboratory and clinical responses, while administration of subcutaneous or oral 5-azacytidine may be less effective. Predictably, the toxicity associated with 5-azacytidine is bone marrow suppression, which limited drug administration in some patients, and was associated with serious infection in a few individuals. Consideration of this and other potential adverse effects of 5-azacytidine shifted interest in the mid-1980s to the use of alternate therapies in patients with thalassaemia.

Hydroxyurea therapy in beta thalassaemia

Clinical responses associated with administration of hydroxyurea in beta thalassaemia have been detailed in a total of 11 patients.[38] Despite increases in fetal hemoglobin, no consistent increases in total hemoglobin during hydroxyurea therapy have been reported. Thus, at this time, there is no evidence to suggest that hydroxyurea increases fetal hemoglobin synthesis to a sufficient extent to significantly modify the phenotype of thalassaemia major.

Recombinant human erythropoietin in beta thalassaemia

The experience of recombinant human erythropoietin therapy in thalassaemia suggests that clinical responses to pharmacologic doses of this agent may be observed in selected patients.[38] A total of 30 patients with thalassaemia have been treated with erythropoietin alone or in combination with hydroxyurea. Of those treated with erythropoietin as a single agent, total hemoglobin concentration has increased in 10 patients, in general without observed effects on fetal hemoglobin synthesis but in parallel with increases in red blood cell counts. The effectiveness and safety of combination therapy with hydroxyurea or other agents, the effect of dose and dosing regimen, and the potential of adverse effects of recombinant human erythropoietin in thalassaemia, all require further study.

Arginine butyrate in beta thalassaemia

Treatment with arginine butyrate has been reported to induce an increase in hemoglobin concentration in one patient with thalassaemia.[40] This pilot study reported that short-term administration of arginine butyrate resulted in increased g globin mRNA synthesis and reduction in globin chain imbalance in all patients with thalassaemia treated with arginine butyrate. One recent study of extended treatment with arginine butyrate suggests that this agent is associated with a response rate lower than predicted on the basis of the pilot trial.[41] Of note, no changes in gamma globin mRNA or in gamma globin chain synthesis was observed in patients in this trial. An explanation for the variability in response to arginine butyrate in these studies is not clear.

Sodium phenylbutyrate in beta thalassaemia

Two related orally active butyric acid compounds, sodium phenylacetate and its pro-drug, sodium-4-phenylbutyrate, have been used for years as effective therapy for children with inherited urea cycle disorders. In the first trial of sodium phenylbutyrate in 11 adults with beta thalassaemia, two patients had very modest increases in hemoglobin concentration during extended therapy with phenylbutyrate. Four of the eight non-transfusion dependent patients, and the three previously regularly transfused patients, had no hematologic response to phenylbutyrate therapy.[42] The response to sodium phenylbutyrate in thalassaemia appears to be modest, may be limited to patients with non-transfusion-dependent beta thalassaemia 'intermedia', and may be correlated with elevations in serum erythropoietin concentration, offering the tantalizing possibility that combination therapy with sodium phenylbutyrate and erythropoietin may have synergistic effects in thalassaemia.

Summary of 'fetal hemoglobin therapy' in thalassaemia

In the relatively few patients in whom clinically significant changes have been observed as summarized above, the factors influencing response to these agents remain unknown. Encouraging changes in laboratory or clinical parameters observed during administration of new compounds in pilot studies should be followed by extended clinical trials to establish effectiveness in larger cohorts. As in chemotherapy for malignant disease, it is likely that combination therapies may prove useful in the augmentation of fetal hemoglobin in the beta hemoglobinopathies. Studies to evaluate the effectiveness of combination therapies in patients with thalassaemia are proceeding.[38]

KEY POINTS FOR CLINICAL PRACTICE

1. Regular transfusions eliminate the complications of anaemia and ineffective erythropoiesis and sustain normal growth and development throughout childhood in thalassaemia major.

2. Progressive iron overload as a result of regular transfusions may be associated with fatal cardiac arrythmias and congestive failure in the second decade of life in patients who do not receive regular iron chelating therapy.

3. Initiation of iron chelating therapy with desferrioxamine should be based upon direct assessment of hepatic iron concentration, and should not be initiated before completion of one year of regular transfusions.

4. The balance between efficacy and toxicity of desferrioxamine can be maintained by regular direct assessment of body iron burden, with maintenance of hepatic iron concentration between 3–7 mg/g dry weight liver tissue.

5. Desferrioxamine doses should never exceed 50 mg/kg body weight/24 h, even in heavily iron loaded patients treated with intravenous regimens.

6. Allogeneic bone marrow transplantation offers an alternative to standard clinical management of thalassaemia. Three characteristics have been significantly associated with survival and event-free survival following marrow transplantation: (i) the degree of hepatomegaly; (ii) the presence of portal fibrosis on liver biopsy; and (iii) the effectiveness of therapy with desferrioxamine prior to allogeneic bone marrow transplantation.

7. Therapy with the orally active iron chelating agent deferiprone is able to reduce and maintain, over 3 years of therapy, hepatic iron at concentrations in some patients with thalassemia major.

8. Clinical trials aimed at augmentation of fetal hemoglobin synthesis in thalassaemia have included short and long term administration of 5-azacytidine, hydroxyurea, recombinant human erythropoietin and butyric acid compounds, as well as combinations of these agents. In the relatively few patients in whom clinically significant changes have been observed, the factors influencing response to these agents remain unknown. Combination therapies may prove useful in the augmentation of fetal hemoglobin.

REFERENCES

1. Weatherall DJ, Clegg JB. The thalassaemia syndromes. 3rd edn. Oxford: Blackwell, 1981
2. Higgs DR. α-Thalassemia. In: Higgs DR, Weatherall DJ. eds The Haemoglobinopathies. Bailliere's Clinical Haematology vol. 6, 1993; 117–150
3. Galanello R. Molecular basis of thalassemia major. Int J Pediatr Hematol Oncol 1995; 2: 383–396
4. Cazzola M, De Stefano P, Ponchio L et al. Relationship between transfusion regimen and suppression of erythropoiesis in beta thalassaemia major. Br J Haematol 1995; 89: 473
5. Collins AF, Dias GC, Haddad S et al. Evaluation of a new neocyte transfusion preparation vs washed cell transfusion in patients with homozygous beta thalassaemia. Transfusion 1994; 34: 517–520
6. Cohen AR. Management of iron overload in the pediatric patient. In: Oski FA, ed Paediatric Hematology. W.B.Saunders, 1987; 521–544
7. Clemente MG, Congia M, Lai ME et al. Effect of iron overload on the response to recombinant interferon-alfa treatment in transfusion-dependent patients with thalassaemia major and chronic hepatitis C. J Pediatr 1994; 125: 123–128
8. Hershko C, Weatherall DJ. Iron-chelating therapy. CRC Crit Rev Clin Lab Sci 1988; 26: 303–346
9. Modell B, Berdoukas V. The clinical approach to thalassaemia. London: Grune and Stratton, 1984
10. Olivieri NF. Iron chelation therapy and thalassaemia. In: Kelton G, Brian M. eds Current Therapy in Hematology/Oncology, 5th edn. 1995; 80–89
11. Brittenham GM, Griffith PM, Nienhuis AW et al. Efficacy of deferoxamine in preventing complications of iron overload in patients with thalassemia major. N Engl J Med 1994; 331: 567–573
12. Olivieri NF, Nathan DG, MacMillan JH et al. Survival of medically treated patients with homozygous β thalassemia. N Engl J Med 1994; 331: 574–578
13. Weintrob NB, Olivieri NF, Tyler BJ, Andrews D, Freedman MH, Holland FJ. Effect of age at the start of iron chelation therapy on gonadal function in β-thalassemia major. N Eng J Med 1990; 323: 713–719
14. Chatterjee R, Katz M, Cox TF, Porter JB. Prospective study of the hypothalamic-pituitary axis in thalassaemic patients who developed secondary amenorrhea. Clin Endocrinol 1993: 39: 287 296
15. Pippard M. Desferrioxamine induced iron excretion in humans. Bailliere's Clin Hematol 1989; 2: 323
16. Brittenham GM, Cohen AR, McLaren CE et al. Hepatic iron stores and plasma ferritin concentration in patients with sickle cell anemia and thalassemia major. Am J Hematol 1993; 42: 81–85
17. Olivieri NF, Grisaru D, Daneman A, Martin DJ, Rose V, Freedman MH. Computed tomography scanning of the liver to determine efficacy of iron chelation therapy in thalassemia major. J Pediatr 1989; 114: 427–430
18. Kaltwasser JP, Gottschalk R, Schalk KP, Hartl W. Non-invasive quantitation of liver iron-overload by magnetic resonance imaging. Br J Haematol 1990; 74: 360–363
19. Olivieri NF, Koren G, Matsui D et al. Reduction of tissue iron stores and normalization of serum ferritin during treatment with the oral iron chelator L1 in thalassemia intermedia. Blood 1992; 79: 2741
20. Liu P, Olivieri NF. Iron overload cardiomyopathies: new insights into an old disease. Cardiovasc Drugs Ther 1994; 8: 101–110
21. Brittenham GM, Farrell DE, Harris JW et al. Magnetic-susceptibility measurement of human iron stores. N Engl J Med 1982; 307: 1671–1675
22. Angelucci E, Baronciani D, Lucarelli G et al. Needle liver biopsy in thalassemia: analyses of diagnostic accuracy and safety in 1184 consecutive biopsies. Br J Haematol 1994; 89: 757–761
23. Cartwright GE, Edwards CQ, Kravitz K et al. Hereditary hemochromatosis: phenotypic expression of the disease. N Engl J Med 1979; 301: 175–179
24. Porter J, Huehns E. The toxic effects of desferrioxamine. Bailliere's Clin Hematol 1989; 2: 459–474
25. DeVirgiliis S, Congia M, Frau F et al. Deferoxamine-induced growth retardation in patients with thalassemia major. J Pediatr 1988; 113: 661–669

26. Hartkamp MJ, Babyn PS, Olivieri NF. Spinal deformities in deferoxamine-treated beta-thalassemia major patients. Pediatr Radiol 1993; 23: 525–528
27. Porter JB, Jaswon MS, Huehns ER, East CA, Hazell JWP. Desferrioxamine ototoxicity: evaluation of risk factors in thalassaemic patients and guidelines for safe dosage. Br J Haematol 1989; 73: 403–409
28. Olivieri NF, Berriman AM, Tyler BJ, Ingram J, Francombe WH. Continuous intravenous administration of deferoxamine in adults with severe iron overload. Am J Hematol 1992; 41: 61–63
29. Lucarelli G, Galimberti M, Polchi P et al. Marrow transplantation in patients with thalassemia responsive to iron chelation therapy. N Engl J Med 1993; 329: 840–844
30. Giardini C, Galimberti M, Lucarelli G et al. Desferrioxamine therapy accelerates clearance of iron deposits after bone marrow transplantation for thalassaemia. Br J Haematol 1995; 89: 868–873
31. Olivieri NF, Koren G, Hermann C et al. Comparison of oral iron chelator L1 and desferrioxamine in iron-loaded patients. Lancet 1990; 336: 1275–1279
32. Hoffbrand AV. Oral iron chelation. Semin Hematol 1996; 33: 1–8
33. Olivieri NF, Brittenham GM, Matsui D et al. Iron-chelation therapy with oral deferiprone in patients with thalassemia major. N Engl J Med 1995; 332: 912
34. Berkoukas VA, Bentley P, Frost H, Schnebli HP. Toxicity of oral iron chelator L1 (Letter). Lancet 1993; 341: 1088
35. Berkovitch M, Laxer RM, Inman R et al. Arthropathy in thalassaemia patients receiving deferiprone. Lancet 1994; 343: 1471–1472
36. Mehta J, Singhal S, Mehta BC. Deaths in patients receiving oral iron chelator L1 (Letter). Br J Haematol 1993; 85: 430
37. al-Refaie FN, Hershko C, Hoffbrand AV et al. Results of long-term deferiprone (L1) therapy. A report by the International Study Group on Oral Iron Chelators. Br J Haematol 1995; 91: 224–229
38. Olivieri NF. Reactivation of fetal hemoglobin in patients with β-thalassemia. Semin Hematol 1996; 33: 24–42
39. Ley TJ, DeSimone J, Anagnou NP et al. 5-Azacytidine selectively increases gamma-globin synthesis in a patient with β+ thalassemia. N Engl J Med 1982; 307: 1469–1475
40. Perrine SP, Ginder GD, Faller DV et al. A short-term trial of butyrate to stimulate fetal-globin-gene expression in the beta-globin disorders. N Engl J Med 1993; 328: 81–86
41. Sher GD, Ginder G, Little JA, Wang SY, Dover G, Olivieri NF. Extended therapy with arginine butyrate in patients with thalassemia and sickle cell disease. N Engl J Med 1995; 332: 106–110
42. Collins AF, Pearson HA, Giardina P, McDonagh KT, Brusilow SW, Dover GJ. Oral sodium phenylbutyrate therapy in homozygous beta thalassemia. Blood 1995; 85: 43–49

5

Congenital hypothyroidism

M. D. C. Donaldson   D. B. Grant

Congenital hypothyroidism can be defined as impairment of thyroid function resulting from any process beginning before birth – although its manifestation may occur some time later – and may be classified according to: the **site of functional impairment** – the thyroid gland itself (primary), pituitary gland (secondary), or hypothalamus (tertiary); the **degree of impairment** – plasma thyroxine (T_4) maintained in the normal range (compensated) or subnormal (decompensated); the **duration** – transient or permanent and the **aetiology**. Hyperthyrotropinaemia and hypothyroxinaemia are merely descriptive terms, often used in the context of transient change in thyroid function during the newborn period. Table 5.1 gives a broad classification of the causes of thyroid stimulating hormone (TSH) elevation arising during the first year.

Table 5.1 Causes of raised TSH in infancy

True permanent congenital hypothyroidism	Transient TSH elevation with normal or low T_4
Thyroid dysgenesis – 80%	**Assay artefact/error**
Athyreosis 30%	**Maternal factors**
Ectopia 30%	Iodine deficiency
Hypoplasia 20%	Amiodarone therapy
Dyshormonogenesis – 20%	Antithyroid drugs (e.g. carbimazole)
Iodine trapping defect	Thyroid autoantibodies
Organification defect	**Perinatal factors**
thyroid peroxidase deficiency	Birth asphyxia
thyroglobulin deficiency/abnormality	Prematurity
Deiodinase deficiency	Sepsis
Other – rare	Respiratory distress syndrome
Receptor defects	**Iodine exposure** (e.g. during sterile
TSH resistance	procedures including surgery)
T_4 resistance	**Syndromes**
Immune damage from maternal antibodies	Down's
Syndromes	
Pendred's (deafness with goitre)	
Pseudohypoparathyroidism	

EPIDEMIOLOGY OF PERMANENT PRIMARY CONGENITAL HYPOTHYROIDISM

Thyroid dysgenesis and dyshormonogenesis combine to give a prevalence of approximately 1 in 4000 live births in those countries where neonatal screening is practised.[1] The prevalence of dyshormonogenesis varies according to the frequency of consanguinity. Thyroid dysgenesis is more than twice as frequent in females as males and seems to be rare in black infants.

DIAGNOSIS OF PRIMARY CONGENITAL HYPOTHYROIDISM

The mainstay of early diagnosis is neonatal screening which should be regarded as an invaluable **adjunct to**, rather than a **substitute for**, clinical detection. The latter is required to detect severe hypothyroidism during the perinatal period before the screening result is available, and remains the only hope of early diagnosis in countries where neonatal screening is not yet established. Thyroid imaging is of value in **confirming** the diagnosis of congenital hypothyroidism and **defining its cause**.

Neonatal screening

Neonatal screening for hypothyroidism began in the mid-1970s, becoming established in most developed countries by the early 1980s.[2,3] Some screening programmes measure capillary T_4 and TSH but most (including those in the UK) measure TSH only. This latter approach is more cost effective, with a lower recall rate, but fails to detect secondary and tertiary hypothyroidism in which both T_4 and TSH will be low. Figure 5.1 shows the Guthrie card collection, TSH processing, and recall procedure for the programme in Scotland, which is broadly similar to that of England and Wales. Recently, we have carried out an audit of the neonatal screening programme for hypothyroidism in Scotland between August 1979 (when the programme started) and December 1993 (Ray et al., in preparation). From 1983 onwards, the median age of Guthrie collection was consistently 6–7 days in infants with definite or probable congenital hypothyroidism, but 5–14 days in infants with transient TSH elevation or uncertain thyroid status (in whom prematurity and sickness were much more frequent). Of the 344 infants in the cohort, as many as 36 (10.5%) had their first Guthrie test after 10 days of age. The apparent reason for this failure to sample between the recommended 4–6 days is the belief that phenylalanine levels will not be correctly interpreted in infants who are not yet receiving milk (e.g. premature, sick babies). However, a child with phenylketonuria who is not receiving milk will tend to have elevated phenylalanine levels anyway due to catabolism. Moreover, there is no reason why Guthrie sampling should not take place between 4 and 6 days in all babies, submitting a second sample later from babies who were not receiving milk at the time of first sampling.

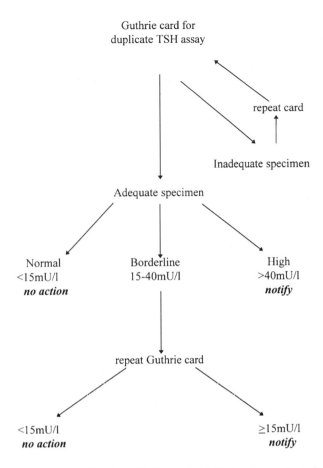

Fig. 5.1 Protocol for the notification of infants with TSH elevation on Guthrie card screening in Scotland.

Clinical evaluation

Figure 5.2 shows the typical signs of hypothyroidism in a severely affected newborn infant. In 235 Scottish infants with definite or probable congenital hypothyroidism, of whom only 18 were on treatment at the time of notification, the commonest features at diagnosis were jaundice (123), poor feeding (68), umbilical hernia (35), coarse facies (34), large or prominent tongue (31), constipation (23), lethargy (20), hoarse cry (19) and hypotonia (11). Only 53 of the infants had no features recorded at diagnosis.

Thyroid imaging

Neonatal TSH screening will identify not only babies with true permanent congenital hypothyroidism, but also those with transient hypothyroidism and

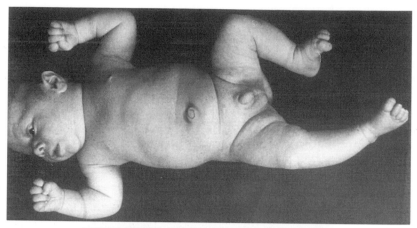

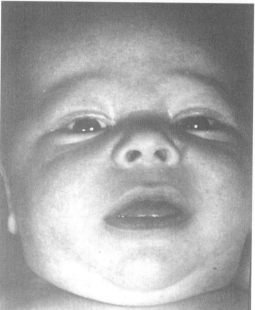

Fig. 5.2 Newborn infant with congenital hypothyroidism due to athyreosis. Note coarse facies and umbilical hernia.

hyperthyrotropinaemia (see Table 5.1). Radioisotope scanning of the thyroid is widely regarded as the gold standard in confirming the diagnosis of true congenital hypothyroidism and defining the cause, but whether, when and how to scan remains controversial. Imaging before or within the first few days of thyroxine therapy will usually distinguish between permanent and transient thyroid dysfunction while also differentiating between thyroid dysgenesis (which is sporadic) and dyshormonogenesis (which carries a 1 in 4 recurrence risk). Technically it is easier to scan a child in the neonatal period than during the toddler and pre-school years when cooperation is required, and often not forthcoming! Those who do not advocate early scanning point to the potential disruption caused by the procedure, especially when babies are preterm and/or sick, or born far away from the nearest isotope scanning department. They argue that in doubtful cases it is simplest and best to begin thyroxine treatment, challenging the diagnosis at a later stage by reduction in thyroxine dosage followed by measurement of plasma TSH. A compromise approach is to discontinue thyroxine therapy and carry out thyroid scanning in all children after the age of 2 years (by which time neuro development is largely complete) but, as mentioned above, this is technically more difficult.

More recently ultrasound scanning has been used. Annette Grüters and her team from Berlin have trained in the practice of thyroid ultrasound and routinely scan newborns with TSH elevation (personal communication). If the thyroid gland is absent on ultrasound they assume dysgenesis due to either athyreosis or ectopia. If the thyroid gland is *in situ* then causes such as hypoplasia, dyshormonogenesis, and transient impairment are considered and actively investigated at a later stage (see below). Clearly this approach requires sufficient exposure to patient numbers for the investigator to become skilled, and is difficult to apply in a District Hospital setting.

AETIOLOGY AND TYPES OF PERMANENT CONGENITAL HYPOTHYROIDISM

Thyroid dysgenesis

Maldescent of thyroid tissue from the tongue to the neck during foetal life results in ectopia and is usually associated with a degree of hypoplasia. The gland may also be hypoplastic *in situ*, or completely absent. The aetiology of thyroid dysgenesis is unknown. A slight increase in other congenital malformation in infants with congenital hypothyroidism raises the possibility of a common teratogenic insult. The preponderance of females with thyroid dysgenesis remains unexplained.

Dyshormonogenesis and receptor defects

Dyshormonogenesis is a term loosely describing a group of biosynthetic disorders, which together with receptor defects and abnormalities of the TSH molecule may result in defective synthesis of thyroxine. These abnormalities include defective iodine uptake by the thyroid gland, unresponsiveness of the thyroid gland to TSH due to a receptor defect or bioinactivity, mutations in the thyroglobulin gene resulting in defective structure of the molecule, and defects in the organification process (including thyroid peroxidase deficiency), and deiodinase deficiency. Recent advances in molecular genetics have resulted in some of these defects being characterised.[4] Figure 5.3 shows the work up of patients with suspected biosynthetic disorders, based on the ^{123}I uptake and response to perchlorate discharge test.

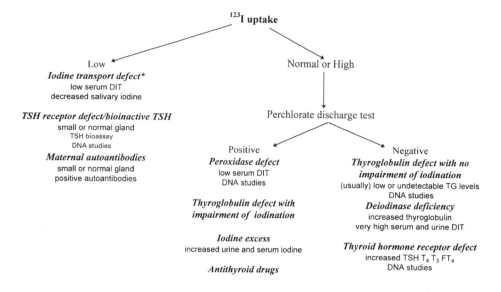

except where otherwise indicated thyroid gland is normal or large
DIT = diiodotyrosine
*DNA studies should soon be available

Fig. 5.3 Work up of patients with congenital hypothyroidism and gland *in situ* (after Grüters et al.[4]).

The thyroid gland will be normal or enlarged in all of these abnormalities with the exception of TSH receptor defect/TSH bioinactivity where it may be normal or small. [123]Iodine uptake will be reduced or absent with iodine transport and TSH receptor defects, normal with thyroglobulin defects, and increased with peroxidase and deiodinase defects. The perchlorate discharge test will be positive not only with thyroid peroxidase deficiency but also with thyroglobulin defects resulting in defective iodination, with antithyroid drugs, and exposure to iodine. In thyroglobulin disorders, plasma levels are usually low or absent but may be normal or high in the defects which result in production of a bioinactive molecule which retains immunoreactivity. Serum and urine diiodotyrosine levels will be low with peroxidase defects and high with deiodinase defects. Finally, the very rare condition of thyroxine unresponsiveness due to a thyroxine receptor defect is suggested by the combination of elevated TSH, thyroxine and T_3 with clinical signs of hypothyroidism and a normal or enlarged gland.

Autoimmune thyroiditis

It is known that thyroid autoantibodies in the mother may cross the placenta and have a blocking effect on the fetal thyroid, leading to transient congenital hypothyroidism (see below). There have also been several reports of permanent congenital hypothyroidism associated with maternal autoantibodies and autoimmune thyroiditis is recognised as a rare cause of permanent congenital hypothyroidism with a small *in situ* thyroid gland.[5]

AETIOLOGY OF TRANSIENT TSH ELEVATION

Mild TSH elevation on the Guthrie sample with subsequent normal venous thyroxine and TSH levels in an apparently healthy term infant may reflect problems with the assay in the screening laboratory, or simply a more vigorous TSH surge following birth than usual. Persistently high TSH levels associated with thyroxine levels which are relatively low (T_4 < 100 nmol/l, or free T_4 < 13 pmol/l) or frankly subnormal (T_4 < 60 nmol/l, free T_4 < 9 pmol/l) are commonly seen in preterm and/or sick infants.[6] Exposure to iodine from neonatal procedures (e.g. umbilical catheter or long-line insertion) or surgery is an important cause,[7,8] but not all preterm infants develop high TSH levels following exposure to iodine, and not all infants with transient TSH elevation have been shown to have raised iodine levels in the blood or urine.[9] The blocking effect of maternal autoantibodies has already been mentioned. Some apparently normal infants have essential hyperthyrotropinaemia, the TSH gradually returning to the normal range after months or years. Finally, infants with Down's syndrome may show transient thyroid dysfunction, often with very mild elevation of the TSH.[10]

DIFFERENTIATION BETWEEN TRUE PERMANENT PRIMARY CONGENITAL HYPOTHYROIDISM AND TRANSIENT TSH ELEVATION

A newborn with clinical features of hypothyroidism (Fig. 5.2), unrecordable plasma thyroxine, grossly elevated TSH, and absent activity on thyroid isotope scan does not pose a diagnostic problem. In some infants, however, the distinction between true permanent congenital hypothyroidism and transient derangement of thyroid function can be difficult. Thyroid isotope scanning is not universally practised in the newborn period and, while generally reliable, may give misleading results in infants who have been exposed to iodine, or to maternal blocking antibodies. As mentioned above, ultrasound scanning of the thyroid can distinguish between the presence or absence of a gland in the neck, but in the former instance cannot differentiate between permanent and transient impairment. Although congenital hypothyroidism in siblings is usually due to a recessively inherited disorder of biosynthesis, maternal thyroid blocking antibodies may also affect successive siblings.[4] TSH elevation after the first year of life on thyroxine treatment is very suggestive of permanent thyroid dysfunction, but maternal blocking antibodies have been reported to exert a reversible effect for a number of years.

Since thyroid scanning is not universal in Scotland (only 96 of the 235 children with definite or probable congenital hypothyroidism had been scanned), we devised other criteria for the 1979–1993 cohort in an attempt to distinguish between permanent and transient derangement of thyroid function. Infants were considered to have definite congenital hypothyroidism if one or more of the following applied: abnormal thyroid scan, initial venous T_4 < 60 nmol/l and TSH > 40 mu/l in an otherwise well term baby, TSH > 10 mu/l after the first year on treatment (whether due to under-dosage or compliance problems), or TSH > 15 mu/l after deliberate withdrawal of thyroxine treatment; sibling of a child known to have dyshormonogenesis. Probable congenital hypothyroidism was diagnosed if the above criteria were not met but there was substantial TSH elevation (> 100 mu/l) with relatively low venous T_4 (60–100 nmol/l) in an otherwise well term infant. Transient TSH elevation was diagnosed when initial Guthrie TSH was > 15 mu/l but normal venous T_4 and TSH (< 5 mu/l) were subsequently found off therapy. Cases which did not meet the criteria for these three categories were classified as thyroid status uncertain, and included infants who were preterm and/or sick at the time of Guthrie sampling, in whom other criteria for definite hypothyroidism were not applicable, and where thyroid reassessment had yet to be performed. Using these criteria, the 344 infants were categorised as having definite (223), and probable (12) congenital hypothyroidism, with transient TSH elevation (86) and uncertain thyroid status (23) in the rest.

RAISED TSH LEVELS AND CONGENITAL MALFORMATION

An association between congenital hypothyroidism and other malformations has been described. Grant and Smith found a 7% incidence of congenital malformation in a cohort of UK babies with established congenital hypothyroidism.[11] Other workers have reported a much higher incidence than this,[12,13] probably due to difficulty in distinguishing between true permanent congenital hypothyroidism and transient TSH elevation. In the Scottish 1979–1993 cohort, the incidence of malformation in true/probable hypothyroidism was 5%, with increased prevalence of dysmorphic syndromes and cardiac defects, while the incidence of non-cardiac malformations was not significantly different to that of the general population (Oakley et al., in preparation). The incidence of malformation in babies with transient TSH elevation was high (12%), and was associated with a much higher incidence of prematurity (27%) and sickness (35%) than in the definite group (7% and 6%, respectively). These findings reinforce the need to challenge the diagnosis of hypothyroidism in infants who were preterm, sick, and/or malformed at the time of initial Guthrie testing. Indeed, the diagnosis of transient TSH elevation was made retrospectively in 21 of the 86 Scottish children only after deliberate withdrawal of thyroxine treatment.

INITIAL MANAGEMENT

At the time of notification by the screening laboratory, most infants with hypothyroidism are being cared for at home by proud parents who are quite unaware that their child has a congenital malformation requiring life-long treatment. While it is desirable to recall the infant for venous sampling and initiation of treatment on an urgent basis, it is also important to notify the family in a manner that will not cause unnecessary distress, and perhaps spoil the parents' perception of their baby. We recommend that the paediatrician notified should speak personally to the general practitioner requesting that the parents be seen and asked to bring their child to hospital on the following day. The GP should inform the family that the child may well have an under-active thyroid gland, requiring tablets for life, but that the outlook is excellent. The delay involved is minimal, and this approach encourages an attitude of calm in the parents, as well as avoiding the ludicrous scenario in which the baby is brought to the hospital by an ambulance with blue flashing lights! In Scotland, the median age of notification by the screening laboratory is currently 11 days, and the median age of starting treatment 12 days.

What initial assessment should the hospital do, and when should treatment be instituted? Following a careful clinical history and examination (including measurement of the baby and, where possible, of parental heights), the minimal investigation requirement is an adequate venous sample for thyroxine and TSH measurement. We also recommend taking extra blood for thyroid autoantibodies, and a maternal sample for thyroid function and autoantibodies. We advocate thyroid isotope scanning within the first few days of notification, but recognise that practice will vary according to the views of the clinician, the radiology department, the geographical location, and the clinical state of the child. We no longer recommend X-raying the knee to measure the severity of intrauterine hypothyroidism.

A well term infant with a TSH of greater than 50 mu/l on Guthrie screening is very likely to have true congenital hypothyroidism. In these (the majority of cases) and in infants with obvious clinical signs of hypothyroidism, treatment can be instituted immediately after the venous sample has been taken. In a preterm, ill, or dysmorphic infant, or where the Guthrie TSH sample is below 50 mu/l, the clinician may prefer to obtain the venous thyroxine and TSH result as quickly as possible before deciding whether or not to commit the child to treatment. If the thyroxine level is normal ($T_4 > 100$ nmol/l or free $T_4 > 13$ pmol/l) it is reasonable to withhold treatment while continuing to monitor the baby carefully. If, however, the thyroxine level is low it is probably advisable to institute treatment without delay, being prepared to re-evaluate the thyroid function at a later stage.

FIRST YEAR MANAGEMENT

Dosage during the first year

There is a surprising lack of consensus as to the appropriate starting dose in an infant with congenital hypothyroidism. One approach is to give 100

$\mu g/m^2$, using the simple weight-based formula of:

$$\frac{\text{Weight (kg)} \times 4 + 7}{\text{Weight} + 90}$$

Using this formula, a new born infant weighing 1.1, 2.2, and 3.3 kg (equivalent to 28, 34, and 40 weeks gestation) would thus have a surface area of 0.12, 0.17, and 0.21 m^2 respectively equating to initial thyroxine doses of 12.5, 17.5, and 25 μg daily (or 11, 8, and 7.5 $\mu g/kg/day$). Some authorities recommend higher initial doses than these – 37.5 or even 50 μg daily for term infants.

There is also controversy as to how the clinician should respond to TSH levels during the first months of life. One approach is to increase the daily thyroxine dose until the TSH is suppressed to below 5 mu/l. Another is to give the desired dose for the child's weight/surface area, encourage optimal compliance, and allow the TSH to normalise spontaneously. Advocates of the first approach believe that high TSH levels reflect under-treatment. Those who recommend the second approach believe that the thyrotrophs in the pituitary gland need time to adjust to the new thyroxine environment after months of intrauterine hypothyroidism, and that 'chasing' the TSH may result in over-treatment with unwanted symptoms such as irritability, restlessness and poor sleeping pattern.

Our current practice is to give 100 $\mu g/m^2/day$ of thyroxine in the first instance, increasing the dose if necessary to keep the plasma T_4 level at or above 150 nmol/l (free $T_4 \geq 20$ pmol/l), and allowing the TSH to subside spontaneously. However, we accept that the ideal approach to first year dosage has not yet been established, and a prospective study currently being organised by the Thyroid Working Group of the European Society for Paediatric Endocrinology should help to clarify the situation.

Frequency of follow up

Substantial neurodevelopment takes place up to the end of the second year, and good compliance is essential during this time. To optimise this, and ensure that the family are properly counselled and educated, we advise seeing newly diagnosed infants fortnightly during the first 6 weeks, then every 2 months until the end of the first year. This amounts to roughly 9 visits during the first year, a considerable commitment for both clinician and family. Clearly the care can be shared with the GP in order to reduce the number of hospital visits, and there must be flexibility between family and clinician to negotiate the number of visits for each individual child.

T_4 and TSH monitoring

Ideally there should be T_4 and sensitive TSH assays for capillary blood spots which could be collected at home between hospital visits and sent directly to the laboratory. In practice, a venous sample is usually required for T_4 measurement, and the lower limit of sensitivity for the TSH assay by Guthrie card method is 10–15 mu/l, inadequate for clinical purposes. We recommend venous sampling on most visits during the first year when growth is rapid and several changes in dose are usually required.

MANAGEMENT AFTER THE FIRST YEAR

Thyroxine dosage after the first year

From one year onwards therapy is relatively straightforward and uncontroversial. Thyroxine replacement at a dose of 100 $\mu g/m^2/day$ will result in a euthyroid, normally growing child. This equates to doses of approximately 50, 62.5, 75, 100, and 150 μg daily at 1, 3, 5, 10, and 15 years, respectively, or roughly 4–5 $\mu g/kg/day$ before the age of 5 years, and 3 $\mu g/kg/day$ thereafter. The dose of thyroxine should be increased to keep pace with the child's growth, using TSH monitoring to confirm reasonable compliance (see below) rather than waiting for the TSH to become elevated.

Monitoring

Once the rapid growth – and changing dose requirements – of infancy are over, the frequency of clinic visits can be much reduced. We advise seeing children twice during the second year, and annually thereafter unless there are problems. At each visit the height and weight are recorded and plotted, the child's development and educational progress are noted, the thyroxine dosage checked for body surface area or weight and a venous blood sample for TSH, total T_4, or free T_4 is taken. Anticipation of a blood test often renders the child unduly fearful, in which case it is kinder to use anaesthetic cream, which parents can be given to apply one hour before the appointment. TSH elevation of greater than 10 mu/l on a reasonable dose of thyroxine for body surface area/weight almost always reflects difficulties with compliance. When this happens, we write to the family asking them to check the tablets and dosage with the family doctor and arrange a repeat blood test 4 weeks later, asking the parents to ensure that tablet taking is faultless. This usually achieves normalisation of TSH and is preferable to recommending an increase in the thyroxine dosage which will result in symptoms of over-treatment if compliance improves. A particular pattern to watch for is that of high total T_4 (>150 nmol/l) or free T_4 (above 20 pmol/l) with grossly elevated TSH (>50 mu/l). This picture is consistent with very poor compliance followed by frantic tablet taking just before the clinic appointment!

We do not routinely assess bone age, since this investigation does not seem to alter our management.

Challenging the diagnosis

When reliable thyroid imaging during the neonatal period has shown an abnormal gland, or when the venous TSH has risen above 10 mu/l beyond the first year while on thyroxine treatment, the diagnosis of permanent hypothyroidism is reasonably secure. If, however, the child was preterm and/or sick at the time of Guthrie sampling, or if there was an associated mal-formation (see above) then re-evaluation of thyroid status is required. Re-evaluation is also desirable in children showing TSH suppression (below 1 mu/l) on a dose of thyroxine which is low for body surface area/weight. The simplest diagnostic challenge is to halve the thyroxine dosage and remeasure TSH after several weeks, stopping treatment altogether unless the TSH has shown a diagnostic rise. A more definitive challenge consists of reducing the thyroxine dosage to zero over a 4–6 week period, or replacing thyroxine with T_3 for 3–4 weeks and then discontinuing for 1–2 weeks. In Glasgow, our cur-rent practice after temporary discontinuation of thyroxine treatment is to cannulate the child and give 200 µg of TRH, measuring TSH at 0, 30 and 60 min. If desired, additional blood for thyroglobulin, DIT, etc. can be drawn at time 0 (see Fig 5.3). Following the TRH test the cannula is kept in and the child transferred to the Radioisotope Department where thyroid scan is per-formed using ^{123}I and (if dyshormonogenesis is suspected) a perchlorate dis-charge test. After the thyroid scan the child resumes thyroxine replacement until the results of the tests are available. It is our practice to offer full thyroid reassessment after the age of 2 years in all cases, and to positively recommend re-evaluation in selected children.

NEUROPSYCHOLOGICAL OUTCOME IN CONGENITAL HYPOTHYROIDISM

Cognitive function

It is now generally accepted that early diagnosis and treatment has com-pletely changed the prognosis for congenital hypothyroidism and all the pub-lished accounts of cognitive function in children identified by neonatal screening indicate quite clearly that early treatment is associated with a marked improvement in outcome, as compared with the impaired intelli-gence which was common in late-treated patients.[14,15] However, there is still debate on whether early diagnosis and treatment can fully reverse the effects of prenatal hypothyroidism on brain development – thus allowing completely normal development – or whether some degree of impairment persists despite early therapy.

While there have now been a fairly large number of follow-up studies in children with early-treated congenital hypothyroidism, relatively few have compared hypothyroid children with healthy control children. Table 5.2 summarises the results of 10 such studies carried out between the ages of 4–10 years, using a variety of tests of cognitive function.[16–25] With one excep-tion, these studies have shown a small deficit in mean IQ score for the hypothyroid children ranging from 4 to 11 IQ points. However, in all the studies the mean IQ score has been within the normal range and in only 3

Table 5.2 Mean IQ scores reported for hypothyroidism and control children

Study	Test age (years)	Number s of subject	Test used	Mean IQ score Hypothyroid children	Control children	Ref no.
New England	10	72	WISC-R	106	109	16
London	10	59	WISC-R	109	115	17
Rotterdam	9	62	WISC-R	97	103	18
Stockholm	7	24 girls	Griffiths	101	98	19
		10 boys		98	95	
Norway	6	27	WPPSI	88*	99	20
Quebec	5	36	Griffiths	102*	106	21
Toronto	5	39	WPPSI	107	111	22
UK	5	344	WPPSI	105*	112	23
Paris	4	49	Terman Merrill	116	118	24
Switzerland	4	40	Snijers Oomen	104	108	25

studies did the difference between the hypothyroid children and the healthy controls reach statistical significance.

While the above findings have encouraged the view that the effect of pre-natal hypothyroidism can be completely eliminated, a number of authors have commented that outcome is less good in children with severe hypothyroidism, as judged by low pre-treatment plasma T_4 or marked retardation of bone age. Table 5.3 gives the results of 4 studies which compare outcome in children with very low pre-treatment plasma T_4 levels with that in children with intermediate pre-treatment plasma T_4.[17,18,26,27] The results show significant differences in favour of the children with less severe disease and further analysis of the findings in a large cohort of hypothyroid children born in the UK indicates that there is evidence of a threshold effect for pre-treatment plasma T_4 at around 35–47 nmol/l with normal outcome in the cases with T_4 levels above this threshold.[27]

The differences in the findings of different studies, particularly the New England follow-up study which has shown a normal distribution for intelli-

Table 5.3 Mean IQ scores reported in children with low and intermediate plasma T_4 levels at diagnosis

Study	Test age (years)	Total number of subjects	Test	IQ in children with low pre-treatment T_4	IQ in children with inter-mediate T_4	Ref. no.
London	10	59	WISC-R	105	115	17
Rotterdam	9	61	WISC-R	95	101	18
Quebec	12	27		89	104	26
UK	5	228	WPPSI	101	110	17

gence with no effect of severity[28,29] and other results from North America and Europe have been attributed to differences in the quality of treatment, particularly thyroxine dosage at the time of diagnosis,[30] and two recent publications support this view.[31,32] Thyroxine dose and patient compliance with treatment in later childhood and adolescence have also been reported to affect the results of tests of cognitive function.[20] However, several other studies have failed to demonstrate any significant association between IQ test score and thyroxine dosage, either at diagnosis or in later childhood.

Age at start of treatment is another possible factor which might account for differences in outcome and this is supported by a collaborative European study[33] which showed significant negative correlation between IQ score and age at start of treatment in a large group of children with thyroid agenesis. However, this correlation is no longer evident when children treated before 6 weeks of age are excluded. In addition, a number of authors have reported no clear association between age at start of treatment and subsequent IQ score and there is little evidence that the timing of treatment during the first weeks of life has a major effect on outcome.

Educational attainments

There is as yet little information on educational outcome in children diagnosed by screening. However, the cohort of children born followed in the New England Collaborative Study had normal educational scores at the age of 12 years.[34] This is in contrast with results from France[35] in which hypothyroid children had a higher class retake rate on entry to school and were also found to have some impairment of mathematical ability, as opposed to school tasks covering language and vocabulary. These latter findings are similar to our own as yet unpublished findings in a group of hypothyroid children in England aged 10 years. Reading skills were essentially normal in these children but those with severe hypothyroidism did significantly less well in mathematics (Fuggle, in preparation). In the Scottish 1979–1993 cohort, a simple audit by questionnaire showed that of 149 children who were of school age in 1994, 121 were attending mainstream schools with no special help, 16 were receiving extra help in normal schools, and 2 children were attending special schools, and information was unavailable in 10 children. This compares favourably with a 17–18% prevalence of learning support amongst control Scottish children recruited in a low birth weight study by Hall et al.[36]

Impaired motor performance

Impaired motor performance was a striking feature of hypothyroid children born before the introduction of screening. Initially considered to be due to cerebellar ataxia, it became clear that the motor problems were related to a wider range of neurological deficits.[37] All available evidence suggests that some relatively minor degrees of motor impairment are still found in children with early-treated hypothyroidism, particularly in patients with low pre-treatment plasma T_4 concentrations.[38–40] However, the motor difficulties found in children identified by screening appear to be much less severe than those formerly encountered in late-diagnosed cases, although it is still not clear whether these motor difficulties are likely to cause any significant long-term handicap.

Behaviour disorders

Prior to neonatal screening, behaviour disorders were very common in children with congenital hypothyroidism.[15,37] Follow-up studies on children diagnosed by screening suggest that disordered behaviour is still a problem in many such children,[41] particularly those who were treated with relatively high doses of thyroxine in the first year of life.

Neuro-otological function

Impaired hearing was a common but often unrecognised problem in children before the introduction of screening,[42] as was disturbance of vestibular function.[43] There have been few published studies of hearing in children with early-treated hypothyroidism but one such study showed only minor degrees of hearing impairment.[44] We have also found a raised incidence of impaired hearing in the threshold range 15–20 dB and mild impairment of vestibular function.[45] However, while raised hearing thresholds may cause some difficulties with conversation against high levels of background noise, severe degrees of deafness now appear to be very uncommon.

Conclusions

The findings described above strongly suggest that children with congenital hypothyroidism – particularly patients with low pre-treatment plasma T_4 values – may still show evidence of minor degrees of brain dysfunction as judged by the presence of deficits in cognitive function and motor skills, behaviour disorders and mild impairment of hearing and vestibular function. It is important that parents, teachers and paediatricians are aware of these difficulties so that early supportive action can be taken to minimise any long-term effects in later life.

KEY POINTS FOR CLINICAL PRACTICE

1. Guthrie sampling for TSH measurement should take place between 4 and 6 days of life irrespective of gestation, clinical condition, and milk intake so as to avoid unnecessary delay in the diagnosis of congenital hypothyroidism. In the minority of children who are not receiving milk at the time of initial Guthrie sampling, a second specimen should be sent for phenylalanine estimation once milk feeding has begun.

2. A Guthrie TSH of > 50 mu/l in an otherwise well infant is highly likely to be due to true congenital hypothyroidism. In these circumstances, it is reasonable to commence thyroxine treatment without delay, having obtained an adequate venous sample for T_4 and TSH measurement.

3. In infants with modest Guthrie TSH elevation, and/or problems such as prematurity and sickness it may be preferable to obtain urgent venous T_4 and TSH results before deciding whether or not to start treatment. If the plasma T_4 is < 100 nmol/l or free T_4 < 13 pmol/l, treatment should be started without delay.

4. The diagnosis of permanent congenital hypothyroidism should be confirmed after the first or second year by temporary reduction or withdrawal of thyroxine treatment, unless (a) diagnostic thyroid scan was carried out in newborn period, (b) venous TSH > 10 mu/l after the first year of life despite thyroxine therapy (reflecting underdosage or poor compliance).

5. Diagnostic challenge is particularly important in children who were preterm, sick, or had other malformation at the time of Guthrie sampling since transient TSH elevation is relatively common in these subjects.

6. The initial dose of thyroxine in newborn infants is controversial. One approach is to give 25 µg in all but the most preterm infants, adjusting the dose during infancy to keep plasma T_4 above 150 nmol/l or free T_4 above 20 pmol/l.

7. After the first year of life a thyroxine dose of 100 µg/m²/day will keep the child euthyroid. The dose should be increased to keep pace with growth, and TSH measurement used to confirm adequate compliance.

8. Children should be seen frequently during infancy to optimise dosage and compliance. After the second year of life annual visits should suffice.

9. High venous TSH values despite an appropriate dose of thyroxine almost always reflect problems with compliance. Repeat sampling 4 weeks after careful supervision of medication will usually show normalisation of TSH.

REFERENCES

1. Toublanc JE. Epidemiological inquiry on congenital hypothyroidism in Europe (1985–1988). Horm Res 1990; 34: 1–3
2. Fisher DA, Dussault JH, Foley TR et al. Screening for congenital hypothyroidism: results of screening one million North American infants. J Pediatr 1979; 94: 700–705
3. Hulse JA, Grant DB, Clayton BE et al. Population screening for congenital hypothyroidism. BMJ 1980; 280: 675–678
4. Grüters A, Finke R, Krude H, Meinhold H. Etiology grouping of permanent congenital hypothyroidism with a thyroid gland in situ. Horm Res 1994; 41: 3–9
5. Van der Gaag R, Drexhage H, Dussault J. Role of maternal immunoglobulins blocking

TSH induced thyroid growth in sporadic forms of congenital hypothyroidism. Lancet 1985; ii: 246
6. Schonberger W, Grimm W, Gempp W, Dinkel E. Transient hypothyroidism associated with prematurity, sepsis, and respiratory distress. Eur J Pediatr 1979; 132: 85–92
7. Grüters A, l'Allemand D, Heidemann PH, Schurnbrand P. Incidence of iodine contamination in neonatal transient hyperthyrotropinemia. Eur J Pediatr 1983; 140; 299–300
8. l'Allemand D, Grüters A, Beyer P, Weber B. Iodine in contrast agents and skin disinfectants is the major cause for hypothyroidism in premature infants during intensive care. Horm Res 1987; 28: 42–49
9. Leger J, Czernichow P. Hyperthyrotropinemie neonatale transitoire. Arch Fr Pediatr 1988; 45: 783–786
10. Fort P, Lifshitz F, Bellisario R et al. Abnormalities of thyroid function in infants with Down's syndrome. J Pediatr 1984; 104: 545–549
11. Grant DB, Smith I. Survey of neonatal screening for primary hypothyroidism in England, Wales and Northern Ireland 1982–4. BMJ 1988; 296: 1355–1358
12. Bamforth JS, Hughes L, Lazarus J, John R. Congenital anomalies associated with hypothyroidism. Arch Dis Child 1986; 61: 608–609
13. Fernhoff PM, Brown AL, Elsas LJ. Congenital hypothyroidism: increased risk of neonatal morbidity results in delayed treatment. Lancet 1987; ii: 490–491
14. Klein AH, Meltzer S, Kenny FM. Improved prognosis in congenital hypothyroidism treated before age three months. J Pediatr 1972; 81: 912–915
15. Hulse JA. Outcome of congenital hypothyroidism. Arch Dis Child 1984; 59: 23–30
16. New England Congenital Hypothyroid Collaborative. Elementary school performance of children with congenital hypothyroidism. J Pediatr 1990; 116: 27–32
17. Simons WF, Fuggle PW, Grant DB, Smith I. Intellectual development at 10 years in early treated congenital hypothyroidism. Arch Dis Child 1994; 71: 232–234
18. Kooistra L, Laane C, Vulsma T et al. Motor and cognitive development in children with congenital hypothyroidism; long-term evaluation of the effects of neonatal treatment. J Pediatr 1994; 124: 903–909
19. Ilichi A, Larsson A. Psychological development at 7 years of age in children with congenital hypothyroidism: timing and dosage of initial treatment. Acta Paediatr Scand 1991; 80: 199–204
20. Heyerdahl S, Kase BF, Lie SO. Intellectual development in children with congenital hypothyroidism in relation to recommended treatment. J Pediatr 1991; 118: 850–857
21. Glorieux J, Dussault, JH, Morisette J, Desjardins M, Letarte J, Guyda H. Follow up at ages 5 and 7 years in mental development in children with hypothyroidism detected by Quebec screening program. J Pediatr 1985; 107: 193–215
22. Rovet JF, Ewstbrook D-L, Ehrich RM. Neonatal thyroid deficiency: early temperament and cognitive characteristics. J Am Acad Child Adolesc Psychiatry 1984; 23: 10–22
23. Fuggle P, Tokar S, Grant DB. Intellectual ability of early treated children with congenital hypothyroidism: results from the UK national study. Horm Res 1991; 35: 16
24. Toublanc JE, Rives S, Acosta A, Chicaud J. Le developpment psychomoteur et intellectuel chez 52 enfants atteints d'hypothroidie congenitale depistee a la naisance. Arch Fr Pediatr 1990; 47: 191–195
25. Illig R, Largo RH, Weber M et al. Sixty children with congenital hypothyroidism detected by neonatal screening; mental development at 1, 4 and 7 years: a longitudinal study. Acta Endocrinol 1986; Suppl 279: 346–353
26. Glorieux J, Dussault J, Van Vliet G. Intellectual development at age 12 years in children with congenital hypothyroidism diagnosed by neonatal screening. J Pediatr 1992; 121: 581–584
27. Tillotson SL, Fuggle PW, Smith I, Ades AE, Grant DB. Relation between biochemical severity and intelligence in early treated congenital hypothyroidism: a threshold effect. BMJ 1994; 309: 440–445
28. New England Congenital Hypothyroidism Collaborative. Effects of neonatal screening for hypothyroidism: prevention of mental retardation by treatment before clinical manifestations. Lancet 1981; ii: 1095–1089
29. New England Congenital Hypothyroidism Collaborative. Neonatal hypothyroidism: status of patients at 6 years of age. J Pediatr 1985; 108: 915–918
30. Mitchell ML, Klein RZ. Motor and cognitive development in children with congenital

hypothyroidism. J Pediatr 1994; 126: 673
31. Dubuis J-M, Richer F, Glorieux J, Deal C, Dussault JH. Should all patients with congenital hypothyroidism (CH) be treated with 10-15 µg/kg/day levothyroxine (T4)? Pediatr Res 1994; 35; 4/part 2 98A.
32. Rovet JF, Ehrich RM. Long term effects of thyroxine for congenital hypothyroidism. J Pediatr 1995: 126: 380–386
33. Illig R, Largo RH, Qin Q. Mental development in congenital hypothyroidism after neonatal screening. Arch Dis Child 1987; 62: 1050–1055
34. New England Congenital Hypothyroidism Collaborative. Correlation of cognitive test scores and adequacy of treatment in adolescents with congenital hypothyroidism. J Pediatr 1994: 124: 383–387
35. Rochiccioli P, Roge B, Alexander F, Taubier MT. School achievement in children with hypothyroidism detected at birth and search for predictive factors. Horm Res 1992; 38: 236–240
36. Hall A, McLeod A, Counsell C, Thomson L, Mutch L. School attainment, cognitive ability and motor function in a total Scottish very low birth weight population of 8 years – a controlled study. Dev Med Child Neurol 1995; 37: 1037–1050
37. McFaul R, Dorner S, Brett EM, Grant DB. Neurological abnormalities in patients treated for from early life. Arch Dis Child 1978; 53: 611–618
38. Fuggle PW, Grant DB, Smith I, Murphy G. Intelligence, motor skills and behaviour at 5 years in early-treated congenital hypothyroidism. Eur J Pediatr 1991; 150: 570–574
39. Rochiccioli P et al. Developpement neurologique des hypothyroides neonatales. Arch Fr Pediatrie 1987; 44: 721–724
40. Gottschalk B, Richman RA, Lewindowski L. Subtle speech and motor deficits of children with congenital hypothyroidism treated early. Dev Med Child Neurol 1994; 36: 216–220
41. Rovet JF, Ehrich RM, Sorboda D-L. Effect of thyroid hormone level on temperament in infants with congenital hypothyroidism detected by screening of neonates. J Pediatr 114: 63–68
42. Vanderscheuren-Lodeweyckx, Debruyne F, Dooms L, Eggermont E, Eeckels R. Sensorineural hearing loss in sporadic congenital hypothyroidism. Arch Dis Child 1983; 58: 419–422
43. Sato T, Ishiguro C, Watanabe Y, Mizukoshi K. Quantitative analysis of cerebello-vestibular function in congenital hypothyroidism. Acta Paediatr Jpn 1987; 29: 121–129
44. Francois M, Bonfils P, Leger J, Czernichow P, Narcy P. Role of congenital hypothyroidism in hearing loss in children. J Pediatr 1994; 124: 444–446
45. Bellman SC, Davies A, Fuggle PW, Grant DB, Smith I. Mild impairment of neuro-otological function in early treated congenital hypothyroidism. Arch Dis Child 1996; 74: 215–218

6

Recent advances in coeliac disease

J. A. Walker-Smith

DEFINITION

Coeliac disease may be defined as follows: it is a disease of the proximal small intestine characterized by an abnormal small intestinal mucosa (small intestinal enteropathy). It is associated with a permanent intolerance to gluten. Removal of gluten from the diet leads to a full clinical remission and restoration of the small intestinal mucosa to normal. Thus coeliac disease is a life-long disorder that affects both children and adults. It may first present either in childhood or adult life.

It is now recognised that the small intestinal enteropathy is an immunologically mediated enteropathy. Symptoms result from structural damage to the small intestinal mucosa, which may cause malabsorption. Although the molecular basis of the immune response has been elucidated,[1] and the primary genetic susceptibility determined,[2] it remains unclear what second trigger is required to initiate this life-long condition. It is the certainty of eventual relapse that differentiates coeliac disease from other childhood enteropathies, such as cows' milk sensitive enteropathy. This suggests some additional property of the gluten molecules that affects either enterocyte function or mucosal antigen presentation. It is difficult to separate the initiating immunological event in coeliac disease from secondary responses. However, recent findings show that the primary response probably occurs amongst the T helper lymphocytes of the mucosal lamina propria.

THE EPIDEMIOLOGY OF CHILDHOOD COELIAC DISEASE

Coeliac disease occurs predominantly amongst those of European origin, with the highest incidence in the children and adults of North Europe and Scandinavia, but it may also occur in the north-west part of the Indian sub-continent. The west coast of Ireland, around Galway Bay, has the highest reported incidence, with coeliac disease affecting over 1 in 300 of the entire population. Southern European populations may also have a high local incidence, and Italy, in particular, has areas in which coeliac disease is one of the most common childhood ailments. Recent Italian work suggests that the true incidence of coeliac disease in susceptible populations may be dramatically higher than has been previously recognised: a serological study of the entire school-age population around Ancona uncovered large numbers of undiagnosed children with coeliac disease, a phenomenon described as the 'tip of the iceberg'.[3]

The practical application of these observations is particular awareness of a child's genetic background, and a low threshold for performing endomyseal antibody tests (see below) in children of Italian, Celtic or Scandinavian origin.

The primary susceptibility to coeliac disease relates to major histocompatibility complex (MHC) status, with a particular Class II allele (HLA-DQ) found in almost all patients.[2] The first recognised genetic association was to a Class I tissue-type, HLA B8. This is now known to be inherited by linkage to the true Class II susceptibility gene. There is an intriguing geographical correlation between the population density of B8 and the pattern of spread of cereal farming across Europe in prehistoric times. This might even suggest that a high intake of grains has shaped human genetic evolution, and raises questions about the extent of interaction between cultivated cereals and the human small intestine. Such a high population density of B8 also occur in north-west Indian sub-continent. It is notable that normal individuals without coeliac disease may show dose-related mucosal damage with high gluten intake. A similar condition may be induced by feeding gluten to Irish setter dogs. Thus there remains the possibility of a dosage effect, and it is striking that there is a much higher incidence of overt disease in Swedish children, who are fed high doses of gluten at weaning, than in the genetically similar Danes, who receive much less gluten.[4] On the face of it, this would argue for restriction of gluten intake in infancy in Sweden, but the concern that this may lead to atypical late presentation has led to caution in initiating any change there. There is known to be an increased risk of small bowel lymphoma in adults presenting with coeliac disease in mid-life.[5] It may thus be advantageous to present early and with classical signs, as a strict gluten-free diet substantially reduces this risk.[5]

Within Europe, there are reports of increasing (Sweden), decreasing (UK) and stable incidence of coeliac disease (Italy).[6] This may reflect environmental change such as age of introduction and dose of gluten rather than a true change in incidence.[7]

GENETIC PREDISPOSITION TO COELIAC DISEASE

The hereditary basis of coeliac disease has been underlined by the finding of classical morphological changes in the small intestinal mucosa of 10% of asymptomatic family members.[8] The MHC type determines the specificity of the peptide binding site on antigen presenting cells. Class I molecules (such as HLA-B8) present antigen to CD8 T-lymphocytes, whereas Class II molecules (HLA-DP, DR or DQ) present to CD4+ T helper cells. Thus it is important to recognise that the initial association with HLA B8 was secondary, due to linkage disequilibrium with HLA DQ2, which is found in over 90% of European patients. This implies that the intestinal CD4 cells, found within the mucosal lamina propria rather than the epithelial compartment, are of central importance for pathogenesis.

The primary association of coeliac disease is to the HLA-DQ dimer DQA1*0501/DQB1*0201.[9] The great majority of patients and first degree relatives (and up to 20% of normals in susceptible populations) may express this dimer on antigen-presenting cells. Yet it is clear from the number of unaffected people that the possession of this haplotype is insufficient in itself to cause gluten-induced changes, and the administration of gluten to HLA-identical siblings of coeliac patients does not always result in small intestinal pathology. The HLA-DQ dimer is also strongly linked to HLA-DR status. If children are of the HLA-DR3 tissue type, they will carry both the X and BDQ molecules on the same chromosome, whereas if they are HLA-DR5 and also DR7 they will carry one molecule on each chromosome. The end result is the same, in that their antigen presenting cells can express together these specific HLA-DQ molecules, and thus present processed gluten peptides to potentially reactive lamina propria CD4 cells. Indeed, a Norwegian group has derived clones of mucosal CD4 cells that respond to gluten only when presented by cells expressing the susceptibility HLA-DQ dimer.[1] This is exciting, because it is now possible to cleave native gluten into small amino acid chains, and thus determine exactly which fraction of the gluten molecule is truly immunogenic. Two possibilities then arise: looking for sequence homology with known viruses or enteric pathogens (defining the unknown second 'hit'), and genetically engineering wheat that does not contain the immunogenic sequence.

THE COELIAC LESION

The proximal small intestinal mucosa of patients with coeliac disease becomes abnormal on gluten ingestion. The abnormality is characterised by stunted or even absent villi associated with an increase in crypt length and cell numbers – the so-called 'flat mucosa'. There is both an increased rate of crypt cell proliferation and a doubling of mucosal lamina propria volume. This latter phenomenon may be analogous to the retro-orbital swelling that occurs in auto-immune thyroid disease, which is known to be mediated by a T cell cytokine (interferon-γ) that is also produced within the coeliac lesion. The flat appearance of the mucosal surface in coeliac disease may thus be caused by increase in volume of the intervillous tissues rather than actual loss of villi. The enterocytes may be abnormal, showing a flattened or vacuolated appearance, with irregularities of the microvilli and mitochondria seen on electron microscopy. This epithelial damage may be unrelated to the mucosal T cell-mediated changes, and there is some evidence that a component of the gluten molecule, wheat germ agglutinin (WGA), may possess lectin-like properties and directly trigger the enterocyte epidermal growth factor (EGF) receptor. This might contribute to the crypt hyperplasia characteristic of the condition. The evolution of gluten-induced changes has been studied by sequential ultrastructural examination after gluten challenge.[10] The changes occurred predominantly within the lamina propria. There was progressive increase of connective tissue spaces with fibril formation, and increase in the density of endothelial and the subepithelial basement membranes. It is noteworthy that these changes evolved in parallel with increasing lamina propria lymphocyte numbers.

All structural damage resolves on gluten withdrawal but recurs if gluten is reintroduced to the diet. Similar intestinal changes are frequently found in dermatitis herpetiformis, in association with a bullous skin eruption due to subepithelial IgA deposition. Both the cutaneous and intestinal lesions regress with gluten exclusion.

THE IMMUNOLOGICAL BASIS OF COELIAC DISEASE

Humoral immunity in coeliac disease

Most physicians are aware of the humoral component of the coeliac lesion, particularly as diagnosis is at least partly based on circulating antibodies. Although the current disease concept is based on T cell activation, it is clear that the mucosal and systemic humoral response is important.[11] There is significant increase of IgA-secreting plasma cells within untreated coeliac mucosa, as well as marked increase of IgM production. In support of a pathological role for antibody, there is also subepithelial deposition of activated complement and IgG. Immune complexes also appear to be released into the circulation in excess, overloading the normal hepatic and splenic clearance mechanisms. Luminal perfusion studies have shown increased amounts of secretory IgA and IgM, with high titres of luminal IgA and IgM anti-gliadin antibodies. Immunohistochemistry of mucosal biopsies has shown IgG, IgM and IgA secreting cells.

Circulating antibodies in coeliac disease

It has long been known that antibodies to gliadin and other food proteins may be found in the serum of coeliac patients. Three types of antibody (anti-gliadin IgA antibodies, anti-reticulin and anti-endomyseal IgA antibodies) are now recognised to be produced in untreated coeliac disease, with titres falling on gluten exclusion.

Circulating levels of IgA anti-gliadin antibodies have been used as sensitive diagnostic markers of coeliac disease. Although they may occur at high levels and increase on gluten challenge, they are not at all specific and may be found in a variety of small intestinal enteropathies. They are relatively inexpensive to perform, however, and thus are still quite widely used.

Anti-reticulin and anti-endomysial IgA antibodies are more specific markers for coeliac disease but may also be seen in healthy first-degree relatives. Both antibodies recognise connective tissue matrix components and could, therefore, be technically considered as autoantibodies. Whether this autoimmune process contributes to the coeliac lesion is unknown. The matrix components recognised by both antibodies occur in reticular connective tissue and appear to be similar. Although more specific, the endomysial antibody in particular providing sufficient specificity to provide a true screening test, they are more difficult to perform. There is an additional logistic problem with the endomysial antibody test, in that it is performed on monkeys' esophagus. Thus recent reports that similar binding patterns can be seen on human umbilical cord are welcome.[12] The reason why sera from coeliac patients should cross-react with primate tissues or umbilical cord matrix is unknown, but likely to be interesting. However, at the moment, it is entirely unclear whether this phenomenon is telling us something important. The presence of anti-endomysial IgA antibodies in a child with villous atrophy strongly supports a diagnosis of coeliac disease, but it is not specific.[13] However, a primary role for humoral immunity in the pathogenesis of the enteropathy of coeliac disease appears doubtful because: (i) these antibodies are found so frequently in latent coeliac patients and first degree relatives; and (ii) coeliac disease has been shown to occur despite severe hypogammaglobulinaemia.[14]

The intraepithelial compartment

Intraepithelial lymphocytes are found in normal small intestinal epithelium with a density of 20–40 per 100 epithelial cells. They are generally situated near the basement membrane, and are effectively separated from luminal contents only by the epithelial tight junctions. Their total numbers are large taking into account the vast intestinal surface area, probably reflecting the degree of luminal antigenic stimulation. They show different patterns of surface marker expression to circulating or lamina propria T cells, as more than 90% express CD8 (the cytotoxic/suppressor phenotype) and less than 10% CD4. About 90% use the $\alpha\beta$ cell receptor and about 10% are $\gamma\delta$ T cell receptor cells. In coeliac disease density of intraepithelial lymphocytes is increased (> 40/100 epithlial cells), the cells are often larger and situated nearer the lumen, there are reduced proportions of CD8+ (60–90%) and $\alpha\beta$-TCR (50–80%) T cells, there is increased density of $\gamma\delta$ T cells. However, even in active disease, neither $\alpha\beta$ nor $\gamma\delta$ intraepithelial lymphocytes express T-cell activation markers such as CD25. Although of diagnostic value, this increase in intraepithelial lymphocytes is not specific for coeliac disease: such increase in density may be seen in cows' milk sensitive enteropathy/post-enteritis syndrome or other causes of small intestinal mucosal damage in infancy.[15] Increased numbers of intraepithelial lymphocytes are also found in many first-degree relatives. High numbers may remain in latent coeliacs or despite gluten-exclusion, during which only the $\alpha\beta$ population decreases, giving a proportionate increase in $\gamma\delta$. The $\gamma\delta$ cells are now thought to represent an evolutionarily early form of T cell, which recognises antigen differently to the more modern $\alpha\beta$ cells, and which shows tropism to mucosal surfaces. They may be recruited in response to tissue damage, specifically to expressed heat shock proteins, which is consistent with the idea that wheat glutens may actually be directly toxic to gut epithelium. The $\alpha\beta$ cells also form part of the extrathymic differentiation pathway, centred round the intestine, in which deletion mechanisms for potentially self-reactive cells are probably not as effective as within the thymus.[16,17]

The interstitial compartment

In contrast to the intraepithelial compartment, there is a diverse inflammatory infiltrate within the lamina propria, including antibody producing plasma cells (IgA, IgG and IgM), mast cells, eosinophils and T lymphocytes. The actual density of T cells is not increased, but overall numbers are, because of the 2-fold increase in lamina propria volume. As in normal small bowel, CD4 T cells dominate this compartment.[18] In striking contrast to the intraepithelial lymphocytes, there may be increased expression of activation markers such as CD25 (the α chain of the interleukin-2 receptor, required for clonal proliferation after antigen recognition), particularly amongst CD4 T+ cells. There are increased concentrations of soluble interleukin-2 receptor in the serum on relapse. The eosinophil infiltrate has been shown to produce cytokines such as interleukin-5, which will contribute to further IgA synthesis, and to secrete toxic products such as major basic protein into the surrounding tissue. There is also evidence of macrophage activation, and high local production of cytokines such as TNFα have been reported.

DIAGNOSTIC CRITERIA

In 1970, the Interlaken or European Society for Paediatric Gastroenterology and Nutrition (ESPGAN) diagnostic criteria were proposed whereby the key diagnostic criterion was the presence of small intestinal mucosal damage, i.e. enteropathy which responded to gluten elimination. The mucosa healed on a gluten-free diet only to relapse again after gluten challenge albeit at variable time intervals, although usually less than 2 years.[19]

Implicit in this complicated diagnostic approach with the performance of at least three small intestinal biopsies related to gluten elimination and challenge, was the conception that another syndrome of gluten intolerance existed which was transient or temporary. Thus the diagnostic category of transient gluten intolerance arose.[20]

More recently ESPGAN revised the diagnostic criteria basically no longer recommending such a complete procedure of gluten elimination and challenge in every case but only: (i) in those who presented under 2 years of age, the age group when transient gluten intolerance occurred; (ii) in those children who wanted to depart from a gluten-free diet; and (iii) in those cases where there was no previous biopsy or the diagnosis was uncertain.[21] This move largely came from the collaborative Italian study published by Guandalini et al.[22]

In recent times, various antibody tests of high diagnostic specificity and sensitivity for coeliac disease have been developed. As already mentioned, the best of these diagnostically are IgA anti-endomyseal antibody (EMA) and IgA anti-gliadin antibody (AGA). Whilst these are of great assistance diagnostically, most authorities have continued to insist that small intestinal biopsy remains the gold standard for diagnosis of coeliac disease. The use of antibodies however has enabled cases of coeliac disease to be recognised that have not been readily diagnosed before, the so-called atypical forms of the disease.

A recent multi-centre study[6] demonstrated that there is an overall increase in the age at diagnosis in children with coeliac disease in Europe. When the symptoms and signs at the time of presentation were studied by dividing children in to two groups: those with typical symptoms and those with atypical, it was found that geographical areas with a high mean age at diagnosis reported high frequencies of atypical symptoms and vice versa.

Amongst children diagnosed as atypical 'coeliac disease' there are those without any symptoms yet a flat mucosa. This concept of 'coeliac disease' in a completely asymptomatic form arose first from studies investigating the relapse of patients treated first with a gluten-free diet and then provoked by gluten challenge, according to the original ESPGAN diagnostic procedure. In the majority of cases, small intestinal mucosal relapse occurred without clinical manifestations. The second way asymptomatic patients were recognised was when first-degree relatives of known patients were biopsied and shown to have an abnormal mucosa. Today we can say that this asymptomatic state is not an exceptional. Instead of the term asymptomatic, it has been suggested that the term 'silent' be used for these children.[23] These patients may have some minor symptoms but these are noted only after diagnosis has been made and treatment started. Then the patients may feel generally better after a gluten-free diet than they did before treatment.

Some investigations have described so-called latent (or potential) coeliac disease. The first observation of such latency was made two decades ago by Weinstein.[24] Many recent observations support this concept. Latency in coeliac disease means that the disease exists but is not currently manifest. This term should be applied only to patients who fulfil the following conditions: (i) have, on biopsy, a normal small intestinal mucosa when on a normal diet; and (ii) at some other time, before or since, have yielded a flat small intestinal mucosa which has recovered on a gluten-free diet.[25] In practice it might be difficult to separate latent coeliac disease from transient gluten intolerance.

CLINICAL FEATURES

Classical symptoms

Chronic diarrhoea

The clinical forms of coeliac diseases are very variable and wide ranging (Table 6.1). Chronic diarrhoea, which may be acute or insidious in onset, is

Table 6.1 Mode of presentation of coeliac disease in 52 coeliac children at The Royal Alexandra Hospital

Diarrhoea	32
Failure to thrive of no apparent cause	7
Vomiting	6
Weight loss	3
Anorexia	2
Short stature	1
Protuberant abdomen	1

the commonest presenting symptom. Classically, most children with coeliac disease have a history of diarrhoea. The stools are characteristically pale, loose and very offensive and may resemble oatmeal porridge, as Gee described in 1888.[26] The child may pass two or three stools a day but often just one large bulky stool. The child may also have recurrent attacks of more severe diarrhoea, sometimes with the stools becoming watery.

Constipation

However, as has been recognised for some time, a few children with coeliac disease may have constipation. These children may have a dilated colon with constipation giving a clinical pattern that may be confused with that of children who have Hirschprung's disease.

Failure to thrive

Failure to thrive is an important way in which coeliac disease may present and coeliac disease needs to be considered in every child with this syndrome regardless of the presence of diarrhoea.

Vomiting

Vomiting can, on occasion, be the sole symptom.

Emotional symptoms

Emotional symptoms are common in children with coeliac disease but they are an uncommon mode of presentation of this condition. Gibbons, in 1889,[27] drew attention to the fact that the child with coeliac disease 'is extremely irritable, fretful, capricious or peevish. Nothing seems to please him and altogether he is quite unlike himself'. The coeliac child is often in a state of close dependence upon the mother, leading to a pronounced exacerbation of fretfulness and irritability when separated from her. There may be sleep disturbance. This state is best described as 'clingingness'. In addition, the coeliac child is often emotionally withdrawn from the environment and this may be described as lassitude; such withdrawal may even resemble autism. Not only may the child have emotional symptoms but the mother may become depressed, anxious and abnormally preoccupied with her child.

Anorexia

Anorexia is classically said to be a common feature of coeliac children, but only about 50% may have this symptom. Some children may in fact have an increased appetite. Short stature and delayed puberty are uncommon but important symptoms of coeliac disease.

Accompanying symptoms

Specific enquiry concerning the symptoms present at the time of diagnosis in a group of children with coeliac disease are indicated in Table 6.2. Their broad range is readily apparent.

Atypical symptoms

Examples of such atypical presentations of coeliac disease include extraintestinal manifestations such as short stature, delayed puberty, mouth ulceration

Table 6.2 Symptoms present at the time of diagnosis in 52 coeliac children at The Royal Alexandra Hospital

Diarrhoea	45
Abdominal distension	23
Vomiting	32
Lassitude	32
Weight loss	31
Irritability	30
Anorexia	25
Abdominal pain	23
Frequent respiratory infection	14
Failure to thrive	14
Sleep disturbance	9
Appetite increased	8
Acute oedema	7
Muscle wasting	7
Pallor	7
Muscle weakness	4
Constipation	3
Mouth ulceration	2
Rectal prolapse	2
Skin infections	2

and iron or folic acid deficiency anaemia as well as non-specific and often rather mild gastrointestinal symptoms such as recurrent abdominal pain.

Physical signs

Although the classic appearance of a miserable child with a distended abdomen and wasted buttocks and shoulder girdles (i.e. proximal limb girdles) does still occur, abnormalities on physical examination of a child with coeliac disease may be much less obvious in the 1990s. Indeed, some abdominal protuberance may be the only physical sign. However, muscle wasting and loss of muscular power with hypotonia may be present and the child may be delayed or have fallen back in his motor milestones. Measurements of height and weight are valuable and the child's height and weight at diagnosis are often found to be below the tenth percentile and sometimes below the third. Nevertheless, single measurements may be within the normal range and so isolated observations may not be useful diagnostically. Knowledge of earlier measurements of height and weight and the plotting of such observations on a percentile chart may prove very helpful diagnostically. Any child whose rate of weight gain has significantly slowed, especially when this is accompanied by a slowed rate of growth and gastrointestinal symptoms, merits considerations for the diagnosis of coeliac disease.

Age of onset

There is considerable variation in the age of onset of symptoms in coeliac disease. Gee originally described symptoms as presenting most often between the age of 1 and 5 years.[26] It may in fact present for the first time at any age from infancy to old age.

In a survey of 110 coeliac children at the Queen Elizabeth Hospital, seen between 1950 and 1969 by Young and Pringle,[28] the onset of symptoms began in most children under the age of a year with a peak between 7–12 months, although most were diagnosed in the second year of life (see Table 6.3). In a further survey at the same hospital of 42 children diagnosed between 1972 and 1975, the majority had an onset of symptoms under 6 months and most were diagnosed under a year (Table 6.4).[30] This trend to earlier diagnosis may have been related to increased awareness of the disease but is also clearly related to the earlier age of presentation of symptoms. Thus

Table 6.3 Age of children with coeliac disease at onset of symptoms

Series	Years studied	No of patients	0–6 months	7–12 months	13–24 months	2–5 years	6 years & over
Young & Pringle 1971[28]	1950–1969	63	25	29	9	0	0
Hamilton et al. 1969[29]	1964–1968	42	10	11	12	8	1
Walker-Smith & Kilby 1977[30]	1972–1975	42	26	9	3	2	2

Table 6.4 Age of children with coeliac disease at time of diagnosis

Series	Years studied	No of patients	0–6 months	7–12 months	13–24 months	2–5 years	6 years & over
Young & Pringle 1971[28]	1950–1969	91	–	33	37	18	3
Hamilton et al. 1969[29]	1964–1968	42	0	6	16	15	5
Walker-Smith & Kilby 1977[30]	1972–1975	42	8	14	10	4	6

in the 1970s there was a trend for symptoms of most children with coeliac disease to begin under the age of 1 year.

A review of 25 years of coeliac disease at Queen Elizabeth Hospital[7] has demonstrated a significant rise in the age of presentation in the late 1970s and 1980s. In fact, in this analysis, the number of children diagnosed as new cases between 1976 and 1985 was very similar to the number diagnosed at the Hospital between 1960 and 1971. However, between 1971 and 1975 there were many more cases diagnosed. When the year of birth of this cohort of patients is examined it is seen that children with coeliac disease studied during this 25 year period were born most often in the late 1960s or early 1970s. Whether this observation does in fact solely relate to the age of introduction of gluten to the diet still remains to be established. It is, however, consistent with the Swedish observations already mentioned.[4] It does seem likely to be the case for bottle fed infants.[7] It is not the case, however, for breast-fed infants. Thus, the frequency of breast feeding as well as the role of gastrointestinal infection and other at present unknown environmental factors must all be taken into account when interpreting the these changes in incidence. Other authors have described a decrease in incidence of coeliac disease in the UK.[31–33] However, it is most important to appreciate this disease does still occur. Atypical cases may be being missed in the UK. There is no epidemiological study available to determine this issue.

There is usually a variable 'latent interval' between the introduction of gluten into the diet and the development of clinical manifestations. The explanation for this interval remains unknown. In some children the interval may be months and in other years but some infants may have symptoms immediately gluten is added to their diet.

Once symptoms have appeared there may be a delay in diagnosis but, with increased awareness of this condition and the ready availability of the technique of small intestinal biopsy in paediatric centres, this interval is becoming less common except for atypical cases.

Modes of presentation

Classical presentation aged 9–24 months

This is sometimes called the 'usual' presentation. There is gradual failure to gain weight or loss of weight after introduction of cereals, the child having been previously well. This is accompanied by anorexia and alteration in stools which are softer, paler, larger and more frequent than usual. There is abdominal distension, muscle wasting and hypotonia. More than half of the 1972–1975 series at Queen Elizabeth Hospital for Children fell into this category. This is still the commonest mode of presentation in London.

Presentation in infants before 9 months

Vomiting is frequent and may be projectile in this age group. Diarrhoea may be severe, especially with intercurrent infections, not necessarily gastroenteritis. Abdominal distension may not be marked. This is now in the 1990s a rare mode of presentation. It is very difficult to distinguish from the post-enteritis/cows' milk sensitive enteropathy syndrome.

Presentation with constipation

These children are often very hypotonic with marked abdominal distension. This is an uncommon presentation.

Presentation at older age

Short stature, iron-resistant anaemia, rickets and personality problems all may occur. Diarrhoea is not a prominent feature. Such a mode of presentation is characteristic for children in Britain originating from the northern part of Indian sub-continent.

Presentation in asymptomatic siblings

After a case of coeliac disease is positively diagnosed, siblings should have clinical history and growth checked. If a suspicion of coeliac disease arises, IgA gliadin antibody or IgA anti-endomyseal antibody and serum immunoglobulins should be done. A small intestinal biopsy should then be performed if there is presence of a circulating antibody.

Ethnicity and coeliac disease

Whilst coeliac disease is chiefly a disease of people originating in Europe for reasons explained earlier, it can occur in patients from the northern part of Indian subcontinent, Arabs and West Indian children of mixed origin.[34] It has not been described in Japanese, Chinese nor in Black Africans.

Clinical associations

For some years it has been known that coeliac disease is often associated with other well known disorders. The best example perhaps is dermatitis herpetiformis, where the rash as well as the coeliac-like small intestinal mucosal damage responds to gluten elimination. Thus dermatitis herpetiformis is a manifestation of coeliac disease which expresses itself outside the gastrointestinal tract and is not just an associated disease. Another manifestation is dental enamel hypoplasia.[35]

The most clearly verified disease association of coeliac disease is juvenile diabetes mellitus.[36] Several screening studies show the prevalence of coeliac disease among diabetic children to be 2–6%. Other associations have been found especially with autoimmune diseases such as thyroiditis, Addisons's disease, vasculitis and chronic liver diseases.

In 1966, Cooke and Smith reported 'unexplained unconsciousness' in 5 adult coeliac patients.[37] Then, in 1978, Chapman and colleagues reported an increase of epilepsy in coeliac disease.[38] Various psychic disturbances and even schizophrenia as well as chronic, progressive neurological disorders have been described in association with coeliac disease.[39]

Sammaritano et al.[40] proposed, in 1988, a specific syndrome associating coeliac disease with intracranial calcification and folic acid deficiency. In the same year Malten et al.[41] described also the association of coeliac disease, epilepsy and intracranial calcification. Since then there have been many Italian studies concerning this issue. The Italian Working Group on Coeliac Disease and Epilepsy[42] have been particularly active with a very large study. 77% of patients with epilepsy and intracranial calcification on computer tomographic (CT) scanning had the characteristic small intestinal lesion of coeliac disease. The observation by Bardella et al.[43] that epilepsy may be preventable in children with coeliac disease who adhere strictly to a gluten-free diet is of particular importance for paediatrics. Not one of 81 patients who adhered to a strict gluten-free diet, compared to 4 of 47 patients on an unrestricted diet, had epilepsy and calcifications. These observation suggest that epileptic patients should be screened by endomyseal antibody testing and, if positive, have a small intestinal biopsy to diagnose coeliac disease.

What is now clear from these and other observations is the concept that coeliac disease may not only be associated with skin disorders, bone disorders and malignancy as well as the classical gastroenterological manifestations but also with significant neurological disease.

TREATMENT

The recommendation of a strict gluten-free diet for life remains as firm as ever,[21] especially in view of the evidence in adults of protection against malignancy by such a diet.[5] Recently, evidence has been produced[44] that oats may not be harmful in adults with coeliac disease. There is no comparable evidence in children. Hence the recommendation that a diet free of wheat, rye, barley and oats must remain for children with coeliac disease until a comparable study has been undertaken in this age group.

KEY POINTS FOR CLINICAL PRACTICE

1. Coeliac disease remains an important clinical entity in the 1990s.

2. Whilst classical forms of the disease are still important, atypical manifestations are also significant. At present, in some countries, these may be unrecognised.

3. IgA anti-endomyseal antibody is a valuable screen for undiagnosed coeliac disease with a high degree of specificity.

4. Small intestinal biopsy remains gold standard for diagnosis, combined with response to a gluten-free diet.

5. Serial biopsies related to elimination challenge are still required for children aged less than 2 years at diagnosis, uncharacteristic cases and for children who wish to abandon the diet.

6. A strict gluten-free diet for life remains a firm recommendation. There is some evidence that this may protect against malignancy.

REFERENCES

1. Lundin KEA, Scott H, Hansen T et al. Gliadin-specific, HLA-DQ (α1*0501 β1*0201) restricted T cells isolated from the small intestinal mucosa of celiac disease patients. J Exp Med 1993; 78: 187–196
2. Sollid LM, Markussen G, Ek J, Gjerde H, Vartdul F, Thorsby E. Evidence for a primary association of coeliac disease to a particular HLA-DQ alpha/beta heterodimer. J Exp Med 1989; 169: 345–350
3. Catassi C, Raetsch IM, Fabiani M, Rossini M, Bordicchia F, Candela F. Coeliac disease in the year 2000: exploring the iceberg. Lancet 1994; 343; 200–203
4. Weile B, Cavell B, Nivenius K, Krasilnikoff PA. Striking differences in the incidence of coeliac disease between Denmark and Sweden: a plausible explanation. J Pediatr Gastroenterol Nutr 1995; 21: 64–68
5. Holmes GKT, Prior P, Lane MR, Pope RN, Allan RN. Malignancy in coeliac disease-effect of a gluten-free diet. Gut, 1989; 30: 333–338
6. Greco L, Maki M, DiDonato F, Visakorpi JK. Epidemiology of coeliac disease in Europe and the Mediterranean area. In: Auricchio S, Visakorpi JK. eds Common Food Intolerances 1: Epidemiology of Coeliac Disease. Basel: Karger, 1992; 25–44
7. Kelly DA, Phillips AD, Elliott EJ, Dias JA, Walker-Smith JA. Rise and fall of coeliac disease: 1960–85. Arch Dis Child 1989; 64: 1157–1160
8. Maki M, Holm K, Kipsanen V et al. Serological markers and HLA genes among healthy first-degree relatives with coeliac disease. Lancet 1991; 338: 1350–1353
9. Sollid LM, Thorsby E. HLA susceptibility genes in celiac disease: genetic mapping and role in pathogenesis. Gastroenterology 1993; 105: 910–922
10. Shiner M. Ultrastructural changes suggestive of immune reactions in the jejunal mucosa of children following gluten challenge. Gut 1973; 14: 1–12
11. Brandtzaeg P. Immunologic basis for coeliac disease, inflammatory bowel disease and type

B chronic gastritis. Curr Opin Gastroenterol 1991; 7: 450–462

12. Ladinsner B, Rossipal E, Pittschieler J. Endomysuium antibodies in coeliac disease: an improved method. Gut 1994; 35: 776–778

13. Chan KN, Phillips AD, Mirakian R, Walker-Smith JA. Endomysial antibody screening in children. J Pediatr Gastroenterol Nutr 1994; 18: 316–320

14. Webster ADB, Slavin G, Shiner M. Coeliac disease with severe hypogammaglobulinaemia. Gut 1981; 22: 153–157

15. Spencer J, MacDonald TT, Diss TC, Walker-Smith JA, Ciclitira PJ Isaacson PG. Changes in intraepithelial lymphocyte subpopulations in coeliac disease and enteropathy associated T cell lymphoma (malignant histiocytosis of the intestine). Gut 1989; 30: 339–346

16. Janeway C, Jones B, Hayday A. Specificity and function of T cells bearing γδ-receptors. Immunol Today 1988; 9: 73–76

17. Murch S, Walker-Smith JA. The immunology of coeliac disease. Ann Nestlé 1993; 51: 59–65

18. Selby WS, Janossy G, Bofill M, Jewell DP. Lymphocyte subpopulations in the human small intestine. The findings in normal mucosa and in the mucosa of patients with adult coeliac disease. 1983; 52: 219–228

19. Meeuwisse GW. Diagnostic criteria in coeliac disease. Acta Paediatr Scand 1970; 59: 461

20. Walker-Smith JA. Transient gluten intolerance: does it exist? Neth J Med 1987; 93: 1356–1362

21. Walker-Smith JA, Guandalini S, Schmitz J, Shmerling DH, Visakorpi JK. Revised criteria for diagnosis of coeliac disease. Arch Dis Child 1990; 77: 891–894

22. Guandalini S, Ventura A, Ansaldi N et al. Diagnosis of coeliac disease: a time for change? Arch Dis Child 1989; 64: 1320–1324

23. Visakorpi JK. Silent coeliac disease: the risk groups to be screened. In: Auricchio S, Visakorpi JK. eds Common Food Intolerances 1: Epidemiology of Coeliac Disease. Basel: Karger, 1992; 84–92

24. Weinstein WM. Latent celiac sprue. Gastroenterology 1974; 66: 489–493

25. Ferguson A, Arranz E, O'Mahoney S. Definitions and diagnostic criteria of latent and potential coeliac disease. In: Auricchio S, Visakorpi JK. eds Common Food Intolerances 1: Epidemiology of Coeliac Disease. Basel: Karger, 1992; 199–127

26. Gee SJ. On the coeliac affection. St Bartholomew's Hosp Rep 1888; 24: 17

27. Gibbons RA. The coeliac affection in children. Edinburgh Med J 1889; 35: 321

28. Young W, Pringle EM. 110 children with coeliac disease. Arch Dis Child 1971; 46: 421

29. Hamilton JR, Lynch MJ, Reilly BJ. Active coeliac disease in childhood. Q J Med 1969; 38: 135–140

30. Walker-Smith JA, Kilby A. Small ontestinal enteropathies. In: Essentials of paediatric gastroenterology. Edinburgh: Churchill Livingstone, 1977

31. Littlewood JM, Crollick AJ, Richards IDG. Childhood coeliac disease is disappearing. Lancet 1980; ii: 1359

32. Dossetor JFB, Gibson AAM, McNcish AS. A recent reduction in the incidence of childhood coeliac disease in the west of Scotland. In: McConnell RB. ed The Genetics of Coeliac Disease. Lancaster: MTP Press, 1990; 41–45

33. Stevens FM, Egan-Michell B, Cryan E, McCarthy CT, McNicholl B. Decreasing incidence of coeliac disease. Arch Dis Child 1987; 62: 465–468

34. Hung JCC, Phillips AD, Walker-Smith JA. Coeliac disease in children of West Indian origin. Arch Dis Child 1995; 73: 166–167

35. Aine L, Maki M, Collin P, Keyrilainen O. Dental enamel defects in celiac disease. J Oral Pathol Med 1990; 19: 241–245

36. Maki M, Hallstrom O, Huupponen T, Vesikari T. Increased prevalence of coeliac disease in diabetes. Arch Dis Child 1984; 59: 739–742

37. Cook WT, Smith WT. Neurological disorders associated with adult coeliac disease. Brain 1966; 89: 683–722

38. Chapman RWG, Laidlow JM, Colin-Jones D, Eade OE, Smith CL. Increased prevalence

of epilepsy in coeliac disease. BMJ 1978; ii: 250–251

39. Hallert C, Derefeldt T. Psychic disturbances in adult coeliac disease. 1. Clinical observations. Scand J Gastroenterol 1982; 17: 17–19
40. Sammaritano M, Andermann F, Melanson D, Guberman A, Tinuper P, Gastant H. The syndrome of intractable epilepsy, bilateral occipital calcification and folic acid deficiency. Neurology, 1988; 38 (Suppl. 1): 239
41. Molteni N, Bardella MT, Baldassarri AR, Bianchi PA. Coeliac disease associated with epilepsy and intracranial calcifications: report of two patients. Am J Gastroenterol 1988; 83: 992–994
42. Gobbi G, Bouquet F, Greco L et al. Coeliac disease, epilepsy, and cerebral calcifications. Lancet 1992; 340: 439–443
43. Bardella MT, Molteni N, Prampolini L et al. Need for follow-up in coeliac disease. Arch Dis Child 1994; 70: 211–213
44. Janatuinen EK, Pikkarainen PH, Kemppainen TA et al. A comparison of diets with and without oats in adults with celiac disease. N Engl J Med 1995; 333: 1033–1037

7

Cholera

N. S. Crowcroft

Cholera became one of the re-emergent diseases in 1991 when the seventh pandemic spread to the Western Hemisphere. An ecological approach is necessary to understand this re-emergence because the causes of cholera lie in the interaction between demographic, social, political and economic factors and the environment.[1] As physicians, we cannot distance ourselves from these factors since we have a responsibility to understand the determinants of health.

Advances have been made in our understanding of cholera that will help predict future patterns of disease. These include contributions from molecular biology, demography, epidemiology and environmental studies. The ability to communicate such information has increased through the development of the information superhighway, the internet. Molecular techniques are helping to explain the pattern of spread[2] and the relationship between competing strains.[3,4] However, we do not yet understand fully how cholera spreads internationally, or how to predict or control its spread.

Cholera vaccine research has generated several new candidate vaccines. Nevertheless, the role of new cholera vaccines in the prevention and control of cholera is not yet clear. There are limits to the high-technology approach. *Vibrio cholerae* is constantly evolving and changing and the emergence of a new epidemic serogroup, *V. cholerae* O139, is a reminder of the capacity of bacterial pathogens to evolve more quickly than their hosts.

CHOLERA IN THE 1990s

Cholera is a toxin-mediated bacterial infection of the gastrointestinal tract caused by *V. cholerae*, a curved and actively motile, oxidase positive, Gram negative rod. Most infections are asymptomatic or mild, but severe cases of cholera, present with rapid onset of watery diarrhoea ('rice water'), vomiting, leg cramps and extreme dehydration. In severe cases ('cholera gravis') death can occur in hours.

The incubation period varies from a few hours to a few days. The El Tor biotype is excreted for 3–20 days compared with 1–7 days for the Classical type, and symptomatic excretion is more common with El Tor. Asymptomatic mild cases can outnumber severe cases by as much as 100 to 1 in endemic areas, and may be important in sustaining epidemics as well as endemic disease.[5]

Some people are more vulnerable to cholera than others. Gastric hypoacidity increases susceptibility; *Helicobacter pylori* infection may increase vulnerability by this mechanism. Cholera gravis occurs more often in those with blood group O.[6] Breast feeding is protective and cystic fibrosis heterozygosity may turn out to be protective.[7]

Case fatality

Differences in mortality between provinces, countries and continents reflect inequalities in levels of education, access to and quality of health services. In the first 3 months of the epidemic in Peru, case fatality was almost 12 times higher in the less accessible inland departments (4.6%) than in the coastal departments (0.4%).[8]

Case fatality can be kept low if cases are managed appropriately. Worldwide, the case fatality has fallen during the seventh pandemic from 49.3% in 1961 to 4.8% in 1981 and 1.7% in 1983.[9] In 1993, Africa had the highest mortality at 3.1%, but this was a fall from 5.1% in 1992, and is part of a downward trend. Rates were lower in Latin America at 1.1%.

Reporting

Cholera is one of only three diseases internationally notifiable to the World Health Organization (WHO). Under International Health Regulations, national health authorities should report the first suspected cases of cholera on their territory as soon as possible. For the purposes of reporting, a 'confirmed case' of cholera is laboratory-confirmed *V. cholera* O1 or O139 infection of any person with diarrhoea (but some countries report asymptomatic patients with laboratory-confirmed cholera infection as 'confirmed cases'). Once a case of cholera has been confirmed in an area where the disease is not already known to be present, all new cases, suspected or confirmed, should be reported to the WHO at least weekly.[10]

Classification of strains

The classification of *V. cholerae* strains can be confusing, and has become more complicated since the advent of O139 cholera. Strains are divided into serogroups on the basis of serology from O1 to O139. The O1 serogroup is further classified into serotypes (Inaba, Ogawa, Hikojima) and biotypes (Classical and El Tor) which can be found in any combination. One strain predominates in an epidemic. Further typing is possible using bacteriophages or, more recently, ribotyping. Ribotyping involves the analysis of restriction fragment polymorphisms of rRNA genes and enables the variation of *V. cholerae* to be studied at a molecular level.[11]

From a clinician's perspective, the most important factor is the capacity of the organism to produce cholera toxin as manifest in clinical disease. From a public health perspective, the epidemic potential of the strain is of greater significance. Only two serogroups, O1 and O139, have caused epidemic or pandemic cholera. Other serogroups may cause sporadic cases of cholera, but not epidemics. The nature of this epidemic capacity is unknown. There is a degree of independence between the factors determining epidemic potential and toxin-production since non-epidemic strains sometimes produce cholera toxin, and epidemic strains sometimes do not produce cholera toxin.

Cholera toxin acts by binding to a monosialganglioside receptor (GM1) on the intestinal mucosa with its B subunit, releasing the A1 subunit which migrates to the basolateral membranes where it permanently activates adenylate cyclase. This causes massive loss of fluid. Cholera toxin seems to have additional actions via prostaglandins and platelet activating factor.[12] The cholera toxin genes for both the A and B subunits are encoded with several other toxin genes on a large transposon-like element called the CTX element. This has been described as a 'virulence cassette' which confers virulence when acquired by non-toxigenic strains.[13] Although necessary, it does not seem to be sufficient for virulence, which also relies on the degree of colonisation. V. cholerae produces a range of toxins in addition to cholera toxin including Zot, Ace, haemolysin/cytolysin and other less-well characterised toxins which are important in deletion mutant vaccine strains in determining tolerability.

Fresh stool or a rectal swab in transport medium should be sent to the laboratory as soon as possible to diagnose cholera. Faeces or rectal swabs are cultured on thiosulphate citrate bile salts sucrose medium and the culture tested for the O1 and O139 antigens. In areas where cholera is rare, it can be helpful to test for the production of cholera toxin. Serological diagnosis can be made by rising titre of vibriocidal antibodies. Once the first cases in an outbreak have been confirmed, further testing of all suspected cases should be discouraged as this is a waste of resources.[10]

Transmission

The mode of transmission of cholera varies from outbreak to outbreak. It is essential to establish the main route of transmission to be able to apply appropriate control measures. Field epidemiologists have an important role in establishing the mode of transmission in an outbreak.[14] There are three main modes of transmission: water, food that has been contaminated during preparation, and seafood that was contaminated by living in infected waters.

During epidemics, V. cholerae has been isolated from rivers and water supplies, but rarely at high concentrations. Another important role for water is as the means of maintaining personal hygiene. Poor sanitation maintains transmission during epidemics: secondary transmission does not usually result from cases imported into countries with good sanitation. Water may be most important as a vehicle by which cholera contaminates salads, fruit and other foods that are eaten uncooked, or vegetables during cultivation, rather than through drinking.

External contamination of food with *V. cholerae* is clearly most important for foods which are insufficiently cooked or eaten raw. In Chile, the outbreak in 1991 was largely confined to Santiago where potable water supplies and sewerage are generally adequate, but raw sewage is used to irrigate vegetables. Melons are often irrigated with untreated waste water in Peru.

Cholera has been caused by consumption of seafood such as crab, oyster and mussels. High concentrations of *V. cholerae* have been found in seawater 500 m from a municipal sewer, and in mussels and the skin and intestines of fish raised in such water.[15] Once again, inadequate cooking can be the problem; in Peru raw fish is popular. The vibrio survives refrigeration to 0°C and heating to 60°C.[5] Acidic foods (pH < 5) have been found to protect against infection, such as tomato sauce in Guinea, Mahewu in Zimbabwe, and citrus juice added to water in Latin America.[14]

Prevention

The simplest message for prevention is 'BOIL WATER, COOK FOOD, WASH HANDS'.[10] *V. cholerae* is easily killed by simple water chlorination or by boiling. The best prevention is through provision of adequate drinking water and sanitation, and safe food preparation. Point-of-use water disinfection and improved domestic water storage may be a less expensive option than building the necessary infrastructure for the universal water and sanitation that prevents cholera epidemics in more affluent countries. Community-based interventions need to be appropriate to the predominant local modes of transmission, but examples include education of street food vendors and modifications of traditional recipes, such as lemon juice marinades.[14]

Surveillance is important for prevention, for distributing treatment and prevention supplies, and in allowing the investigation of new outbreaks. Surveillance allows estimations of incidence and fatality rates, assessment of the movement of the epidemic and determination of the effectiveness of control measures.

Antibiotic prophylaxis is only cost-effective when there is a high rate (15–25%) of secondary cases among family contacts or selected individuals (e.g. mothers of children with cholera). Mass chemoprophylaxis is ineffective and leads to the emergence of resistant organisms.

Treatment

The WHO provides guidance on control and treatment of cholera.[10] Most cases can be adequately treated with oral rehydration solution (ORS). Antibiotics are only recommended in the case of severe dehydration. Antimicrobials reduce the duration of diarrhoea, bacterial shedding and the

Table 7.1 Pandemic cholera

Pandemic	Origin	*V. cholerae*	Duration
First pandemic	Bangladesh	Classical	1817–1823
Second pandemic	Bangladesh	Classical	1826–1851
Third pandemic	Bangladesh	Classical	1852–1859
Fourth pandemic	Bangladesh	Classical	1863–1879
Fifth pandemic	Bangladesh	Classical	1881–1896
Sixth pandemic	Bangladesh	Classical	1899–1923
Seventh pandemic	Indonesia	El Tor	1961–
Eighth pandemic	India	O139	1992–

volume of fluid replacement needed, and can be given orally as soon as vomiting stops; there is no advantage to them being given intravenously. WHO guidelines recommend doxycycline for adults and cotrimoxazole for children, with furazolidine, erythromycin and chloramphenicol as alternatives.[10] However, resistant strains are being reported;[16] *V. cholerae* O139 has been found to be resistant to cotrimoxazole and furazolidine.[17]

PANDEMIC CHOLERA

The first six pandemics

The history of cholera is typified by pandemics which have spared only the northernmost and southernmost parts of the planet. The first six pandemics originated in Bangladesh and were caused by the Classical biotype (Table 7.1). They were associated with massive movements of people, such as military operations or pilgrimages, and followed commercial routes over sea and land. Millions died, with a case fatality frequently of 50% and sometimes as high as 70%.

By 1900, cholera had disappeared from the Western hemisphere, and between 1923 and 1965, 90–99% of the deaths due to cholera worldwide occurred in India, where the disease had become endemic.

The seventh pandemic

The seventh pandemic started in 1961 and has not receded. It differs from the previous ones in many respects. It started in Indonesia, rather than Bangladesh, and it is caused by *V. cholerae* O1 El Tor, not the Classical biotype. The epidemic has progressed more slowly than its predecessors; it took 10 years to reach Africa and 30 years to reach the Americas. The pattern of spread has also been erratic and unpredictable, perhaps because of the advent of cheap air travel and increased shipping which moves potentially contaminated ballast water and sewage around the oceans.[18] The mortality

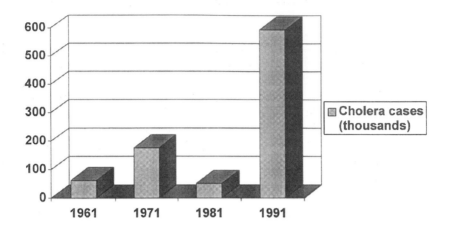

Fig. 7.1 Number of cholera cases notified to WHO, 1970–1991

has been lower than previous pandemics but the organism has a greater tendency to become endemic than the Classical biotype.

1991 was the year that cholera re-emerged, when the seventh pandemic spread to the Western hemisphere, starting in Peru at the end of January that year (Fig. 7.1). In 1991, 595,000 cases of cholera were reported to the WHO – more than in the previous 5 years combined.[9] 70% were in Latin America.

It is not known how cholera was imported into Peru, but possibilities include the discharge of a ship's sewage or contaminated ballast water. It spread along 2000 km of coast in 2 weeks and rapidly caused 12,000 cases. Between 17th February and 20th March 1991, an average of 2,550 cases were reported per day in a country with a population of 22 million.[8] In one area, the cholera vibrio was isolated from 87% of the children and 77% of the adults presenting with non-dehydrating diarrhoea. Ecuador was reached in less than 5 weeks, Colombia in less than 6 weeks followed by Chile and Brazil. In November 1991, cholera reached the mouth of the Amazon river, having crossed the South American continent. By the end of 1994, more than 1 million cases and 10,000 deaths had been reported to the Pan American Health Organisation (PAHO).[19]

The speed with which the epidemic spread was due to several factors. Large municipal water systems are poorly maintained and chlorination is often absent or ineffective. Sewers discharge adjacent to shellfish beds and fishing docks. Fish and shellfish are often eaten raw or partly cooked. Other factors also played a part. Firstly, the population had not been exposed to cholera this century so was non-immune. A high prevalence of infection with *Helicobacter pylori* may have increased susceptibility to cholera. Finally, at least 75% of Peruvians are blood group O.[6] The Latin American strain has now been isolated from shellfish in the Gulf Coast, possibly contaminated from discharge of ballast water.[20]

In 1991, resurgences of cholera were also seen in Africa and South-East Asia as well as Latin America. In 1992, 339,561 cholera cases and 2321 deaths were reported to the WHO from 21 countries in the Western hemisphere. In 1993, the incidence of cholera worldwide had fallen further, although still well above previous years, largely because of falling numbers in most countries in the Americas.

Countries of the Adriatic sea have also been affected by the spread of the seventh pandemic in 1994, with a water-borne outbreak of cholera in Albania, a foodborne outbreak in Italy and *V. cholerae* El Tor isolated from squid from the Adriatic sea and from sewage water.[21]

V. cholerae O139: the eighth pandemic

Until recently, *V. cholerae* serogroup O1 was considered the only bacterium that could cause epidemic cholera. However, an epidemic of non-O1 cholera started in southern Asia in 1992.[22] The organism is *V. cholerae* synonym Bengal serogroup O139 and causes disease that is indistinguishable from O1 cholera.

The first confirmed outbreak occurred in October 1992 in Madras and spread to Madurai and Vellore. In early 1993, similar epidemics began in Calcutta and southern Bangladesh. Adults cases have predominated, suggesting that populations in cholera endemic areas are not immune.[17] The organism has spread more quickly than the El Tor serogroup. It took the El Tor scrogroup about 2 years to displace endemic Classical cholera in India between 1964–66. It took less than 2 months for O139 cholera to become the dominant strain in India, although the El Tor biotype has not been completely displaced.

The amount of toxin produced by this strain corresponds to that produced by *V. cholerae* O1, which is unusual for non-O1 groups. The O139 serogroup shares some characteristics of both O1 and non-O1 strains.[4,23]

SURVEILLANCE OF CHOLERA: NEW WARNING SYSTEMS

Notifications alone are not sufficient to follow the progress of pandemics because cholera is not notified by serogroup or biotype. Although one strain will usually predominate during an epidemic, cholera is endemic in much of the world, and different serogroups and biotypes are found coexisting, such as the El Tor biotype alongside the Classical biotype and the O139 serogroup in Bangladesh and India.[24] Bacteriophage typing and, more recently, molecular techniques allow the epidemiology to be refined. Typing based on restriction fragment length polymorphism of rRNA (ribotyping) has demonstrated that there are different clones of Classical and El Tor *V. cholerae* and that specific ribotypes are associated with particular countries.[11] This technique allows us to study quite precisely the way in which different strains which co-exist in the same geographical area compete with each other.[3] Ribotyping and cholera toxin genes have shown that the Latin American epidemic is probably part of the seventh pandemic and is distinct from strains found in the gulf of Mexico.[2] However, the Latin American epidemic clone is also distinct from other seventh pandemic strains and new strains, particularly drug resistant ones, are appearing.

Electronic systems allow information about cholera to be rapidly disseminated across the planet. The internet is a rapidly growing forum for the exchange of information which is also suited to an international audience as it circumvents the problem of international time differences. There are a multitude of internet sites and groups interested in infectious diseases such as cholera. The WHO have a World Wide Web (WWW) site where information about new and ongoing outbreaks and guidance on dealing with emergencies is available (http://www.who.ch). Similarly, the internet can be used to search for information from other organisations such as the UK Communicable Disease Surveillance Centre (http://www.open.gov.uk/cdsc/cdschome.htm), US Centre for Disease Control (http://www.cdc.gov) and the Pan American Health Organisation (http://www.paho.org). Clinical and non-clinical questions about cholera can be posed to an international audience through various internet groups such as ProMED. Furthermore, medical journals, such as *Emerging Infectious Diseases*, are increasingly publishing on the internet.

POPULATION GROWTH, POVERTY AND ENVIRONMENTAL ASPECTS

Social factors are crucial in promoting the persistence of cholera.[25] Urbanisation and the impact of international debt with continued population growth have, especially during the 1980s, increased the numbers of people vulnerable to cholera and sustained the conditions which help the organism to flourish. War and political unrest also continue to take their toll, as illustrated in the Rwandan refugee crisis. To predict future cholera trends it is important to understand the future trends in the social influences on the disease, including population growth and poverty, as well as the changes in the environment that are projected.

Population growth

It is becoming increasingly difficult to envisage a high-technology solution to diseases of poverty such as cholera and other diarrhoeal diseases that will be effective in the absence of an integrated approach to all the influences that make diarrhoeal diseases kill 3 million children per year. Population growth is one of those influences. More children have been born in the past 40 years than existed in all history prior to the middle of the 20th century.[26] This problem is not restricted to certain parts of the world: it is no longer possible to think in those terms, and ecological concerns must impact on the rights of individuals.[27] Although the rate of increase of the population has been slowing since the 1960s, fertility is not likely to reach low levels until some decades into the next century. By that time, the population of the world will have doubled or perhaps trebled. Many countries or communities have exceeded the carrying capacity of their environment and cannot migrate to improve their standard of living – they are 'demographically entrapped'.[28] The impact of this population pressure was illustrated by events in Rwanda in 1994 where the highest fertility in the world contributed to genocide, and the resultant population migration caused an epidemic of cholera. Migration has been recognised risk factor for cholera since the time of John Snow but what has changed is the scale of migration. There were over 22 million refugees and 25 million displaced persons in the world in 1994[1] and most have fled from one developing country to another that can ill-afford to offer them shelter. Refugee camps may offer living conditions ideally suited only to pathogens such as *V. cholerae*.

Control of cholera will depend in part on dealing with the problems of population growth, through family planning, investing in the health of children, education, and raising the status of women. As demonstrated at the 1994 Cairo International Conference on Population and Development, this is not an easy topic – easier by far to work on a vaccine than to address an issue that is simultaneously personal, cultural and political.[29]

Poverty

Poverty, population growth and the environment are inextricably linked. In a fixed system it is a truism to say that expansion cannot be sustainable. Yet the global economy is in its essence expansionist. The richest countries of the world have formed economic protectionist alliances which sustain poverty.[30] The bare facts about the choices which will face us in the future in standards of living and health are not a topic for general discussion. The idea of stationary economics has not been accepted, and is not even being debated, in mainstream politics. Clearly, sustained population growth makes the task of creating necessary infrastructure such as water treatment and supply systems all the harder. The impact of international debt is an inexcusable evil. The most consumerist societies need to learn to be more frugal and more fair.

The 1980s saw increased poverty and inequality in the developing world. The maintenance and replacement of the existing infrastructure for the provision of drinking water and sanitation has been hard hit, and this infrastructure tends to be available to a few, neglecting rural and marginal urban areas. In Latin America and the Caribbean alone, 130 million people have no access to potable water and the waste produced by 300 million (not so far from the population of the whole European Community) is contaminating water resources used both for drinking water and in irrigation.[31] The 1990s cholera epidemic in the Americas has been attributed to the breakdown of the sanitary infrastructure.[31] In 1990, the World Bank estimated that 1.3 billion people in the developing world lack safe drinking water and nearly 2 billion lacked the means to dispose of faeces.[32]

Advances have been made in attempts to monitor the environment. Routinely collected environmental health indicators relevant to sanitation-related diseases such as cholera are currently inadequate, focusing on aspects of downstream water quality that do not bear directly on faecal-oral disease.[33] Measures need to be developed which include data on the quality and quantity of water supplied, disposal of excreta from adults and children, personal hygiene behaviour, and health outcome data that can be linked to the other indicators.[33]

Various agencies are taking the lead in trying to bring about change. For instance, the PAHO has produced a Regional Plan for Latin America and the Caribbean which recognises the central importance of investment in provision of drinking water and sanitation for health. Support from affluent countries and from international agencies including the World Bank and the United Nations is clearly vital.

Environmental change

It has been accepted only relatively recently that an environmental reservoir of cholera not only exists but is necessary for the maintenance of endemic cholera. The ecological niche is in the aquatic environment, but questions remain about how *V. cholerae* survives. An environmental influence is suggested by the clear seasonality of cholera in endemic areas. This is not explained by temperature, since the peak time for cholera in Bangladesh is the coolest season.[34] It may be linked to seasonality in an environmental niche. Seasonal appearance of non-O1 *V. cholerae* has been found to be predictive of cholera epidemics in endemic areas.[35] An environmental reservoir would explain the occurrence of simultaneous outbreaks in unconnected villages. Free-living *V. cholerae* do not survive well in water in unfavourable conditions, but at the right conditions of temperature, pH and salinity they can survive for months. Survival is further enhanced by association with algae and other aquatic flora and fauna, and survival is promoted in seawater by association with the exoskeleton of marine organisms, in particular with chitin.[34,36,37] *V. cholerae* may survive in unfavourable conditions in a dormant and non-culturable state. There may be environmental niches for cholera outside the aquatic environment, such as earthworms.[36]

Global climate change is forecast to increase the impact of cholera directly and indirectly. Marine organisms such as zooplankton which can serve as reservoirs of *V. cholerae*, feed on marine algae. In the past decade, there has been an unusual spread of algae (phytoplankton) worldwide, such as previously unaffected waters in South America.[38] The spread of algal blooms in coastal and inland waters has been attributed to a combination of poor agricultural management, fertilisers and coastal sewage release. These changed patterns of algal blooms in sea and inland waters worldwide allow cholera to survive in previously unfavourable conditions.[39] Global warming augments these effects by promoting the survival of all the organisms which promote the survival of cholera in the environment. These coastal algal blooms may well have contributed to the Latin American pandemic.[38]

Another important factor is the evolution of the organism; the El Tor biotype is more resistant to the environment than the Classical type and has become endemic even in desert regions. *V. cholerae* O139 appears to survive even better in the environment than *V. cholerae* O1, perhaps explaining its evolutionary advantage.[40]

Climate change also acts indirectly. Rising sea levels will mean falling land mass for some of the most densely populated and poorest regions of the world, exacerbating the risk of cholera epidemics. At the same time, extremes such as droughts and floods can trigger epidemics in the wake of the destruction of infrastructure and of population displacement.[1] Increased UV radiation secondary to stratospheric ozone depletion may be immunosuppressant and may increase vulnerability to all infectious disease.[38]

There are many questions about environmental and demographic change, and projections are likely to be inaccurate. However, there are also certainties. The interactions between society, population growth, the environment and health need to be understood so that interventions can be developed to minimise the harm. Physicians, social scientists, microbiologists, epidemiologists, climatologists and politicians will need to collaborate in the interests of both individual and societies. Physicians should be familiar with the impact of population increase, pollution and poverty on health, and with the global nature of the threat, and help to educate the public and politicians about these issues.[41]

The history of human society is a story about a species adapting its environment to its needs. However, there is a limit to the carrying capacity of the environment. Population growth can be seen as a global experiment which may define what that limit is, and cholera epidemics a warning signal that the limit is being reached. Some believe that the carrying capacity of the planet has already been exceeded.[30]

VACCINES

Inactivated whole-cell parenteral vaccine is not effective in controlling cholera.[10] The place of new cholera vaccines for prevention and control is not yet established.[10,42] Nevertheless, cholera vaccine research has yielded many important advances in the understanding of gastrointestinal mucosal immunity, in the use of adjuvants, in the generation of genetically engineered attenuated strains and in the issues surrounding the release of such strains into the environment.

Immunity to cholera is serotype specific with a stronger response to Ogawa than Inaba antigens,[43] and is antibacterial rather than antitoxin.

Infection with the Classical type of cholera confers almost complete immunity for several years, but immunity following an El Tor infection is virtually non-existent.[44] Furthermore, populations that live in cholera endemic areas lack immunity to the new serogroup *V. cholerae* O139. Similarly, vaccines have varied in their efficacy depending on the infecting biotype, serogroup and serotype of *V. cholerae*.

The B subunits of cholera toxin have been used as adjuvants both in cholera vaccines and others because they resist degradation by proteolytic enzymes and bind avidly to intestinal receptors.

Oral inactivated vaccines consisting of whole cells have been developed with and without recombinant B subunit. These have, like the inactivated parenteral vaccine, been of limited efficacy and duration of protection especially in children under 6 years, and may require boosters to maintain immunity.[45,46]

Since the 1980s, progress has been made with live oral vaccines; live attenuated vaccines for cholera were the first to be produced using recombinant DNA methods. The first recombinant strain to be sufficiently well tolerated to be used in field trials is CVD 103-HgR. Although 94% of the gene encoding for the active moiety of the A subunit of cholera toxin is deleted in this strain, this does not fully explain its attenuation since it does produce other cholera toxins.[13] Controlled studies of safety, immunogenicity and efficacy have been encouraging and large field trials are ongoing.[46] While protection against El Tor strains does not appear to be as good compared with Classical strains, and the duration of immunity is unknown, CVD 103-HgR does appear to elicit a higher antibody response in people with blood group O, who are at increased risk from cholera.[47]

The probability of CVD103-HgR to re-acquire the gene for the toxic moiety is low, but has been demonstrated under experimental conditions.[13] The impact of a revertant strain in a cholera-endemic area might be small, but in a cholera-free area it is more difficult to predict the outcome. Vaccine strains have been derived from highly toxigenic strains of *V. cholerae*. Since we do not understand why biotypes and serogroups emerge, persist or are displaced in nature, we cannot be so confident about releasing new strains into the environment. It has been suggested that live vaccines should be only be used in cholera-endemic areas and should be of the same biotype as that prevalent in that environment.[13] It may be that further genetic engineering will be able to produce mutants which are highly resistant to reversion by genetic recombination, extremely sensitive to UV light and also effective and tolerable cholera vaccines.[13]

The parenteral and oral vaccines that have been produced for *V. cholerae* O1 do not protect against O139, and a prototype oral live attenuated *V. cholerae* O139 is under development.[48]

These new vaccines are not deemed to be cost-effective for travellers.[42] In the case of refugees, there may not be the time or the resources to intervene with vaccination, and it is hard to justify diverting scarce resources to this end. Further cost-effectiveness studies of the new vaccines as an emergency intervention are needed, but will be very difficult to carry out. Emergency relief is a highly skilled task in which several non-governmental agencies are expert. Current recommendations in situations such as the Rwandan refugee crisis remain that appropriate management relies upon low-technology measures delivered by experienced trained personnel – adequate quantities of disinfected water, basic sanitation, active case finding and adequate use of oral rehydration.[49,50]

CONCLUSIONS

Although the first six pandemics of cholera lasted a few years to two decades, the seventh cholera pandemic is showing no signs of retreat. In addition, a new serogroup of epidemic *V. cholerae*, O139, has appeared. Understanding the interaction between the environment, social and demographic factors and cholera is becoming increasingly important. Cholera remains an indicator of social and economic problems. The challenge cholera presents to the world is simple in concept but the solutions, low-technology and political, will not be easily or quickly reached. Such low-technology interventions to prevent cholera have many wider-ranging benefits.

The challenge taken up by the scientific community has been to develop a better vaccine and this process has involved some of the most refined methods available in medical research. Great advances have been made in examining the molecular basis of disease and the molecular epidemiology of *V cholerae*. Out of this research has come new cholera vaccines. We do not yet know what the value of such vaccines will be.

KEY POINTS FOR CLINICAL PRACTICE

1. Cholera is amongst the re-emergent infectious diseases of the 1990s.

2. Since the appearance of O139 cholera in 1992, *V. cholerae* O1 is no longer the only epidemic serogroup.

3. Projected growth in human populations and environmental change, including faecal pollution and global warming, indicate that cholera will persist as a threat to health into the 21st century.

4. Vaccine research is yielding exciting advances in oral vaccines to *V. cholerae* O1 and O139. However, their role in the prevention and control of cholera remains unclear.

5. The internet now allows rapid global exchange of information about and surveillance of cholera.

REFERENCES

1. Wilson ME. Infectious diseases: an ecological perspective. BMJ 1995; 311: 1681–1684
2. Wachsmuth IK, Evins GM, Fields PI et al. The molecular epidemiology of cholera in Latin America. J Infect Dis 1993; 167: 621–626
3. Faruque SM, Alim ARMA, Rahman MM, Siddique AK, Sack RB, Albert MJ. Clonal relationships among Classical *Vibrio cholerae* O1 strains isolated between 1961 and 1992 in Bangladesh. J Clin Microbiol 1993; 31: 2513–2516
4. Faruque SM, Alim ARMA, Roy SK et al. Molecular analysis of rRNA and cholera toxin genes carried by the new epidemic strain of toxigenic *Vibrio cholerae* O139 synonym Bengal. J Clin Microbiol 1994; 32: 1050–1053
5. Glass RI, Claeson M, Blake PA, Waldman RJ, Pierce NF. Cholera in Africa: lessons on transmission and control for Latin America. Lancet 1991; 338: 791–795
6. Tauxe RV, Blake PA. Epidemic cholera in Latin America. JAMA 1992; 267: 1388–1390
7. Gabriel SE, Brigman KN, Koller BH, Boucher RC, Stutts MJ. Cystic fibrosis heterozygote resistance to cholera toxin in the cystic fibrosis mouse model. Science 1994; 266: 107–109
8. World Health Organization. Cholera in Peru. Wkly Epidemiol Rec 1991; 66: 141–145
9. World Health Organization. Cholera. Wkly Epidemiol Rec 1994; 69: 13–17
10. World Health Organization. Guidelines for cholera control. Geneva: WHO, 1993
11. Popovic T, Bopp C, Olsvik O, Wachsmuth K. Epidemiologic application of a standardised ribotype scheme for *Vibrio cholerae* O1. J Clin Microbiol 1993; 31: 2474–2482
12. Guerrant RL. Lessons from diarrhoeal diseases: demography to molecular pharmacology. J Infect Dis 1994; 169: 1206–1218
13. Mekalanos JJ. Live bacterial vaccines: environmental aspects. Curr Opin Biotechnol 1994; 5: 312–319
14. Tauxe RV, Mintz ED, Quick RE. Epidemic cholera in the New World: translating field epidemiology into new prevention strategies. Emerg Infect Dis 1995; 1: 1–8
15. Tamplin ML, Parodi CC. Environmental spread of *Vibrio cholerae* in Peru. Lancet 1991; 338: 1216–1217
16. Threlfall EJ, Said B, Rowe B. Emergence of multiple drug resistance in *Vibrio cholerae* O1 El Tor from Ecuador (Letter). Lancet 1993; 342: 1173
17. World Health Organization. Surveillance of cholera due to *Vibrio cholerae* O139. Wkly Epidemiol Rec 1994; 69: 52
18. McCarthy SA, McPhearson RM, Guarino AM, Gaines SL. Toxigenic *Vibrio cholerae* O1 and cargo ships entering Gulf of Mexico. Lancet 1992; 339: 624–625
19. Pan American Health Organisation. Cholera in the Americas. Epidemiol Bull 1995; 16: 11–13
20. Morris JG. Non-O group 1 *Vibrio cholerae*: a look at the epidemiology of an occasional pathogen. Epidemiol Rev 1990; 12: 179–190
21. Greco D, Luzzi I, Sallabanda A, Dibra A, Kacarricy E, Shapo L. Cholera in the Mediterranean: outbreak in Albania. Eurosurveillance 1995; 9: 1–2
22. Nair GB, Ramamurthy T, Bhattacharya SK et al. Spread of *Vibrio cholerae* O139 Bengal in India. J Infect Dis 1994; 169: 1029–1034
23. Hall RH, Khambaty FM, Kothary M, Keasler S. Non-O1 Vibrio cholerae (Letter). Lancet 1993; 342: 430
24. Jesudason MV, Samuel R, John TJ. Reappearance of *Vibrio cholerae* and concurrent prevalence of O1 and O139 in Vellore, South India. Lancet 1994; 344: 335–336
25. Levine MM, Levine OS. Changes in human ecology and behavior in relation to the emergence of diarrhoeal diseases, including cholera. Proc Natl Acad Sci USA 1994; 91: 2390–2394
26. Bongaarts J. Population policy options in the developing world. Science 1994; 263: 771–776
27. McMichael AJ. Contemplating a one child world. BMJ 1995; 311: 1651–1652
28. King M. Demographic entrapment. Trans R Soc Trop Med Hygiene 1993; 87 Suppl. 1: 23–28
29. Johnson BR. Implementing the Cairo Agenda. Lancet 1995; 345: 875–876
30. Loening UE. The ecological challenges to population growth. Trans R Soc Trop Med Hygiene 1993; 87 Suppl. 1: 9–12
31. Pan American Health Organisation. Regional plan for investment in environment and health. Bull Pan Am Health Org 1993; 27: 82–86

32. World Bank. World Development Report 1993. New York: Oxford University Press, 1993
33. Kolsky PJ, Blumenthal UJ. Environmental health indicators and sanitation-related disease in developing countries: limitations to the use of routine data sources. World Health Stat Q 1995; 48: 132–139
34. Islam MS, Drasar BS, Sack RB. The aquatic environment as a reservoir of *Vibrio cholerae*: a review. J Diarrhoeal Dis Res 1993; 11: 197–206
35. Ventura G, Roberts L, Gilman R. *Vibrio cholerae* non-O1 in sewage lagoons and seasonality in Peru cholera epidemic. Lancet 1992; 339: 937–938
36. Nalin DR. Cholera and severe toxigenic diarrhoeas. Gut 1994; 35: 145–149
37. Huq A, Parveen S, Qadri F, Sack DA, Colwell RR. Comparison of *V. cholerae* serotype O1 strains isolated from patients and the aquatic environment. J Trop Med Hygiene 1993; 96: 86–92
38. Patz JA, Epstein PR, Thomas TA, Balbus JM. Global climate change and emerging infectious diseases. JAMA 1996; 275: 217–223
39. Epstein PR. Algal blooms in the spread and persistence of cholera. Biosystems 1993; 31: 209–221
40. Islam MS, Hasan MK, Miah MA, Yunus M, Zaman K, Albert MJ. Isolation of *Vibrio cholerae* synonym Bengal from the aquatic environment in Bangladesh: implications for disease transmission. Appl Environ Microbiol 1994; 60: 1684–1686
41. Leaf A. Potential health effects of global climatic and environmental changes. N Engl J Med 1989; 321: 1577–1583
42. Steffen R. New cholera vaccines – for whom?. Lancet 1994; 344: 1241–1242
43. Preston NW. Corresponding type-specificity of vibriocidal and agglutinating activities of *Vibrio cholerae* antisera: relevance to vaccine immunogenicity. Epidemiol Infect 1993; 110: 489–497
44. Clemens JD, Van Loon F, Sack DA et al. Biotype as determinant of natural immunising effect of cholera. Lancet 1991; 337: 883–884
45. Begue RE, Castellares G, Cabezas C et al. Immunogenicity in Peruvian volunteers ot a booster dose of oral cholera vaccine consisting of whole cells plus recombinant B subunit. Infect Immun 1995; 63: 3726–3728
46. Cryz SJ, Kaper J, Tacket C, Nataro J, Levine MM. *Vibrio cholerae* CVD 103-HgR live oral attenuated vaccine: construction, safety, immunogenicity, excretion and non-target effects Dev Biol Stand 1995; 84: 237–244
47. Lagos R, Avendano A, Prado V et al. Attenuated live cholera vaccine strain CVD 103 HgR elicits significantly higher serum vibriocidal antibody titers in persons of blood group O. Infect Immun 1995; 63: 707–709
48. Coster TS, Killeen KP, Waldor MK et al. Safety immunogenicity and efficacy of live attenuated *Vibrio cholerae* O139 vaccine prototype. Lancet 1995; 345: 949–952
49. Goma Epidemiology Group. Public health impact of Rwandan refugee crisis: what happened in Goma, Zaire in July 1994? Lancet 1995; 345: 339–343
50. Siddique AK, Salam A, Islam MS et al. Why treatment centres failed to prevent cholera deaths among Rwandan refugees in Goma, Zaire. Lancet 1995; 345: 359–361

Nitric oxide: physiology, pathophysiology and potential clinical applications

R. H. Mupanemunda   A. D. Edwards

Nitric oxide (NO) is an endogenous biological mediator in many vertebrate organ systems, involved in functions as diverse as central and autonomic neurotransmission, hormonal release, bacterial and tumour cell killing, platelet inhibition and smooth muscle cell relaxation.[1] Although NO has a biological role in life forms up to half a billion years old,[2] it is only in the last 10 years that these functions have been elucidated.

In 1980, Furchgott and Zawadzki demonstrated that vascular endothelial cells released a highly unstable vasodilator substance which they named endothelium-derived relaxing factor.[3] Many other endogenous vasoactive substances were found to act through the release of endothelium-derived relaxing factor and to elicit endothelium-dependent-vasodilation.[4] Endothelium-derived relaxing factor was later identified as NO and subsequently shown to be generated from L-arginine.[5-7]

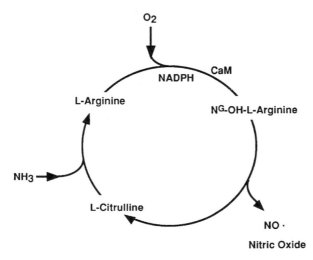

Fig. 8.1 Biosynthesis of nitric oxide from L-arginine. Nitric oxide synthase catalyses the hydroxylation of the nitrogen in the guanidino group of L-arginine and incorporates molecular oxygen into nitric oxide and citrulline in the presence of calmodulin and NADPH. Citrulline is recycled back to L-arginine by incorporating one nitrogen. This modified urea cycle regenerates L-arginine for nitric oxide synthesis and eliminates excess nitrogen created by the cellular metabolism.

BIOSYNTHESIS AND RELEASE OF NITRIC OXIDE

NO is synthesised from L-arginine by the enzyme nitric oxide synthase (Fig. 8.1). Three isoforms of nitric oxide synthase (encoded for by different genes) have been identified and these may be subdivided into constitutive nitric oxide synthase or inducible nitric oxide synthase.[8] There are two constitutive isoenzymes: endothelial nitric oxide synthase; and the neuronal nitric oxide synthase localised to certain central neurons and peripheral non-adrenergic non-cholinergic neurons.

Constitutive nitric oxide synthase is cytosolic, dependent on Ca^{2+} and calmodulin, and releases small amounts of NO for short periods in response to receptor and physical stimulation.[9] Inducible nitric oxide synthase is induced by endotoxin, inflammatory cytokines and lipopolysaccharides resulting in the release of larger amounts of NO.[10] This reaction is slower, requires gene transcription, and can be blocked by glucocorticosteroids, but results in the continuous release of large amounts of NO for long periods. Inducible nitric oxide synthase is functionally calcium independent and can be expressed in a wide variety of cells including macrophages, neutrophils, mast cells, endothelium and vascular smooth muscle cells. Whereas neuronal nitric oxide synthase and inducible nitric oxide synthase are largely cytoplasmic, endothelial nitric oxide synthase is associated with cell membranes, allowing direct NO delivery to underlying smooth muscle and to the blood-endothelial interface.

EFFECTS OF NITRIC OXIDE

NO is soluble both in water and lipid and is, therefore, freely diffusible in biological tissue. It has several actions: in smooth muscle, NO binds to the haem moiety at the active site of soluble guanylate cyclase initiating a conformational change which increases the production of cyclic guanosine 3′5′ monophosphate (cGMP) and facilitates protein phosphorylation by the cGMP-dependent protein kinase which leads to muscle relaxation (Fig. 8.2).[1,11] In the brain, the excitatory neurotransmitter glutamate acts at the N-methyl-D-aspartate subtype of receptor to open Ca^{2+} channels causing an influx of Ca^{2+}- stimulating nitric oxide synthase activity and elevating cGMP levels.[40] NO may also act independently of cGMP by directly activating smooth muscle potassium channels.[12]

At high concentrations, NO has toxic effects including inactivation of iron-sulphur centred enzymes, impairing mitochondrial enzymes, and damaging DNA.[9] One striking feature of nitric oxide synthase is its ability to produce superoxide, in the absence of arginine, as well as NO.[13] Reaction of NO with superoxide may lead to the formation of more toxic radicals including peroxynitrite and hydroxyl radicals which may mediate cytotoxic reactions.[9]

The NO generated by nitric oxide synthase remains effective for only a few seconds as it is readily oxidised to nitrogen dioxide (NO_2) which, in an aqueous solution, is transformed into nitrite which, in turn, is rapidly converted to nitrate in whole blood and eliminated in the urine with a half-life of 5 h. Basal nitrite concentrations in blood are low and those of nitrate are 100-fold higher (30 mmol/l).[14]

In the blood, NO is rapidly inactivated by binding to haemoglobin forming methaemoglobin. However, haemoglobin is rapidly regenerated by red blood cell methaemoglobin reductase with nitrate as a by-product.[8] The high affinity of NO for haemoglobin and its rapid inactivation on combining with methaemoglobin means that its physiological actions remain localised to the site of its generation and its actions are in general rapidly terminated.

However, recent work has shown that NO activity can be prolonged. Haemoglobin is S-nitrosylated in the lung, and S-nitrosothiols are released during arterial-venous transit, thus allowing vasodilation and optimising matching of perfusion to oxygenation (Fig. 8.3).[15] Endogenous NO may also form nitrosothiols with serum albumin which act as an NO carrier.[8] Nitrosothiols may, therefore, act as a store, prolonging the actions of released NO or as additional biological sinks for nitric oxide which regulate the concentration of free NO.

PHYSIOLOGICAL ROLES OF NITRIC OXIDE

Cardiovascular system

NO plays a major role in the regulation of blood flow and pressure as well as the general homeostatic control of the vasculature (Table 8.1). Nitric oxide

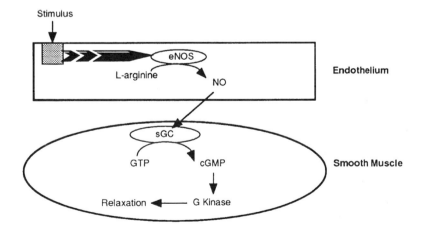

Fig. 8.2 Physiological actions of nitric oxide. The synthesis of nitric oxide by endothelial nitric oxide synthase is triggered by an increase in intracellular Ca^{2+} following stimulation of endothelial cells by mechanical or pharmacological stimuli. The nitric oxide formed diffuses to the subadjacent smooth muscle cells where it activates soluble guanylate cyclase resulting in enhanced synthesis of cyclic guanosine monophosphate from guanosine triphosphate. Cyclic guanosine monophosphate activates protein kinases and leads ultimately to the dephosphorylation of myosin light chains and muscle relaxation.

synthase activity is present in the endothelium of human arteries and veins and the enzyme has been isolated, sequenced and cloned from human umbilical vein endothelium.[9] Systemic administration of nitric oxide synthase inhibitors increases systemic and pulmonary arterial pressure by inhibiting NO synthesis of small arteries.[8] Administration of N^G-mono-methyl-L-arginine, a nitric oxide synthase inhibitor, into the brachial artery of healthy volunteers reduces

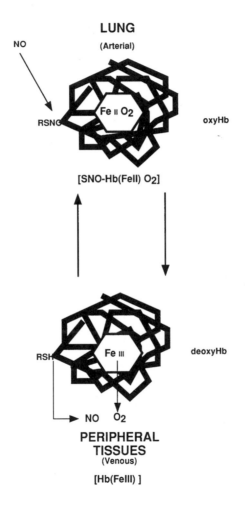

Fig. 8.3 The dynamic activity of blood in vascular control. Haemoglobin is S-nitrosylated in the lung when red blood cells are oxygenated and the nitric oxide group is released during arterial-venous transit. Nitric oxide scavenging by the metal centre of oxy-nitrosohaemoglobin results in conversion of the metal centre to the ferric state which promotes nitric oxide release. Changes in oxygen tension also regulate nitric oxide delivery as nitric oxide release is facilitated by deoxygenation. Nitric oxide released from the sulphydryl groups of haemoglobin possesses nitrosonium character which protects the nitric oxide group from auto-inactivation at the metal centre. Thus haemoglobin has evolved both electronic and allosteric mechanisms to promote the efficient utilisation of oxygen (as nitric oxide controls mitochondrial respiration) and regulate capillary blood flow (by releasing nitric oxide during arterial-venous transit).

Table 8.1 Physiological and pathological actions of nitric oxide

Organ system	Physiological actions	Pathological actions
Cardiovascular	Antithrombotic, antiadhesive, coronary perfusion, inhibition of smooth muscle proliferation, negative inotropic effect	Hypertension, pulmonary hypertension, vasculopathy, microvascular leak, septic shock, myocardial stunning
Respiratory	Hypoxic pulmonary vasoconstriction, ventilation-perfusion matching, airways ciliary motility, immune defense, mucus secretion	Asthma, cystic fibrosis, bronchopulmonary dysplasia, bronchiectasis, immune complex mediated alveolitis, adult respiratory distress syndrome, rhinitis
Central and peripheral nervous system	Cerebral blood flow regulation, neuroendocrine secretion, memory formation, vision, smell	Convulsions, migraine, hyperalgesia, neurotoxicity
Endocrine	Pancreatic exocrine and endocrine secretion adrenocorticoid release, renal renin secretion	Destruction of β islet cells
Immune	Inflammation, antimicrobial, antitumour	Inflammation, tissue injury, septic shock, graft versus host disease, allograft rejection
Gastrointestinal	Gut perfusion, peristalsis, mucosal protection, antimicrobial, exocrine secretion	Gut dysmotility syndromes (achalasia, pyloric stenosis, Hirschsprung's), mucosal injury, inflammatory bowel disorders (ulcerative colitis), carcinogenesis
Genitourinary and reproductive	Glomerular perfusion, glomerulotubular feedback, bladder control, male erection	Acute renal failure, glomerulonephritis uterine quiescence, pre-eclampsia, intrauterine growth restriction, bladder dysfunction, erectile impotence

forearm blood flow by 40%, indicating that resistance vessels are in a continuous state of endogenous NO-mediated vasodilatation. However, veins have a low basal output of NO[9] and their resting tone may be independent of the basal endogenous NO release.[8]

Basal endothelial nitric oxide synthase activity is regulated by several mechanisms: paracrine mediators such as bradykinin and acetylcholine act on endothelial cell surface receptors to generate inositol 1,4,5-trisphosphate production via the phosphoinositide second-messenger system and elicit Ca^{2+} release which activates nitric oxide synthase; shear stress and deformation of vascular endothelium which accompany pulsatile flow through blood vessels stimulate NO release.[9,13] Chronic exercise induces endothelial nitric oxide synthase expression which may account for some of the beneficial effects of regular exercise.[8] Similarly, the induction of endothelial nitric oxide synthase by oestrogen may account for the physiological vasodilation of pregnancy.[9] Cardiac nitrergic neurons innervate the pacemakers and myocardium to mediate negative-inotropic autonomic influences.

NO released from endothelium inhibits platelet aggregation and leukocyte adhesion via a cGMP-dependent mechanism and is synergistic with prostacyclin.[1,9] Platelets also generate NO which may act as a negative feedback mechanism regulating platelet aggregation.[1] NO may also inhibit the proliferation of vascular smooth muscle, the precursor of vascular remodelling.[16]

Respiratory system

Nitric oxide synthase has been identified in airway epithelial cells, autonomic neurons, smooth muscle cells, fibroblasts, macrophages, neutrophils, mast cells and endothelial cells. Endogenous pulmonary NO is involved in airway and vascular smooth muscle relaxation, pulmonary neuro-transmission and host defence.

The epithelial cells of the paranasal sinus produce concentrations of NO close to the highest permissible atmospheric pollution levels. As NO has both a bacteriostatic and bronchodilator properties, it may aid sterility in human paranasal sinuses, condition the inspired air, regulate airway tone and improve ventilation-perfusion matching (V/Q).[9] Endogenous NO modulates mucociliary clearance by increasing ciliary beat frequency in the ciliated epithelial cells.[17]

NO acts as a bronchodilator through its action on soluble guanylate cyclase.[9] In normal individuals, NO inhalation at concentrations of up to 80 ppm has little or no direct effect, but does reduce methacholine induced bronchoconstriction.[17] In asthmatics, NO inhalation produces a small (though inconsistent) bronchodilator effect.[17] There is no evidence for tolerance after prolonged NO administration and the effect of NO is additive with β-adrenoceptor agonists. NO may also stabilise mast cells as it reduces histamine release.[17]

NO functions as a neurotransmitter at inhibitory non-adrenergic non-cholinergic nerves (Fig. 8.4). Neuronal nitric oxide synthase has been localised in nerves supplying bronchial vessels, airway smooth muscles and submucosal glands in humans[17] and in sympathetic, parasympathetic and sensory ganglia supplying the respiratory tract, being more abundant in proximal than in distal airways. Following stimulation, these nerves release NO and have thus been renamed 'nitrergic' nerves.[18] Bronchodilator nitrergic nerves are the only neural bronchodilator pathway in humans, although NO also modulates reflex bronchoconstriction in vivo.[18]

The role of NO in the regulation of the pulmonary circulation has been extensively investigated. Although the first description of the effects of hypoxia on the pulmonary circulation was made over a 100 years ago, the mechanism of hypoxic pulmonary vasoconstriction has remained largely unexplained. Current evidence suggests that reduced pulmonary endothelial NO release may be the mechanism underlying hypoxic pulmonary vasoconstriction.[19] Nitric oxide synthase inhibitors enhance hypoxic pulmonary vasoconstriction, while inhalation of NO abolishes hypoxic pulmonary vasoconstriction in humans.[8] In addition, NO may also be involved in neurogenic vasodilator responses in the pulmonary circulation.[20] These observations are the basis of the therapeutic use of inhaled NO in disorders characterised by severe hypoxaemia and pulmonary vasoconstriction.

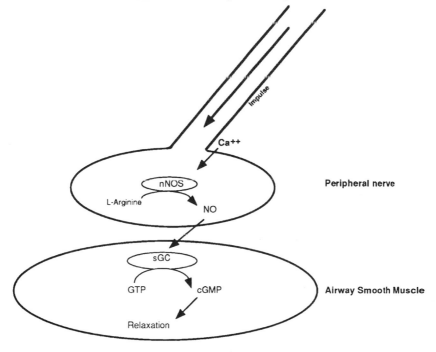

Fig. 8.4 Physiological action of nitric oxide in airway nitrergic nerves. Depolarisation of nitrergic nerves results in an influx of calcium ions and activation of neuronal nitric oxide synthase to synthesise nitric oxide. The released nitric oxide diffuses into airway smooth muscle cells to activate soluble guanylate cyclase resulting in increased cyclic guanosine monophosphate and relaxation.

Central nervous system

Immunostaining of the brain for neuronal nitric oxide synthase has revealed a small number of nitric oxide synthase-positive cells with an extensive distribution throughout the brain, particularly in the cerebellum, superior and inferior colliculi and granule cell layer of the olfactory bulb.[9] The cerebral cortex, hippocampus, posterior pituitary and autonomic fibres in the retina also contain neuronal nitric oxide synthase-positive cells. Stimulation of the excitatory N-methyl-D-aspartate glutamate receptor leads to the release of NO, an effect that is inhibitable by nitric oxide synthase inhibitors.[8] NO has been proposed to play several roles: a mediator of long-term potentiation (hippocampus) and long-term depression (cerebellum); the physiological basis of memory; a mediator of short term electrocortical activation; an alerting response important in control of the arousal state; and a modulator of nociception.[9,21] In addition, NO may also have physiological roles in vision, perception of smell, feeding behaviour, and in modulating cerebral blood flow. After cerebral injury, inducible nitric oxide synthase can be detected in immune cells within the brain.

Gastrointestinal system

In the human gut, nitrergic nerves have been demonstrated in the myenteric plexus of the stomach and intestine, sphincter of Oddi and duodenal sphincter.[9] NO dependent neurotransmission has been demonstrated in the lower oesophageal, ileocolic and anal sphincters. Release of NO mediates gastric adaptive relaxation, peristalsis and relaxation of specialised internal sphincters,[9] and mice lacking the gene for neuronal nitric oxide synthase develop pronounced gastric enlargement.

High concentrations of free NO (up to 6 ppm) are present in the intragastric air in humans. This intragastric NO production is probably non-enzymatic, requiring an acidic environment, as NO in expelled air is reduced by 95% following pretreatment with the proton pump inhibitor omeprazole.[22] NO may be important for the integrity of the gastric mucosa in health and disease both through its antimicrobial action and by influencing mucus production by the gastrointestinal mucosa.[21]

Immune system

Following exposure to endotoxins or cytokines such as tumour necrosis factor-α, interleukin-1β and interferon-γ, macrophages express inducible nitric oxide synthase, leading to increased synthesis and release of NO. NO is involved in the killing of intracellular (e.g. bacteria) and extracellular microorganisms (e.g. parasites). NO mediates some cytotoxic reactions against tumour cells and non-specific immunity,[23] and has immunomodulatory effects via its inhibitory effect on certain subsets of T helper cell lymphocytes, neutrophils and macrophages.[20] The mechanism of NO-mediated cytotoxicity is inhibition of enzymes involved in energy metabolism or synthesis, free radical damage through interaction with superoxide radicals, or other less well characterised methods. Anti-inflammatory glucocorticosteroids inhibit induction of inducible nitric oxide synthase but are ineffective once the enzyme is expressed.[9]

Endocrine system

NO may act as a mediator for hormone release. NO can cause insulin secretion from pancreatic β cells and a constitutive nitric oxide synthase has been demonstrated in pancreatic β cells.[8,9] The release of renin from the kidney and thyroid hormone production may also be influenced by NO.[9] In the adrenal gland, nitric oxide synthase is highly concentrated in a network of neurons that stimulate adrenaline release. Other recent studies have linked NO with: the pancreatic and parotid gland secretion of amylase; pituitary secretion of adrenocorticotropin, luteinizing hormone, growth hormone, oxytocin and antidiuretic hormone; hypothalamic secretion of corticotropin-releasing hormone, luteinizing hormone-releasing hormone and somatostatin and the mesenteric secretion of adrenaline.[21]

Genitourinary and reproductive system

NO mediates functions in the kidney, bladder and reproductive organs. In the rat kidney, the macula densa synthesises NO in response to sodium reabsorption and this dilates the afferent arteriole, thereby increasing the glomerular filtration rate.[9] In the urinary tract, nitrergic neurons regulate bladder function and, in particular, control bladder outflow.[9] NO relaxes upper and lower urinary tract smooth muscle.

NO is the physiological mediator of penile erection. Nitric oxide synthase has been demonstrated in pelvic nerve neurons innervating the corpus cavernosum and in neuronal plexuses of the adventitial layer of the penile arteries.[3] The local application of NO donors, such as glyceryl trinitrate, promotes erection in humans while nitric oxide synthase inhibitors abolish erection.[9] NO also relaxes uterine smooth muscle and nitric oxide synthase is present in the human uterus.[9] Glyceryl trinitrate suppresses active labour in sheep and NO may promote uterine quiescence during pregnancy, as nitric oxide synthase expression is markedly reduced during parturition.[21]

PATHOLOGICAL ROLES OF NITRIC OXIDE

Cardiovascular disease

Vascular endothelium is a major site of NO production, platelet-endothelial-leukocyte interactions and also a regulator of vascular smooth muscle proliferation. Endothelial damage or dysfunction with reduced NO synthesis or release readily leads to cardiovascular disease. Familial hypercholesterolaemia leads to deposition of low density lipoproteins in the subintimal space and endothelial dysfunction which can be reversed by administration of arginine.[8] In animals, arginine administration results in a reduction in the thickness of the intimal lesions.[8] Endothelium-dependent vasodilatation is also impaired in patients with essential hypertension suggesting that impaired NO release may contribute to their hypertensive state.[14]

Pulmonary vascular disease is one of the most serious complications of congenital heart disease. Once established, it is progressive and irreversible, despite correction of the underlying defect. The pathogenesis of pulmonary vascular disease is poorly understood but recent studies suggest that endothelial dysfunction is an early event in the pathophysiology of pulmonary vascular disease. Endothelium-dependent (in contrast to endothelium-independent) pulmonary artery relaxation is impaired in young children with increased pulmonary flow secondary to congenital heart disease, but without established pulmonary vascular disease.[24] Endothelial cells have been demonstrated to be abnormal in the first years of life in children with congenital heart disease and pulmonary hypertension.[24,25] This may account for the predilection of these patients to develop pulmonary hypertension and pulmonary hypertensive crises following corrective surgery, particularly when cardiopulmonary bypass is employed.

Lung disease

Severe hypoxaemic respiratory failure secondary to lung disease (e.g. surfactant deficiency or bacterial pneumonia) is common in the perinatal period. This may lead to the development of persistent pulmonary hypertension of the newborn which is characterised by pulmonary hypertension with right-to-left shunting of blood across the ductus arteriosus and foramen ovale.[25] Although the causal mechanism of persistent pulmonary hypertension of the newborn is not known, recent reports suggest that endogenous NO synthesis and/or release is impaired in this condition. Furthermore, L-arginine, may also be deficient in some infants with persistent pulmonary hypertension of the newborn.[25] Impaired NO synthesis may also contribute to the pathophysiology of severe respiratory distress syndrome and bronchopulmonary dysplasia.[26]

The role of NO in asthma is complex.[27] Expired NO concentrations are higher in asthmatics than in controls and immunohistochemical studies of human lungs reveal that airway epithelial inducible nitric oxide synthase is increased in bronchial biopsies from asthmatics relative to those from normal subjects.[20,27] This could well be accounted for by the known upregulation of proinflammatory cytokines in asthma and raises the possibility of monitoring lung inflammation and directing anti-inflammatory treatment by measuring expired NO levels in asthma.

In the early stages of asthma, NO may act as an endogenous bronchodilator. However the high concentrations of NO produced by inducible nitric oxide synthase may downregulate the activity of constitutive nitric oxide synthase and interfere with the mechanism which normally counteracts constriction of the airways. In established asthma, high concentrations of NO may have adverse effects on capillary permeability causing oedema and plasma leak. Indeed, inhibition of endogenous NO production reduces inflammation and plasma exudation in the airways. Furthermore, the cytotoxic effect of NO may contribute to epithelial shedding, mucosal hyperaemia, airway narrowing and bronchoconstriction. During exercise, there is increased NO release in expired air, which may account for exercise-induced bronchoconstriction in asthmatics.[20] Excessive NO generation may be common in generalised inflammatory disorders of the airways such as cystic fibrosis, bronchiectasis and bronchopulmonary dysplasia. In addition, patients with seasonal rhinitis also have elevated oropharyngeal expired NO concentrations compared to controls.[20]

Corticosteroids inhibit inducible but not constitutive nitric oxide synthase. Steroids may, therefore, exert their anti-inflammatory effect by reducing the formation of NO and thus dampening the pulmonary vascular inflammatory response. The development of selective inducible nitric oxide synthase inhibitors might provide agents with desirable anti-inflammatory effects but without the systemic side effects of steroids.

NO not only modulates pulmonary vascular tone but also inhibits the proliferation of vascular smooth muscle.[16] Impaired NO production may thus contribute to the development of pulmonary hypertension and vascular remodelling seen in chronic respiratory disorders such as cystic fibrosis.

Central nervous system disorders

A proportion of the neuronal death caused by hypoxia-ischaemia is mediated by excess secretion of the excitatory neurotransmitter glutamate which acts, at least in part, by increasing NO release. In cell culture, NO antagonists protect effectively against glutamate induced cell death but, unfortunately, in animal models of hypoxia-ischaemia NO, inhibitors have proved remarkably ineffectual, frequently exacerbating cerebral damage.[28,29] This may reflect the more complex biology of an intact organ system compared to isolated cells.

In inhibiting the action of glutamate, nitric oxide synthase inhibition protects against epilepsy, enhances the action of certain anaesthetic agents, and impairs learning in rats.[9] Inducible nitric oxide synthase expressed by microglial cells has been implicated in the pathogenesis of several conditions including AIDS dementia, multiple sclerosis and other neurodegenerative states.[14]

Gastrointestinal disorders

In biopsy specimens from infants with hypertrophic pyloric stenosis or Hirschsprung's disease and adults with achalasia, a selective lack of nitric oxide synthase has been demonstrated.[9] The loss of action by NO may,

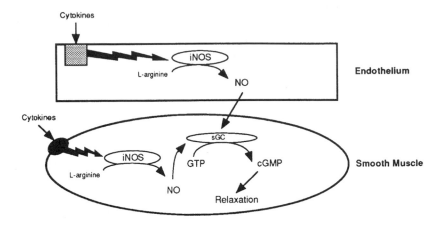

Fig. 8.5 Pathological actions of nitric oxide. The interaction of cytokines or bacterial toxins with receptors on smooth muscle or endothelial cell receptors results in the induction of inducible nitric oxide synthase gene expression. Once induced, nitric oxide synthase produces nitric oxide continuously, resulting in sustained activation of soluble guanylate cyclase, prolonged smooth-muscle relaxation, reduced responsiveness to vasoconstrictors and tissue damage.

therefore, be implicated in the impaired motility observed in these conditions. NO may also have a pathogenic role in ulcerative colitis where inducible nitric oxide synthase activity in superficial mucosal layers is increased.[30] Inhibitors of nitric oxide synthase ameliorate experimentally induced chronic ileitis and the colonic distension and toxic megacolon of severe ulcerative colitis may, at least in part, be secondary to the elevated luminal NO concentrations. Nitric oxide synthase inhibition has been suggested as the mechanism of opiate-induced constipation.[9,14]

Immunological and inflammatory disorders

NO plays a significant role in acute and chronic inflammation. NO interacts with reactive oxygen intermediates to produce molecular species with enhanced cytotoxicity, and excessive production of NO contributes to the vasodilation, vascular leakiness and tissue damage which characterise many inflammatory conditions. Nitric oxide synthase inhibitors reverse several of the classic signs of inflammation, including erythema and vascular leakage. NO plays a role in the immune rejection of allografted organs and in graft versus host disease.[21]

Septic shock is associated with NO overproduction; septic patients and animals lose peripheral vascular tone, and the responsiveness of vessels to constricting agents is diminished (Fig. 8.5).[38] Endotoxin induces inducible nitric oxide synthase in endothelium, vascular smooth muscle and myocardium, and infusion of nitric oxide synthase inhibitors to animal models of septic shock can lead to a rapid and reproducible rise in systemic resistance where other vasoconstrictors are ineffective.[31] NO mediates the cytokine-induced negative inotropic effects on the heart which accounts for the depressed myocardial contractility observed in endotoxemia, cardiomyopathies associated with inflammation as well as the myocardial stun syndrome.[13] Selective inhibitors for inducible nitric oxide synthase are now available and are the subject of intense investigation.

Endocrine disorders

Although NO may have a role in the physiological secretion of insulin, other studies suggest that it plays a role in the pathogenesis of type I diabetes mellitus. Pancreatic β cells have a limited capacity for free radical scavenging and are, therefore, highly sensitive to NO cytotoxicity. Induction of nitric oxide synthase in the islets may therefore contribute to the destruction of pancreatic β cells. In nonobese diabetic mice and experimental models of type I diabetes, progressive insulitis, dysfunction and eventual killing of pancreatic β cells correlate with the induction of inducible nitric oxide synthase.[21] Administration of nitric oxide synthase inhibitors reduces the pancreatic infiltration with macrophages, prevents hyperglycaemia and, in some reports, completely prevents pancreatic dysfunction.[14,21] It has, therefore, been suggested that specific inhibitors of nitric oxide synthase could retard the progression of type I diabetes by preventing the immune-mediated destruction of pancreatic islets.

Both laboratory animals and humans with type I diabetes demonstrate impaired endothelium-dependent vasodilation, suggesting that endogenous NO synthesis and/or release is impaired.[9] Impaired NO biosynthesis may, therefore, be an important pathogenic factor in diabetic microangiopathy.

Genitourinary and reproductive disorders

In chronic renal failure, endogenous inhibitors of nitric oxide synthesis (e.g. N^G-N^G-dimethylarginine) accumulate in plasma and may contribute to the white cell dysfunction and hypertension which characterise this condition.[9] In contrast, platelets from uraemic patients demonstrated elevated NO synthesis which may account for the bleeding diathesis in these patients.[9] There is evidence of nitric oxide synthase induction in immune complex glomerulonephritis.[9]

Musculoskeletal disorders

Patients with rheumatoid arthritis have raised NO concentrations in their plasma and synovial fluid.[14] An inducible nitric oxide synthase, expressed following treatment with interleukin-1β has been cloned from human chondrocytes.[9] Inducible nitric oxide synthase immunoreactivity was found localised in the synovial tissue from rats with adjuvant-induced arthritis, while untreated controls exhibited no inducible nitric oxide synthase staining. Two selective inducible nitric oxide synthase inhibitors, aminoguanidine and N-iminoethyl-L-lysine, suppressed the increase in plasma nitrite levels and joint inflammation associated with adjuvant-induced arthritis in a dose-dependent manner.[32] This suggests novel potential therapeutic approaches to the treatment of this disabling condition.

POTENTIAL CLINICAL APPLICATIONS OF NITRIC OXIDE

Endogenous NO plays many different biological roles. Both deficient and excess NO is linked to disease, and thus pharmacological interventions must be proposed with some caution. However, manipulation of NO has been a safe and effective therapy in several clinical situations. Nitrovasodilators were in clinical use for a century before the underlying mechanism was identified, and experience is accumulating with direct administration of NO to the lungs, although trials to determine whether the treatment reduces mortality are yet to be reported. Many other areas, such as the role of dietary supplementation with L-arginine, are under intense investigation.

Inhaled nitric oxide therapy

Inhaled NO diffuses across the alveolar epithelial cells into the pulmonary vascular smooth muscle cells where it stimulates the production of cGMP, thereby causing pulmonary vasodilation. Inhaled NO thus differs from other pulmonary vasodilator agents in being delivered only to ventilated lung regions where vasodilation will improve V/Q matching. Inhaled NO, therefore, improves oxygenation both by increased pulmonary blood flow and improved V/Q matching. The rapid inactivation of NO results in selective pulmonary vasodilation without systemic hypotension.

In contrast, systemically administered vasodilators dilate all vascular beds. Efforts to dilate the pulmonary vasculature often result in systemic vasodilation and hypotension which worsens co-existing right-to-left shunting. Within the lungs these agents dilate vessels in non-ventilated lung regions, increasing intrapulmonary shunting and impairing gas exchange.

Although NO gas is now available as a medical quality gas, it remains an investigational drug and is not yet licensed. Nonetheless, a series of reports have suggested beneficial effects in disorders characterised by pulmonary vasoconstriction and V/Q mismatch.[25,27] Major outcome trials currently in progress will define the role of this therapy in paediatric and neonatal critical care. The current indications for inhaled NO are as part of intensive therapy for severe hypoxaemia or diagnostic studies in patients with altered pulmonary haemodynamics. The conditions listed below represent current areas of major interest.

Persistent pulmonary hypertension of the newborn

There have been several reports confirming the beneficial role of NO in persistent pulmonary hypertension of the newborn.[33,34] Increasingly, doses of < 20 ppm are being employed, and concentrations of < 1 ppm may maintain sustained improvements in oxygenation.

Congenital heart disease

Inhaled NO at concentrations as low as 1 ppm have been successfully used to treat pulmonary hypertension, and acute pulmonary hypertensive crises, especially following corrective surgery on cardiopulmonary bypass.[25,35]

Respiratory distress syndrome

Pulmonary vascular resistance is elevated in neonates with severe respiratory distress syndrome. Inhaled NO at 5–40 ppm significantly improved oxygenation in preterm infants with severe respiratory distress syndrome.[25]

Bronchopulmonary dysplasia

Inhaled NO at concentrations of 3–40 ppm improved oxygenation in infants with bronchopulmonary dysplasia.[25] However, some infants with severe bronchopulmonary dysplasia who receive prolonged inhalational NO therapy, become dependent on NO presumably due to suppression of endogenous nitric oxide synthase in these infants.

Paediatric acute hypoxaemic respiratory failure

Children with the adult respiratory distress syndrome have severe hypoxaemia associated with marked V/Q mismatch, pulmonary hypertension and decreased cardiac performance. Inhaled NO (3–20 ppm) improved oxygenation, lowered pulmonary arterial pressure, decreased intrapulmonary shunting, and improved cardiac performance in these children.[39]

Primary pulmonary hypertension

Children with primary pulmonary hypertension demonstrate impaired endothelium-dependent pulmonary artery relaxation.[24] Low dose inhaled NO produces selective and sustained pulmonary vasodilation in infants with primary pulmonary hypertension when treatment with other vasodilators has failed.[36]

Asthma

Although the initial studies of inhaled NO in animals suggested a potential role for NO as a therapeutic bronchodilator, the bronchodilator effect of NO in humans has been disappointing. Inhaled NO at 40 ppm has no bronchodilatory effect in children with asthma and mild airways disease.[37] At present, inhaled NO does not appear to have a therapeutic role in the management of asthma.

Diagnostic studies to determine the reversibility of pulmonary hypertension

If increased pulmonary vascular resistance can be lowered with inhaled NO it is unlikely to be fixed. Inhaled NO is being increasingly used to evaluate pulmonary vascular responsiveness in the cardiac catheterisation laboratory and to aid decisions about surgery in children with cardiac shunts and evidence of pulmonary hypertension.[35]

TOXICOLOGY OF INHALED NITRIC OXIDE

Although inhaled NO therapy appears to be a useful therapeutic agent, there are concerns regarding its potential toxicity. Although NO inhalation at concentrations of < 50 ppm appears to have no toxic effects, immature subjects may be more vulnerable.

NO may cause injury itself, or as a consequence of spontaneous oxidation to more toxic oxides of nitrogen such as NO_2 which has an established record of pulmonary toxicity.[38] Furthermore, reactive oxygen intermediates may combine with NO to form peroxynitrite and hydroxyl radicals which may cause oxidative tissue injury.[38] NO may also have immunomodulatory effects, be pro-inflammatory, genotoxic and prolong bleeding time.[38] For these reasons, the lowest effective concentrations of NO should be used. The US Occupational Safety and Health Administration has listed the 8 h time-weighted average safe level at 25 ppm for NO and 5 ppm for NO_2.[38]

STRATEGIES TO DECREASE PRODUCTION OR EFFECT OF NITRIC OXIDE

Therapeutic inhibition of NO synthesis has been attempted in patients with septic shock: the nitric oxide synthase inhibitor N^G-mono-methyl-L-arginine restores blood pressure although its effects on mortality and morbidity have not been fully evaluated.[16] Inhibition of neuronal nitric oxide synthase as therapy for epilepsy or hypoxic-ischaemic cerebral injury or of inducible nitric oxide synthase for asthma, diabetes, inflammatory bowel disorders or rheumatological disorders is at an early investigational stage.

KEY POINTS FOR CLINICAL PRACTICE

1. Nitric oxide is an important messenger molecule in mammals.

2. Nitric oxide has important physiological regulatory roles in many organ systems.

3. Both the excessive and diminished production of nitric oxide is associated with disease.

4. Inhaled nitric oxide is an experimental therapy of great promise for severe hypoxaemia associated with increased pulmonary vascular resistance.

5. Development of agents that modify the production or effect of nitric oxide may provide new approaches to the management and treatment of several disease states.

6. Levels of products of the L-arginine-nitric oxide pathway (such as nitric oxide, nitrate or citrulline) in expelled air or biological fluids may become clinical markers for monitoring certain diseases and the effects of therapy.

7. Finally, for those taking examinations, nitric oxide may be invoked to account for the pathophysiology of almost any disease process in medicine!

REFERENCES

1. Moncada S, Palmer RMJ, Higgs EA. Nitric oxide: physiology, pathophysiology and pharmacology. Pharmacol Rev 1991; 43: 109–142
2. Radomski MW, Martin JF, Moncada S. Synthesis of nitric oxide by the hemocytes of the American horseshoe crab (*Limulus polyphemus*). Philos Trans R Soc Lond 1991; 334: 129–133
3. Furchgott RF, Zawadzki JV. The obligatory role of endothelial cells in the relaxation of arterial smooth muscle by acetylcholine. Nature 1980; 288: 373–376
4. Furchgott RF, Vanhoutte PM. Endothelium derived relaxing and contractor factors. FASEB J 1989; 3: 2007–2018
5. Palmer RMJ, Ferrige AG, Moncada S. Nitric oxide release accounts for the biological activity of endothelium-derived relaxing factor. Nature 1987; 327: 524–526
6. Ignarro LJ, Buga GM, Wood KS, Byrns RE, Chaudhuri G. Endothelium-derived relaxing factor produced and released from artery and vein is nitric oxide. Proc Natl Acad Sci USA 1987; 84: 9265–9269
7. Palmer RMJ, Rees DD, Ashton DS, Moncada S. L-arginine is the physiological precursor for the formation of nitric oxide in endothelium-dependent relaxation. Biochem Biophys Res Commun 1988; 153: 1251–1256
8. Anggard E. Nitric oxide: mediator, murderer, and medicine. Lancet 1994; 343: 1199–1206
9. Vallance P, Moncada S. Nitric oxide – from mediator to medicines. J R Coll Phys Lond 1994; 28: 209–219
10. Vallance P, Moncada S. Role of endogenous nitric oxide in septic shock. New Horizons 1993; 1: 77–87
11. Ignarro LJ. Endothelium-derived nitric oxide: actions and properties. FASEB J 1989; 3: 31–36
12. Bolotina VM, Najibi S, Palacino JJ, Pagano PJ, Cohen RA. Nitric oxide directly activates calcium-dependent potassium channels in vascular smooth muscle. Nature 1994; 368: 850–853
13. Dinerman JL, Lowenstein CJ, Snyder SH. Molecular mechanisms of nitric oxide regulation. Potential relevance to cardiovascular disease. Circ Res 1993; 73: 217–222
14. Moncada S, Higgs A. Mechanism of disease: the L-arginine nitric oxide pathway. N Engl J

Med 1993; 329: 2002–2012
15. Jia L, Bonaventura C, Bonaventura J, Stamler J. S-nitrosohaemoglobin: a dynamic activity of blood involved in vascular control. Nature 1996; 380: 221–226
16. Adnot S, Raffestin B, Eddahibi S. NO in the lung. Respir Physiol 1995; 101: 109–120
17. Barnes PJ, Belvisi ME. Nitric oxide and lung disease. Thorax 1993; 48: 1034–1043
18. Rand MJ. Nitrergic transmission: nitric oxide as a mediator of non-adrenergic, non-cholinergic neuro-effector transmission. Clin Exp Pharmacol Physiol 1992; 19: 147–169
19. Sprague R, Thiemermann C, Varve JR. Endogenous endothelium-derived relaxing factor opposes hypoxic pulmonary vasoconstriction and supports blood flow to hypoxic alveoli in anaesthetised rabbits. Proc Natl Acad Sci USA 1992; 89: 8711–8715
20. Zoritch B. Nitric oxide in asthma. Arch Dis Child 1995; 72: 259–262
21. Schmidt HHHW, Walter U. NO at work. Cell 1994; 78: 919–925
22. Lundberg JO, Weitzberg E, Lundberg JM, Alving K. Intragastric nitric oxide production in humans: measurements in expelled air. Gut 1994; 35: 1543–1546
23. Hibbs Jr JB. Synthesis of nitric oxide from L-arginine: a recently discovered pathway induced by cytokines with antitumour and antimicrobial activities. Res Immunol 1991; 142: 565–569
24. Celermajer DS, Cullen S, Deanfield JE. Impairment of endothelium-dependent pulmonary artery relaxation in children with congenital heart disease and abnormal pulmonary haemodynamics. Circulation 1993; 87: 440–446
25. Mupanemunda RH, Edwards AD. Treatment of newborn infants with inhaled nitric oxide. Arch Dis Child 1995; 72: F131–F134
26. Mupanemunda RH. Nitric oxide in the perinatal period. Contemp Rev Obstet Gynaecol 1995; 7: 210–214
27. Gaston B, Drazen JM, Loscalzo J, Stamler JS. The biology of nitrogen oxides in the airways. Am J Respir Crit Care Med 1994; 149: 538–551
28. Marks KA, Mallard C, Roberts I, Williams C, Gluckman P, Edwards AD. Nitric oxide synthase inhibition attenuates delayed vasodilation and increases injury following cerebral ischaemia in fetal sheep. Pediatr Res 1996; In press
29. Blumberg RM, Cady EB, Wigglesworth JS, McKenzie JE, Edwards AD. Relation between delayed impairment of cerebral energy metabolism and infarction following transient focal hypoxia ischaemia in the developing brain. Exp Brain Res 1996; In press
30. Lundberg JON, Hellstrom PM, Lundberg JM, Alving K. Greatly increased luminal nitric oxide in ulcerative colitis. Lancet 1994; 344: 1673–1674
31. Curzen NP, Griffiths MJD, Evans TW. Role of the endothelium in modulating the vascular response to sepsis. Clin Sci 1994; 86: 359–374
32. Connor JR, Manning PT, Settle SL, et al. Suppression of adjuvant-induced arthritis by selective inhibition of inducible nitric oxide synthase. Eur J Pharmacol 1995; 273: 15–24
33. Roberts JD, Polaner DM, Lang P, Zapol WM. Inhaled nitric oxide in persistent pulmonary hypertension of the newborn. Lancet 1992; 340: 818–819
34. Kinsella JP, Neish SR, Ivy DD, Shaffer E, Abman SH. Clinical responses to prolonged treatment of persistent pulmonary hypertension of the newborn with low doses of inhaled nitric oxide. J Pediatr 1993; 123: 103–108
35. Lunn RJ. Inhaled nitric oxide therapy. Mayo Clin Proc 1995; 70: 247–255
36. Kinsella JP, Toews WH, Henry D, Abman SH. Selective and sustained pulmonary vasodialatation with inhalational nitric oxide therapy in a child with idiopathic pulmonary hypertension. J Pediatr 1993; 122: 803–806
37. Pfeffer KD, Ellison G, Robertson D, Day RW. The effect of inhaled nitric oxide in pediatric asthma. Am J Respir Crit Care Med 1996; 153: 747–751
38. Edwards AD. The pharmacology of inhaled nitric oxide. Arch Dis Child 1995; 72: F127–F130
39. Abman SH, Griebel JL, Parker DK, Schmidt JM, Swanton D, Kinsella JP. Acute effects of inhaled nitric oxide in children with severe hypoxaemic respiratory failure. J Pediatr 1994; 124: 881–888
40. Bredt DS, Snyder SH. Nitric oxide mediates glutamate-linked enhancement of cGMP levels in the cerebellum. Proc Natl Acad Sci USA 1989; 86: 9030–9033

Strategies to assist breastfeeding in preterm infants

P. Meier   L. Brown

Breastfeeding affords mothers and their preterm infants with substantial bene-fits that are specific to this vulnerable population. For preterm infants, moth-ers' milk provides unique nutritional and immunologic components that improve both short- and long-term health outcome. For mothers, breastfeed-ing represents a contribution to infant care that only they can make. This con-tribution is especially meaningful when all other infant caretaking activities are assumed by nurses and physicians.

Although the advantages of breastfeeding in preterm infants are well-docu-mented, mothers of preterm infants initiate and maintain lactation at lower rates than do mothers of healthy, term infants. These low rates reflect the numerous barriers to breastfeeding that are encountered routinely by mothers of preterm infants. Many of these barriers evolved because physicians and nurses have not had access to research-based information that could be applied to clinical breastfeeding problems for this population. As a result, breastfeeding strategies for mothers and preterm infants have been adapted from the bottle feeding literature and from clinical interventions that are effective with healthy term infants. In many instances, these strategies are ineffective or inappropriate in meeting the specific breastfeeding needs of mothers and preterm infants.

The purpose of this chapter is to review knowledge about breastfeeding for preterm infants, and to summarize those strategies that are effective in provid-ing breastfeeding guidance for this population. The focus throughout will be upon distinguishing between research-based and non-research based princi-ples, and upon delineating breastfeeding strategies that are specific to the needs of mothers and preterm infants.

BENEFITS OF BREASTFEEDING FOR PRETERM INFANTS AND MOTHERS

Health benefits of breastfeeding for preterm infants

In the historic literature on premature care, human milk feeding was associ-ated with greater post-discharge weight gain, fewer infections, and a lower incidence of retrolental fibroplasia than were other infant milks.[1-3] In more recent clinical trials, these and other health outcomes of human milk feeding for preterm and/or low birth weight (LBW) infants have been studied, and the findings suggest that human milk confers protection from necrotizing entero-colitis, protection from infection, greater enteral feed tolerance, reduced risk of later allergy, improved retinal function and enhanced neurocognitive develop-ment. A comprehensive description of the studies addressing these health ben-efits is beyond the scope of this chapter, and this body of research has been summarized in recent review papers.[4,5] Although more research is needed in this area, especially in the establishment of causal relationships, several conclu-sions from these studies can be used to guide clinical practice.

First, these studies support the hypothesis that the feeding of human milk to preterm and/or LBW infants affords selected health benefits that are in addi-tion to those that are documented for healthy term infants. This conclusion is especially significant because the research variable, 'human milk feeding' was not standardized among the studies. Some infants received donor milk and others received own-mothers' milk that was produced at various stages of lac-tation. In most, but not all of the studies, human milk was administered by gavage or bottle, rather than the infant's feeding at breast. From a research per-spective, the evidence for health benefits of human milk feeding is especially strong, given that these outcomes were consistent across studies in which het-erogenous samples of human milk were used.

Second, although many of these findings have evolved from one principal research program,[6] recent studies have been conducted in other countries with different groups of preterm infants. The findings from recent studies support those of the principal research program, lending support to the original hypoth-esis of selected, specific health advantages of breastfeeding for preterm infants.

What does this mean to the paediatrician or nurse who is the primary source of information when mothers ask whether they should breastfeed their preterm infants? The answer to this question is complicated and troublesome for many clinicians because they fear that mothers will feel coerced to breastfeed, or that they will feel guilty if they elect to formula feed. This professional perspective is probably outdated, given the recent research advances in this field. With breastfeeding management as with other practice-related issues, the clinician is obliged to inform patients about the most efficacious treatment alternatives, so that patients can make decisions on the basis of this information. Thus, it is appropriate for paediatricians and nurses to discuss these health benefits with mothers who are deciding whether to breastfeed their preterm infants.

Another principle for the clinician to consider when counselling mothers about the decision to breastfeed a preterm infant is that the mothers do not have to commit to a lengthy breastfeeding experience for their infants to enjoy selected health benefits. This means that the paediatrician or nurse can encour-age the mother to initiate lactation, with the understanding that breastfeeding efforts can be discontinued within a week or two if the mother prefers. Establishing a plan such as this has several advantages; mothers initiate lactation immediately after birth when the physiologic triggers are optimal, infants receive colostrum, which contains high concentrations of anti-infective properties, and it is easy for mothers to discontinue lactation efforts after a week or two, with the knowledge that they have contributed uniquely to their infant's care.

Benefits of breastfeeding for mothers of preterm infants

Few systematic studies have addressed the benefits of breastfeeding for mothers of preterm infants, and no causal relationships have been established between breastfeeding and enhanced psychological outcomes for mothers of preterm infants. However, reports in the clinical and research literature suggest that breastfeeding enhances maternal involvement and control over the preterm infant's care.[7,8]

One study provides strong evidence for the maternal role-enhancing effect of breastfeeding.[8] This study involved the conduct of semi-structured interviews in mothers' homes approximately one month after the preterm infant's discharge from the neonatal intensive care unit. The 20 mothers, who had received intensive in-hospital breastfeeding services, were asked to describe the experience of breastfeeding their preterm infants during the early post-discharge period. In the course of the audiotaped interviews, mothers described the 'meaning' of breastfeeding, providing examples from their own experiences. Among the examples was one mother's perception that breastfeeding was the 'only tangible hold' that she had on her preterm infant when the infant was in the neonatal intensive care unit. Other mothers described specific infant behaviors that communicated to them that infants 'enjoyed' breastfeeding, or 'preferred' breast to bottle feeding, perceptions that contributed to their sense of competence and adequacy. Although this study does not confirm that breastfeeding enhances the maternal-infant relationship, it supports the clinical and anecdotal reports of this outcome.

BARRIERS TO BREASTFEEDING FOR MOTHERS AND PRETERM INFANTS

Although few international data addressing the incidence and duration of breastfeeding for mothers and preterm infants are available, two conclusions can be made. First, mothers of preterm infants initiate and sustain breastfeeding at lower rates than do mothers of term healthy infants.[9-11] Second, of those mothers of preterm infants who do initiate lactation, as many as 75% will have abandoned breastfeeding efforts prior to the infant's discharge from the neonatal intensive care unit.[12] An overview of the barriers to breastfeeding for mothers of preterm infants provides an understanding of why these initiation and duration rates are so much lower for this population.

Mothers of preterm infants must initiate lactation with a breast pump because their infants are either too small or too sick to suckle at breast. The expressed milk must be transported to the neonatal intensive care unit so that it can be fed to the preterm infant by gavage or bottle once enteral feedings are introduced. Techniques for initiating and managing feeding at the breast for preterm infants and mothers are highly specific to this population, are not widely disseminated, and have not been standardized into routine clinical practice. As a consequence, many mothers of preterm infants are successful in initiating and sustaining lactation with a breast pump, but never make the transition to feeding their infants at the breast.[10,11]

RESEARCH-BASED STRATEGIES TO ASSIST WITH BREASTFEEDING

The paediatrician and nurse must recognize that supporting breastfeeding for this population encompasses much more than assisting the mother with feeding at breast. In a recent research report,[12] investigators proposed that the delivery of breastfeeding services in the neonatal intensive care unit be categorized into four temporal phases: expression and collection of mothers' milk; gavage feeding of mothers' milk; in-hospital breastfeedings; and post-discharge breastfeeding management. In this research report, interventions within each of the four categories were detailed, and the amount of time involved in providing the interventions was calculated. This model for providing breastfeeding services can serve as an organizing framework for paediatricians and nurses who assist mothers and preterm infants in establishing and sustaining breastfeeding efforts.

Milk expression and collection

Mothers of preterm infants must initiate and sustain lactation with a breast pump for several days, weeks, or months until infants can consume all feedings at breast. Although some mothers can produce adequate volumes of milk during this time, many will experience diminished milk volume over the course of milk expression. Several well-documented factors compromise optimal milk production: fatigue, stress, anxiety, and irregular or incomplete emptying of the breasts.[13-15] Unfortunately, these problems are near universal among mothers of preterm infants, who frequently become discouraged with their milk expression efforts, and elect to discontinue breastfeeding.

Although the physiology of lactation has been studied extensively for mothers and healthy term infants, few studies have focused on optimizing milk yield when mothers must use a breast pump. The available literature supports the practice of initiating milk expression with an electric breast pump as early post-birth as is possible, with some investigators proposing that there may be a 'critical period' early in lactation during which the breasts must be emptied and stimulated adequately to assure a sufficient milk volume.[16] The idea of a 'critical period' supports to the clinical recommendation that mothers of preterm infants initiate milk expression, even if they are undecided about their long-term breastfeeding plans.

The clinician must develop a milk expression plan with the mother of the preterm infant that will be specific to her needs and schedule. With few exceptions, these mothers will need access to a hospital grade electric breast pump, with a milk collection kit that enables them to express milk from both breasts simultaneously. Studies have shown that simultaneous breast emptying results in higher serum prolactin levels and greater milk yield than does single breast pumping.[16,17]

Mothers will need to know how frequently to use the breast pump, and approximately how long they should express their milk at each pumping session. Although this area of clinical practice does not have a strong scientific base, some physiologic principles of breastfeeding for healthy term infants may be applicable. First, in order to capitalize on the idea of a 'critical period' for the lactation hormones, mothers should pump very frequently during the first week post-birth. A schedule that allows 10–12 pumpings per day of 15 minutes' duration in the first week is ideal, if the mother is able to adhere to such a regimen. This frequent, aggressive breast emptying should initiate an excellent milk supply after a week or 10 days, and the mother can decrease the number of milk expressions to 8 per day thereafter. In one study, investigators proposed that optimal milk production was associated with at least 5 daily milk expressions, and a total daily pumping time that exceeded 100 minutes.[15]

The challenge for the clinician is to individualize these data to the particular mother-infant pair. Some mothers will produce large volumes of milk with as few as four or five daily milk expressions, whereas others will produce only small volumes with more frequent pumping. Invariably, mothers will experience difficulty with organizing milk expression, travel to and from the neonatal intensive care unit, and other family responsibilities. A clinical goal should be to sustain a milk supply that will exceed the preterm infant's needs by about 50% at the time of neonatal intensive care unit discharge. The details of the milk expression plan can then be modified to help the individual mother accomplish this goal.

Gavage feeding of expressed mothers' milk

The mother's expressed milk can be fed to the preterm infant by gavage until breastfeedings are initiated. However, to be suitable for infant feeding, the milk must be handled by mothers and nurses in a manner that minimizes bacterial contamination and growth, and that preserves the nutritional and immunological properties of human milk. According to research reports, expressed mothers' milk is seldom sterile,[18,19] and the bacteria that are normally present in the milk can multiply quickly, especially during slow-infusion gavage feedings.[18] Additionally, many nutrients, especially calorie-rich milk lipids, adhere to the lumen of the gavage tube,[20–22] rather than being delivered to the infant. These conditions can compromise infant growth and other health outcomes if not closely monitored.

The available literature supports the practice of feeding colostrum, and then fresh milk from the infant's own mother, using frozen milk only when fresh milk is unavailable. When feasible, the mother's milk should be administered by intermittent gavage, rather than by slow-infusion continuous feedings.[20–22]

Breastfeeding in hospital

Undoubtedly, the major barrier to breastfeeding success for mothers and preterm infants is accessing appropriate information and assistance when it is time to begin feedings at the breast. These mothers require assistance from a clinician with expertise in breastfeeding for preterm infants, who can provide specific information about positioning techniques, milk transfer, and selected breastfeeding devices. In the absence of such individualized support, mothers may express adequate amounts of milk with a breast pump, but be unable to make the transition to feeding at breast.[4,10,11] Strategies that are effective in preventing breastfeeding failure during this time are early introduction of breastfeeding opportunities and providing the mother with assistance specific to the preterm infant.

THE SCIENCE OF EARLY BREASTFEEDING FOR PRETERM INFANTS

In developed countries, breastfeedings are not routinely introduced until preterm infants have demonstrated the ability to consume entire bottle feedings without distress. This practice is based on the undocumented assumption that breastfeeding is 'more work' than is bottle feeding, and will result in infant fatigue or slow weight gain. Unfortunately, the prolonged use of bottles in the absence of breastfeeding can result in an infant feeding mechanism that does not transfer readily to the breast. Mothers become frustrated with subsequent breastfeeding efforts, and frequently elect to discontinue breastfeeding, or to administer their expressed milk by bottle. Earlier introduction of breastfeedings would prevent or minimize this series of problems, but until recently, there were no scientific data to support this clinical practice.

A series of recent research reports has suggested that, contrary to widely held assumptions, early breastfeedings may be less stressful physiologically than are early bottle feedings for preterm infants.[23-26] These studies are of small samples, but the cumulative evidence supports the hypothesis that preterm infants remain more stable physiologically during breast than bottle feedings.

In early research reported by Meier[24] and Meier and Anderson,[26] preterm infants served as their own controls for the measurement of physiologic variables during breast and bottle feedings. During breastfeedings infants demonstrated higher $TcPO_2$ values and higher body temperatures than during comparable bottle feedings. Recently, Blaymore-Bier and colleagues[23]

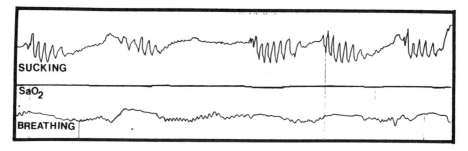

Fig. 9.1 Polygraphic recording demonstrating suck-breathe patterning and oxygenation during bottle feeding for a preterm infant. In this recording the infant alternates short sucking bursts with breathing, but does not breathe within sucking bursts. Oxygen saturation remains stable. (From Meier PP. Suck-breathe patterning during bottle and breastfeeding for preterm infants. In: David TJ. (ed.) Major Controversies in Infant Nutrition; International Congress and Symposium Series No. 215. London: Royal Society of Medicine Press, 1996; 9–20.)

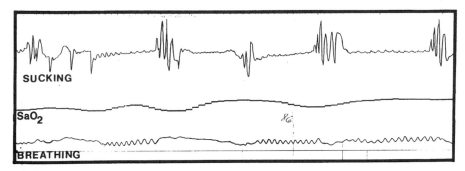

Fig. 9.2 Polygraphic recording demonstrating suck-breathe patterning and oxygenation during bottle feeding for a preterm infant. Oxygen saturation fluctuates, with values as low as 78%, during short sucking bursts. (From Meier PP. Suck-breathe patterning during bottle and breastfeeding for preterm infants. In: David TJ. (ed.) Major Controversies in Infant Nutrition; International Congress and Symposium Series No. 215. London: Royal Society of Medicine Press, 1996; 9–20.)

confirmed the finding of higher oxygen saturation during breast than bottle feeding for a sample of 20 preterm infants. More recently, Meier and colleagues[25] demonstrated differences in the patterning of sucking and breathing when infants served as their own controls for bottle and breast feeding sessions. These patterns revealed that during bottle feeding, preterm infants do not breathe within sucking bursts; instead they alternate short bursts of sucking with breathing (Figs 9.1 & 9.2). In contrast, during breastfeeding, breathing is integrated within sucking bursts (Fig. 9.3). These different patterns of sucking and breathing for the two feeding methods would explain the previous finding that oxygenation remains more stable during breast than bottle feedings for this population.

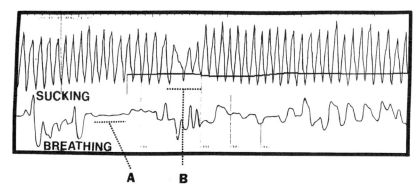

Fig. 9.3 Polygraphic recording demonstrating suck-breathe patterning and oxygenation during breastfeeding for an infant of 33 weeks' gestation. The infant breaths within this long (104 sucks) sucking burst until phase A, when breathing is interrupted for several sucks. In phase B, the infant alters the duration and amplitude of individual sucks, apparently to reinstitute a more regular breathing pattern, which continues through the remainder of the burst. (From Meier PP. Suck-breathe patterning during bottle and breastfeeding for preterm infants. In: David TJ. (ed.) Major Controversies in Infant Nutrition; International Congress and Symposium Series No. 215. London: Royal Society of Medicine Press, 1996; 9–20.)

These data lend support to the practice of introducing breast before bottle feedings for preterm infants, but several important clinical questions about early breastfeeding remain unanswered. First, no universally accepted criteria about when to initiate breastfeeding have been identified. Instead, the literature supports not using traditional criteria such as infant weight, a specific gestational age, or the ability to bottle feed successfully. A useful clinical guideline is to introduce breastfeeding when bottle feeding would have been started, and delay the initiation of bottle feeding for a week or so. As the paediatrician and nurse become increasingly comfortable with breastfeeding for small infants, they will probably find that breastfeeding can be started earlier in the hospital stay. In their small sample of preterm infants, Meier and colleagues[25] noted that some infants demonstrated the ability to consume significant amounts of milk during breastfeeding by 32 weeks of gestation, whereas others did not. The absence of specific breastfeeding readiness guidelines underscores the importance of having a clinical expert who can individualize these scientific data to a specific mother-preterm infant pair.

Techniques for positioning the preterm infant at breast

The mother of the preterm infant should be assisted with positioning techniques that support the infant's head and torso more completely than those that are used commonly for term infants. The preterm infant's head is heavy in relation to the weak neck musculature, and should be encircled and supported by the mother's hand during early breastfeeding experiences. This can be accomplished by using the 'football hold' in which the infant is held like a football, under the mother's arm, with one hand encircling the infant's head, and

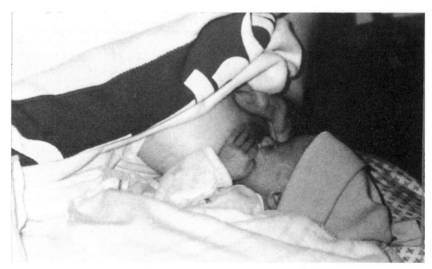

Fig. 9.4 Support during breastfeeding. The infant lies abdomen-to-abdomen across the mother's lap and with her free hand she supports the breast. It is important that the infant not be twisted, and that the head remains aligned with the torso.

the other providing support to the breast. As an alternative, the mother may achieve the same degree of support by use of the position depicted in Figure 9.4, where the infant lies abdomen-to-abdomen across the mother's lap with her free hand supporting the breast. In both positions, it is important that the infant is not twisted, and that the head remains aligned with the torso.

Finally, the mother will probably require assistance in achieving correct placement of the infant's lips and gums on the breast. Although the gums should be placed over the lactiferous sinuses, this position may represent an anatomical challenge for the smallest preterm infants, especially those whose mothers have large and/or flat areolae. According to studies of bottle feeding, preterm infants have lower intraoral suction pressures than do term, healthy infants.[27] Clinically, this means that the preterm infant may be unable to draw the maternal nipple into an ideal position for breastfeeding, a consideration that may influence the volume of milk that the infant ingests. However, intraoral suction pressure increases with maturity of the infant, so this problem should be transient.

Measuring and/or optimizing milk intake

After initial breastfeedings have been established for the mother and preterm infant, the focus of care should be the evaluation and facilitation of milk transfer. Milk transfer is the movement of milk from the breast to the infant, and necessitates an adequate maternal milk supply, maternal milk ejection, and organized infant suckling.[28] Low volumes of milk intake in the preterm infant can result from problems in any of these three functions, singly or in combination.

Although a variety of observational tools have been developed to score 'breastfeeding effectiveness',[29] no published research could be located in which either the reliability or validity of these tools was established for term or preterm infants. Of special concern is the lack of validation research that links the concept of 'breastfeeding effectiveness' to volume of milk intake by the infant.[30,31] Thus, if the paediatrician or nurse needs to know the volume of milk intake for a preterm infant, the available research supports the use of the test-weighing technique. Test-weighing involves weighing the clothed infant pre- and post-breastfeeding under the same conditions; milk intake represents the difference between the pre- and post-feed weights (in g), where 1 g of weight gain equals 1 ml of milk intake.[32] Numerous studies have demonstrated the concurrent validity of test-weighing for both term and preterm infants when electronic scales are used to measure the infant weights.[28,32,33]

Research has demonstrated that milk intake during in-hospital breastfeedings is highly variable for preterm infants, and that infants frequently consume greater volumes of milk during bottle than breastfeeding.[23,28,30,34] Several clinical papers suggest that selected breastfeeding aids may be helpful in maximizing milk intake during breast feeding; among these are the supplemental nurser system, the nipple shield, and breast pump stimulation of the opposite breast during infant feeding.[7,34] Use of these devices must be based on a specific milk transfer problem for the preterm infant, and should be managed by a clinician with expertise in both lactation and preterm infants.

Breastfeeding after discharge from hospital

Considerably less research has been conducted about post-discharge management of breastfeeding for preterm infants than for other phases of the breastfeeding experience. Typically, principles of breastfeeding that are appropriate for term, healthy infants, such as not complementing breastfeedings with additional milk or feeding completely on demand, are generalized to preterm infants. However, there is no indication that these principles are effective or even safe for more vulnerable infants.[28,30,34,35] An emerging body of literature suggests that the early post-discharge period may be especially stressful for mothers of preterm infants, and that these infants' immature feeding patterns may predispose them to temporary underconsumption of milk by breastfeeding alone.

Stresses of breastfeeding in the early post-discharge period

The available research suggests that mothers of preterm infants have breastfeeding concerns in the early post-discharge period that are unlike those they experienced during their infants' hospitalization, and that are different from those reported for mothers of healthy term infants.[31,36,37] The most common concern of these mothers is whether their infants are 'getting enough' milk by breastfeeding alone, even though the mothers are able to express adequate volumes of milk with a breast pump.

The distinction between 'getting enough' and producing an adequate volume of milk for the infant has significant clinical implications, and underscores differences between breastfeeding for preterm and term infants. The available research suggests that mothers of term healthy infants are concerned about an adequate milk supply, whereas mothers of preterm infants are concerned about milk transfer to the infant.[37] This distinction means that mothers of preterm infants can produce enough milk, but they perceive that their infants do not consume all the milk that is available to them. As a result, mothers often elect to give their infants extra milk by bottle or some alternative feeding method.

Underconsumption of milk by breastfeeding alone

The paediatrician needs to know whether these maternal concerns reflect actual or perceived underconsumption of milk. The few data that are available on this topic suggest that when preterm infants are discharged prior to achieving term, corrected age, they may be vulnerable to underconsumption of milk by breastfeeding alone.[28,30,37,38] However, this conclusion cannot be applied indiscriminately to all preterm infants because of variability in the milk transfer mechanism.

When preterm infants are discharged prior to term, corrected age, the data suggest that immature feeding patterns, such as difficulty latching onto the breast or falling asleep early in the feeding, may persist.[31,36,37] These feeding patterns are temporary, but may compromise daily milk intake until the feeding patterns become more like those of a term, healthy infant. However, the milk transfer mechanism is complex, in that these immature feeding patterns may not affect milk intake if the mother's milk supply and milk ejection reflex can compensate for the infant's immature suck. This principle exemplifies the importance of the mother's establishing a milk supply that exceeds the infant's demand by the time of hospital discharge.

The paediatrician should advise the mother to augment her milk supply by using the breast pump in addition to breastfeeding her infant during the early post-discharge period. Use of the breast pump stimulates the breasts to produce more milk than does the preterm infant's sucking alone. The paediatrician can help the mother determine the frequency of breast pump usage, mindful of the goal that she should strive to produce approximately 50% more milk than the infant requires. The mother should continue to express milk until the paediatrician has determined that the infant's rate of weight gain on complete breastfeedings is satisfactory.

Measurement of milk intake in the home

In the US, preterm infants are frequently discharged prior to term, corrected age, and before complete breastfeeding is established. These infants present unique challenges to paediatricians who want to support breastfeeding, but who must also ensure that infants consume an adequate volume of milk for hydration and growth during the early post-discharge period. A new device, the BabyWeigh™ scale, may facilitate in-home breastfeeding management for this population of infants.[28] The scale, which is battery-operated, portable, and calculates milk intake automatically from pre-and post-feed weights, can be rented for short-term home use by mothers of preterm infants. The scale can be used to measure infant milk intake during breastfeeding and/or monitor daily weight gain.

The accuracy of the test-weighing with BabyWeigh scale was described in a recent report. The test-weights with the scale provided an extremely accurate measure of milk intake for a large range of infant weights and volumes of milk consumed.[28] Mothers were able to use the scale accurately, and reported anecdotally that they would like to have this scale for use in the early post-discharge period with their own infants.

Clinicians who provide breastfeeding services for mothers of term, healthy infants may feel that performing in-home test-weights is unnecessary, and that a focus on 'numbers' may undermine mothers' breastfeeding efforts.[35,39] However, mothers of preterm infants have reported that they are not able to use routine clinical indices of milk intake to determine whether their infants have consumed an adequate volume of milk, and frequently administer extra milk 'just to be sure'.[37] The inability of mothers of preterm infants to use these clinical indices of intake accurately was confirmed in recent research.[28]

While outcome studies involving the in-home test-weights are underway,[40] there are no scientific data available at this time that link the use of this technique to favorable breastfeeding outcome. However, clinical experience in our institution suggests that the use of in-home test-weights permits earlier hospital discharge for some preterm infants, because milk intake can be evaluated in the home. Additionally, measurement of milk intake and/or daily weight gain provide mothers and paediatricians with the objective information necessary to make the final transition to breastfeeding during the early post discharge period.

KEY POINTS FOR CLINICAL PRACTICE

1. Breastfeeding provides specific benefits for mothers and preterm infants that are in addition to those that are documented for term, healthy infants. The clinician should share this information with mothers as they make feeding decisions for their preterm infants.

2. Mothers of preterm infants initiate and sustain lactation at lower rates than do mothers of term, healthy infants. These low rates reflect numerous barriers to successful breastfeeding for this vulnerable population.

3. The clinician should help the mother of a preterm infant develop a milk expression plan that includes early, frequent pumping. Ideally, the mother's milk supply should exceed the volume requirements of the preterm infant by approximately 50% at the time of infant discharge from the neonatal intensive care unit.

4. Until the preterm infant is able to feed at breast, the mother's expressed milk can be fed by gavage. When available, fresh, rather than frozen, milk should be fed.

5. Many mothers of preterm infants express adequate amounts of milk with a breast pump, but are unable to make the final transition to breastfeeding. Strategies to prevent breastfeeding failure during this period include introducing breastfeedings before (or instead of) bottle feedings, and assistance from a clinician who has expertise with breastfeeding preterm infants.

6. Recent studies suggest that preterm infants remain more stable physiologically during breast than bottle feedings; the underlying mechanism may be different patterning of sucking and breathing for the two feeding methods.

7. The post-discharge period is extremely stressful for mothers of preterm infants, whose major concern is whether their infants are consuming an adequate volume of milk during breastfeeding. This concern is different from mothers of term infants, who are concerned about producing enough milk for their infants.

8. There may be a vulnerable period with respect to adequate milk intake for preterm infants who are discharged prior to achieving term, corrected age, and before breastfeeding is completely established. This temporary under-consumption of milk may represent immature feeding behaviors on the part of the preterm infant.

9. The milk transfer mechanism is dependent upon an adequate milk supply, milk ejection, and infant suckling. Infants with immature feeding behaviors can consume adequate volumes of milk if a mother's milk supply and milk ejection reflex function optimally.

10. Test-weighing is an accurate technique for estimation of milk intake during breastfeeding, and can be completed in the hospital or in the home during the early post-discharge period.

REFERENCES

1. Crosse VM, Hickmans EM, Howarth BE et al. The value of human milk compared with other feeds for premature infants. Arch Dis Child 1954; 29: 178–195
2. Ford FJ. Feeding of premature babies. Lancet 1949; 1: 989–994
3. Hepner WR, Krause AC. Retrolental fibroplasia: clinical observations. Pediatrics 1952; 10: 433–443
4. Meier PP, Brown LP. State of the science: breastfeeding for mothers and low birth weight infants. Nurs Clin North Am 1996; 31: 351–365
5. Brown LP, Meier PP, Spatz DL et al. Use of human milk for low birth weight infants. On Line J Knowl Synth Nurs 1996; 3: (27)
6. Lucas A. Does early diet program future outcome? Acta Pediatr Scand Suppl 1990; 365: 58–67
7. Cohen S. High tech-soft touch: breastfeeding issues. Clin Perinatol 1987; 14: 187–196
8. Kavanaugh KL, Zimmerman B, Meier PP et al. The rewards outweigh the efforts: Breastfeeding outcomes for mothers of preterm infants. J Hum Lact; In press
9. Ryan A, Pratt W, Wysong J et al. A comparison of breast-feeding data from the national surveys of family growth and the Ross laboratories' mothers survey. Am J Public Health 1991; 81: 1049–1052
10. Lefebvre F, Ducharme M. Incidence and duration of lactation and lactational performance among mothers of low-birth-weight and term infants. Can Med Assoc J 1989; 140: 1159–1164
11. Kaufman K, Hall L. Influences of the social network on choice and duration of breast-feeding in mothers of preterm infants. Res Nurs Health 1989; 12: 149–159
12. Meier P, Engstrom J, Mangurten H et al. Breastfeeding support services in the neonatal intensive care unit. J Obstet Gynecol Neonatal Nurs 1993; 22: 338–347
13. Brown L, Hollingsworth A, Armstrong C. Factors affecting milk volume in mothers of VLBW infants. In: Abstracts of the 1991 Scientific Sessions of the 31st Biennial Convention. Indianapolis: Sigma Theta Tau Int, 1991; 46
14. deCarvalho M, Anderson D, Giangrecco A et al. Frequency of milk expression and milk production by mothers of non-nursing premature neonates. Am J Dis Child 1985; 139: 483–485
15. Hopkinson J, Schanler R, Garza C. Milk production by mothers of premature infants. Pediatrics 1988; 81: 815–820
16. Neifert M, Seacat J. Milk yield and prolactin rise with simultaneous breast pump. Proceedings of the Ambulatory Pediatric Association Annual Meeting, Washington, D.C., May 7–10, 1985
17. Auerbach K. Sequential and simultaneous breast pumping: a comparison. Int J Nurs Studies 1990; 27: 257–265

18. Botsford K, Weinstein R, Boyer K et al. Gram-negative bacilli in human milk feedings: quantitation and clinical consequences for premature infants. J Pediatr 1986; 109:707–710
19. Meier P, Wilks S. The bacteria in expressed mothers' milk. MCN Am J Matern Child Nurs 1987; 12: 420–423
20. Brennan-Behm M, Carlson E, Meier P et al. Caloric loss from expressed mother's milk during continuous gavage infusion. Neon Netw 1994; 13: 27–32
21. Greer F, McCormick A, Loker J. Changes in fat concentration of human milk during delivery by intermittent bolus and continuous mechanical pump infusion. J Pediatr 1984; 105: 745–749
22. Stocks R, Davies D, Allen F et al. Loss of breastmilk nutrients during tube feeding. Arch Dis Child 1985; 60: 164-166
23. Blaymore-Bier J, Ferguson A, Anderson L et al. Breastfeeding of very low birth weight infants. J Pediatr 1993; 123: 773–778
24. Meier PP. Bottle and breastfeeding: effects on transcutaneous oxygen pressure and temperature in preterm infants. Nurs Res 1988; 37 :36–41
25. Meier PP. Suck-breathe patterning during bottle and breastfeeding for preterm infants. In: David TJ. (ed.) Major Controversies in Infant Nutrition; International Congress and Symposium Series No. 215. London: Royal Society of Medicine Press, 1996; 9–20
26. Meier PP, Anderson GC. Responses of small preterm infants to bottle and breast feeding. MCN Am J Matern Child Nurs 1987; 12 :97–105
27. Anderson GC, Vidyasagar D. Development of sucking in premature infants from 0–7 days postbirth as measured with a suck scoring system. In: Anderson GC, Raff B. (eds) Newborn Behavioral Organization: Nursing Research and Implications. National Foundation March of Dimes. Birth Defects: Original Article Series 15. New York: Liss, 1979: 145–171
28. Meier P, Engstrom J, Crichton C et al. A new scale for in-home test-weighing for mothers of preterm and high risk infants. J Hum Lact 1994; 10: 163–168
29. Riordan J, Auerbach K. (Eds) Breastfeeding and Human Lactation. Boston: Jones & Bartlett, 1993
30. Meier P, Engstrom J, Fleming B et al. Estimating milk intake of hospitalized preterm infants who breastfeed. J Hum Lact 1996; 12: 21–26
31. Hill PD, Ledbetter RJ, Kavanaugh KL. Breastfeeding patterns of low birthweight infants at hospital discharge and four weeks after birth. J Obstet Gynecol Neonatal Nurs; In press
32. Woolridge MW, Butte N, Dewey KG et al. Methods for the measurement of milk volume intake of the breast-fed infant. In: Jensen RC, Neville MC. (Eds) Human Lactation: Milk Components and Methodologies. New York: Plenum, 1985; 5–20
33. Meier P, Lysakowski TY, Engstrom JL et al. The accuracy of test weighing for preterm infants. J Pediatr Gastrol Nutr 1990; 62–65.
34. Meier PP, Mangurten HH. Breastfeeding the preterm infant. In: Riordan J, Auerbach K. (eds): Breastfeeding and Human Lactation. Boston: Jones & Bartlett, 1993; 253–278
35. Meier PP. Caution needed in extrapolating from term to preterm infants: author's reply: letter to the Editor. J Hum Lact 1995; 11: 91–92
36. Hill PD, Hanson KS, Mefford AL. Mothers of low birthweight infants: breastfeeding patterns and problems. J Hum Lact 1994; 10: 169–176
37. Kavanaugh K, Mead L, Meier P et al. Getting enough: mothers' concern about breastfeeding a preterm infant after discharge. J Obstet Gynecol Neonatal Nurs 1995; 24: 23–32
38 Ramasethu J, Jeyaseelan L, Kirubakaran C. Weight gain in exclusively breastfed preterm infants. J Trop Pediatr 1993; 39: 152–159
39. Walker M. Test-weighing and other estimates of breastmilk intake (Letter to the Editor). J Hum Lact 1995; 11: 91
40. Brown LP. Breastfeeding services for LBW infants: Outcomes and cost. NINR Grant #NR03881, DHHS

Persistent pulmonary hypertension of the newborn

M. Rabinovitch

Persistent pulmonary hypertension of the newborn (PPHN) may be the result of underdevelopment of the lung and pulmonary vascular bed, maladaptation of the pulmonary vascular bed to extrauterine life as a result of postnatal stress, or maldevelopment of the pulmonary vascular bed in utero from a known or unknown cause (Fig. 10.1). The use of inhaled nitric oxide as a specific pulmonary vasodilator has been a major breakthrough, particularly in the treatment of PPHN secondary to maladaptation. Recent advances in understanding the developmental biology of the pulmonary circulation should lead to novel strategies to induce new growth in the size and number of vessels, when there is underdevelopment or maldevelopment. This chapter will review what is known about normal vascular growth and development, including new insights into cellular and molecular mechanisms related to functional as well as structural maturation.

IN UTERO AND PERINATAL VASCULAR REMODELING AND GROWTH

Considerable work in the 1960s and 1970s was directed at understanding the normal features of pulmonary vascular development (reviewed in[1]). In the fetus, it was determined that all preacinar arteries are present by the 16th week of gestation and, thereafter, respiratory units are added with accompanying as well as supernumerary arteries. The preacinar arteries and those at the terminal bronchiolus level are muscular, whereas the intraacinar arteries, i.e. those accompanying respiratory bronchiolus, alveolar duct, and alveolar wall, are nonmuscular. The preacinar arteries are thick-walled and appear to change little in wall thickness relative to external diameter throughout the fetal period.

In the immediate postnatal period, there is likely rapid recruitment of small alveolar duct and wall vessels and dilatation of muscular arteries. Within a few days, the smallest muscular arteries dilate, and their walls thin to adult levels; by 4 months of age, this process has included the largest muscular pulmonary arteries and is complete. With increasing age, muscle is observed in arteries located more peripherally within the acinus. At first, nonmuscular arteries become partially muscular and later they become fully

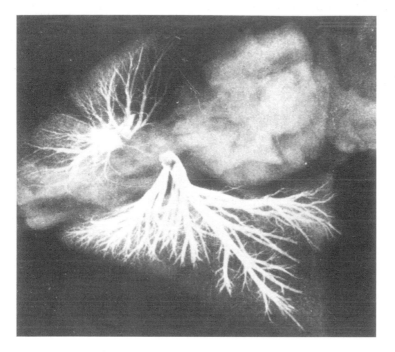

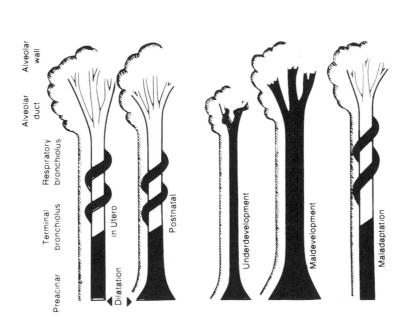

Fig. 10.1 Left, Schema showing normal arterial dilation during transition from fetal to neonatal circulation. When the lung is underdeveloped, the vascular bed is hypoplastic and abnormally muscular. When it is maldeveloped, the vascular bed is abnormally muscular; when it is maladapted, it has not dilated appropriately at birth. Right, Arteriogram showing a small right lung with a distorted and even smaller left lung. Arteries in both lungs are reduced in size and number. (From Kitagawa M, Hislop A, Boyden EA, Reid L. Lung hypoplasia in congenital diaphragmatic hernia. A quantitative study of airway, artery, and alveolar development. Br J Surg 1971; 58: 342–346.)

muscularized. For example, in early infancy, vessels at alveolar duct level are still largely nonmuscular, but in childhood, they become partially muscularized and, in the adult, are fully muscularized. Clinical as well as experimental studies have suggested that the muscularization of these peripheral pulmonary arteries may be related to the differentiation of pericytes, as well as to the recruitment of fibroblasts. Alveolar wall arteries remain largely nonmuscular, even in the adult. Arteries grow both in number and size, and they grow most rapidly in infancy. While alveoli also proliferate, the ratio of alveoli to arteries actually decreases from the newborn value of 20:1 to the value of 8:1, which is achieved first in early childhood and persists. The growth and development of the pulmonary circulation is also likely influenced by the trophic effects of neuropeptides released from nerve endings, as well as neuroendocrine bodies associated with accompanying airways.[2]

Experimental studies have indicated how changes in connective tissue, especially elastin and collagen[3] and cellular arrangement[4] govern the normal adaptation to postnatal life. In addition, it has been recognized that there are smooth muscle cells with differing proliferative potentials.[5] Moreover, the high proliferative potential demonstrated in neonatal bovine pulmonary artery smooth muscle cells is reflective of a difference in activation of protein kinase C.[6]

FUNCTIONAL MATURATION OF THE PULMONARY CIRCULATION

The mediators responsible for maintaining the increased pulmonary vascular tone in the constricted fetal circulation, and for the normal fall in pulmonary vascular resistance in the newborn, have been the subject of much study, both experimentally and clinically.[7] Studies in isolated peripheral pulmonary arteries from fetal and neonatal lambs have shown that endothelin is a powerful vasoconstrictor[8] and first indicated that it may be responsible for the increase in pulmonary vascular resistance in the fetus. This also appears to be related to the availability of specific receptors.[9,10] Moreover, endothelial cells in culture release endothelin under the influence of hypoxia.[11]

Dilator prostaglandins partially influence the fall in pulmonary vascular resistance, since indomethacin retards but does not prevent the decrease observed with oxygen.[12] Current thinking, however, suggests that vasodilation of the newborn pulmonary circulation is largely the result of increased production of endothelial-derived relaxing factor, nitric oxide (NO).[13,14] This may be further accentuated by inhibition of phosphodiesterases.[15] Repression of potassium channels may also play an important role in the early postnatal pulmonary vasodilation.[16,17] It is also important to consider that the mechanical properties of fetal pulmonary vascular smooth muscle cells are different from those of the neonate and adult, owing to differences in the myosin content and actin : myosin ratio.[18]

A

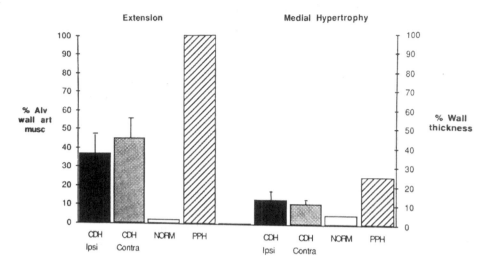

C

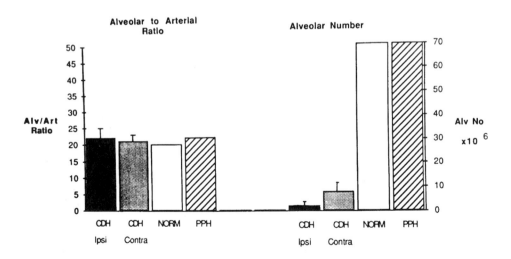

Fig. 10.2 A (upper left) Morphometric data from nine patients with congenital diaphragmatic hernia (CDH), compared with published values in normal newborns and in infants with idiopathic persistent pulmonary hypertension of the newborn (PPH). Infants with CDH had greater smooth muscle extension into peripheral arteries and increased medial hypertrophy than normal infants, but less than infants with PPH. **C** (lower left) Morphometric data from six infants with CDH compared to normal neonates and infants with PPH. Alveolar/arterial ratio was similar to that in normal infants, but total alveolar number was severely reduced in both ipsilateral and contralateral lungs. (From Bohn D, Tamura M, Perin D et al. Ventilatory predictors of pulmonary hypoplasia in congenital diaphragmatic hernia, confirmed by morphometric assessment. J Pediatr 1987; 111: 423–431.)

B

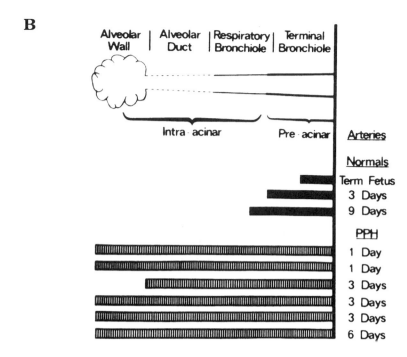

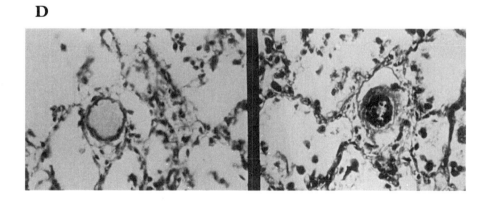

Fig. 10.2 (continued) **B** (upper right) Diagrammatic location of muscle in the walls of the intraacinar arteries. In normal infants less than 1 week of age, no muscular arteries are found within the acinus. All the patients with persistent pulmonary hypertension (PPH) had 'extension' of muscle into the small intraacinar arteries. **D** (lower right) Photomicrographs of alveolar wall arteries distended with the barium gelatin suspension from (left) a 3-day-old with normal lungs and (right) a 3-day-old with persistent pulmonary hypertension. The normal artery (left) is nonmuscular, with a single endothelial cell lining surrounded by a thin layer of connective tissue. The artery wall (right) consists of smooth muscle (darkly stained) two cell layers thick, surrounded by a thick connective tissue sheath enclosing a dilated lymphatic (located superiorly). Elastin-van Gieson stain, × 160. (From Murphy JD, Rabinovitch M, Goldstein JD, Reid LM. The structural basis of persistent pulmonary hypertension of the newborn infant. J Pediatr 1981; 98: 962–967.)

ABNORMAL PULMONARY VASCULAR GROWTH AND REMODELING

Underdevelopment of the lung

One of the most common causes of PPHN is underdevelopment of the lung (reviewed in[1]) associated with congenital diaphragmatic hernia or as a feature of isolated hypoplastic or dysplastic lungs, scimitar syndrome, or secondary to oliogohydraminos seen in renal agenesis and dysplasia. Pulmonary hypoplasia is also related to prematurity, absence of the phrenic nerve, asphyxiating thoracic dystrophy, or rhesus isoimmunization and has been described experimentally with amniocentesis,[19] and smoking.[20]

The accompanying derangement and/or hypoplasia of the pulmonary vascular bed will be, depending upon its severity, either incompatible with life or result in reversible or irreversible pulmonary artery hypertension and right-to-left shunting from birth. In addition to the structural changes in the vessels, the severity of the impaired gas exchange (hypoxia, hypercarbia) due to abnormalities in the airways no doubt also contributes greatly to the pulmonary hypertension.

Reversal of the pulmonary hypertension postoperatively in infants with congenital diaphragmatic hernia has been achieved with tolazoline and also with the extracorporeal membrane oxygenator (ECMO)[21] or high-frequency oscillation,[22] NO alone or in combination with phosphodiesterase inhibitors.[23] An interesting study showed that NO after ECMO could be useful in the treatment of infants with PPHN and hypoplastic lungs, including diaphragmatic hernia that had been refractory prior to ECMO.[23] In some cases, however, the hemodynamic abnormality is irreversible.

While the degree of arterial muscularity may predict whether the pulmonary vascular bed will be reactive, in our studies of infants who succumbed after attempt at repair of congenital diaphragmatic hernia, a striking decrease in the number of alveoli and associated arteries[22] appears to be the major determinant of mortality (Fig. 10.2). This is probably why many attempts to reverse severe pulmonary hypertension with NO have been less successful in this group of patients.

In lungs studied at postmortem from infants with pulmonary hypoplasia or dysplasia, pulmonary hypertension seems to be associated with a reduced number of arteries appropriate to the reduced number of airways. Often, but not always, the arteries are also small, but not incompatible with the size of the lung. Also, while the arteries, both centrally and peripherally, may be more muscular than normal, as in congenital diaphragmatic hernia,[22] there may be hypoplasia of the pulmonary musculature, as in renal agenesis. There are also dysplasias of the lung associated with PPHN, the most recently reported being alveolar capillary dysplasia (Fig. 10.3).[24] This abnormality is currently refractory to treatment, so a biopsy should probably be done to guide clinical management.

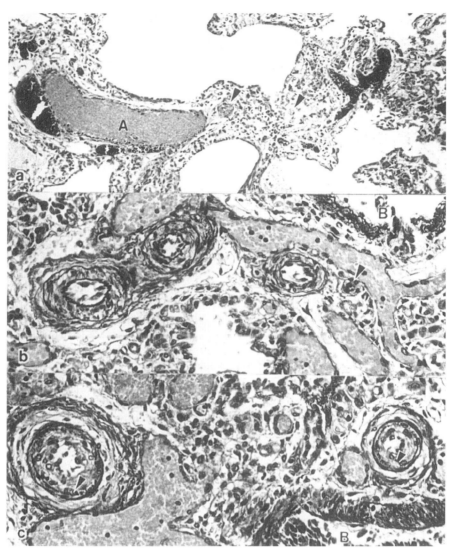

Fig. 10.3 Lung micrographs from the left (a) and right (b, c) lungs of case 2. (**a: top**) Barium distends the lumen of a preacinar artery (A) but does not enter the anomalous vein to the left of the artery. Intraacinar arterial branches that contain barium are identified (arrowheads) but intraacinar veins and venules are distended with red cells, presumably forced ahead of the barium by the postmortem angiogram. Airspaces are lined by cuboidal epithelium and no luminal capillaries are seen, all vessels lying centrally in the airspace walls. Hematoxylin and eoxin ×85. (**b: middle**) Intraacinar pulmonary arteries showing medial muscular thickening that forms a continuous layer even in the smallest branch (arrow), which is 20 μm in external diameter. Media is demarcated by external and internal elastic laminae, stained black in this elastic stain. A bronchiole is identified (B). Elastic-van Gieson, ×210. (**c: bottom**) Intraacinar arteries, the smaller measuring 60 μm in external diameter, with concentric intimal fibrosis; the latter is overlaid by arrowheads that mark the internal elastic laminae. The media is narrow in these branches, but note that the lumen (containing festooned endothelial cells) is the same size as in the similar-sized arteries seen in (b). Elastic-van Gieson, ×210. (From Cullinane C, Cox PN, Silver MM. Persistent pulmonary hypertension of the newborn due to alveolar capillary dysplasia. Pediatr Pathol 1992; 12: 499–514.)

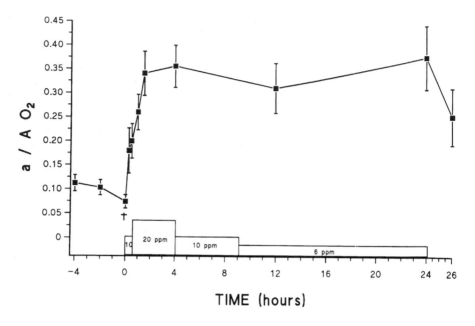

Fig. 10.4 Response to inhalation of nitric oxide. A persistent and sustained improvement in a/AO$_2$ gradient is seen even at a low dose. (From Kinsella JP, Neish SR, Shaffer E, Abman SH. Effect of low-dose inhalational nitric oxide in pulmonary hypertension of the newborn. Lancet 1992; 340: 819–820.)

Experimental studies showing that heparin can stimulate remodeling of the pulmonary circulation were carried out in newborn lambs and rabbits. In both species, infusion of heparin was shown to accelerate maturation of the pulmonary circulation by inducing an increase in the number of peripheral pulmonary arteries relative to alveoli.[25] This might prove of clinical benefit in inducing the growth of peripheral arteries and, thereby, in reducing pulmonary vascular resistance.

MALADAPTATION OF THE PULMONARY VASCULAR BED

Infants with perinatal stress from a variety of causes, e.g. hemorrhage, hypoglycemia, aspiration, or hypoxia, may fail to demonstrate the normal drop in pulmonary vascular resistance at birth (reviewed in[1]). The normally muscular vessels fail to dilate and left ventricular dysfunction likely contributes as well. Of all the types of persistent pulmonary hypertension, this, in theory, should be the most amenable to improvement following treatment of the pulmonary disorder and general hemodynamic state of the infant with hyperventilation or with vasodilators. The use of inhaled NO has been of major benefit in reversing persistent pulmonary hypertension of the newborn secondary to maladaptation (Fig. 10.4).[26] There is evidence, at least experimentally, that

L-arginine is also effective,[27] as are strategies to maximize dilator effects due to cyclic guanosine monophosphate by inhibiting phosphodiesterases which cause degradation of guanylate cyclase.[28,29]

Increased production of endothelin may underlie the pathophysiology of PPHN secondary to maladaptation, as well as mal- and underdevelopment. That is, increased circulating levels of endothelin have been shown in PPHN secondary to a variety of etiologies and there is an associated decrease with resolution of the PPHN.[30] The use of endothelin receptor blockade or endothelial converting-enzyme inhibition[31] may, therefore, also prove beneficial in this regard, especially if specificity could be controlled to maximize dilatory activity. That is, endothelin A receptors and endothelin B constrictor as opposed to dilator receptors should be targeted.

Maldevelopment of the pulmonary vascular bed

Murphy et al. observed,[32] through structural studies of the lung at postmortem from fatal cases of meconium aspiration, that the latter, while appearing to be a postnatal stress, is often the manifestation of intrauterine dysfunction. In 1 of 6 infants studied, there was evidence of failure of normally muscular peripheral arteries to dilate appropriately at birth; in all the others, the nature and severity of the vascular abnormalities suggested an intrauterine insult of some duration (Fig. 10.2).

Newborns in whom there is no apparent reason for persistent pulmonary hypertension are the most perplexing of all. Clinical studies have suggested a relationship between maternal ingestion of prostaglandin synthetase inhibitors, either aspirin or indomethacin, and subsequent PPHN (reviewed in[1]). In some cases the symptoms were transient, whereas in others, the outcome was more severe or fatal. There is, however, a large population of women who take aspirin during pregnancy and a low incidence of persistent pulmonary hypertension in their newborns and, conversely, in the majority of infants with PPHN, no history of maternal ingestion of these compounds can be documented.

Experimental studies in lambs have shown that prostaglandin synthetase inhibitors will constrict the ductus arteriosus in utero. Chronic indomethacin treatment in pregnant rats will produce structural changes in the pulmonary vascular bed of the newborn. Thus, it seems likely that, in an occasional susceptible human fetus, there may be a relationship between prostaglandin synthetase inhibitors and persistent pulmonary hypertension. In morphometric studies in lungs from fatal cases of persistent pulmonary hypertension of the newborn, the most striking feature is the presence of muscle in arteries small and peripheral in location and normally nonmuscular. The muscle cells are surrounded by darkly-stained elastic laminae, suggesting that they formed several weeks prior to death and, therefore, in utero.

In differentiating PPHN due to maldevelopment, it is important to exclude causes of combined mal- and underdevelopment, such as alveolar capillary dysplasia, and also congenital heart defects, especially isolated pulmonary vein stenoses, as well as more common lesions readily diagnosed by ultrasound. These include total anomalous veins, transposition of the great arteries, and more complex left- or right-sided obstructive lesions.

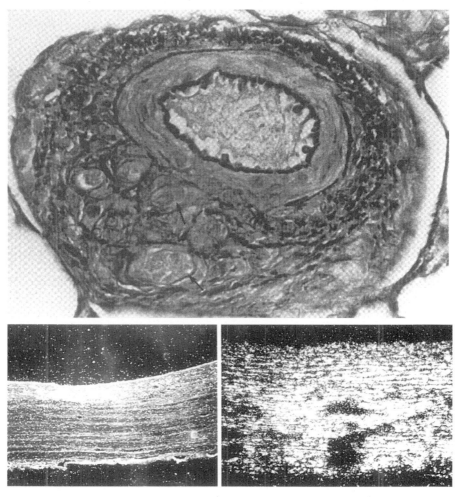

Fig. 10.5 (Upper), An artery from the lung of a 2-week-old calf raised at a simulated altitude of 4300 m from birth. Pulmonary artery systolic pressure was 100 mmHg. There is marked medial hypertrophy (m) and adventitial thickening with neovascularization (arrow). Elastic tissue stain, × 275. (Kindly supplied by K. Stenmark.) (Lower), In situ hybridization localization of tropoelastin mRNA in control and hypertensive vessels from neonatal calves. White staining over areas indicates tropoelastin mRNA labeling. In normotensive vessels (left), labeled cells (^{35}S-labeled T66–T7) were confined to the inner media. Minimal signal is noted in the outer vessel wall. In vessels from hypertensive animals (14 days of hypoxia) (right), intense autoradiographic signal was observed throughout the media, albeit in a patchy distribution. (From Prosser I, Stenmark K, Suthar M et al. Regional heterogeneity of elastin and collagen gene expression in intralobar arteries in response to hypoxic pulmonary hypertension as demonstrated by in situ hybridization. Am J Pathol 1989; 135: 1073–1088.)

Experimental studies

The structural and physiologic changes of PPHN of the newborn have not been reproduced in experimental guinea pigs by chronic maternal hypoxemia. In lambs, the clinical syndrome has been produced by administration of a cytokine associated with inflammation, i.e. tumor necrosis factor alpha. Relatively short periods of hypoxia in the fetal lamb will result in sustained elevation of pulmonary artery pressure and structural changes in the pulmonary arteries.

In utero closure of the ductus arteriosus has proven to simulate the structural changes and the initial hemodynamic picture of persistent pulmonary hypertension.[33,34] In these studies there was evidence of impaired endothelial-dependent vasodilatation.

Since NO can induce angiogenesis and endothelin may be a mitogen for smooth muscle cells, one might speculate that increased production of endothelin or reduced production of NO in utero might lead to an increase in muscularity of peripheral pulmonary arteries and a reduction in their number.

Numerous studies are also addressing whether the abnormalities observed with PPHN my be related to cytoskeletal changes and whether there are sub-populations of smooth muscle cells which may clonally proliferate in response to an abnormal mitogenic stimulus.[5,6] These cells may also show a different potential for the production and accumulation of extracellular matrix connective tissue components such as collagen, elastin, and proteoglycans.[2] Increased adventitial thickening demonstrated in a calf model of hypoxia-induced neonatal pulmonary hypertension (Fig. 10.5) may prevent the access of NO to the vascular smooth muscle cells.[35]

Chronic in utero hypoxia, hyperoxia or abnormally increased pulmonary blood flow and pressure or inflammation may also stimulate the cascade of structural changes observed postnatally which include muscularization of normally nonmuscular peripheral arteries, medial hypertrophy of muscular arteries and reduced number of peripheral vessels, as has been shown postnatally.

A UNIFYING HYPOTHESIS

Our own studies have suggested that increased activity of an endogenous vascular elastase might play a pivotal role in inducing the structural changes in the pulmonary circulation. We have shown experimentally that a variety of pulmonary hypertension-producing stimuli can increase pulmonary artery elastase and that inhibition of elastase activity with a variety of inhibitors can prevent or retard the progression of pulmonary vascular changes and associated pulmonary hypertension.

We envision the pathophysiologic sequence of events as follows (summarized in Fig. 10.6). In response to a pulmonary hypertension-producing stimulus, the first casualty is the endothelial cell. The subsequent structural and functional changes associated with the perturbed endothelium result in loss of the barrier function. We speculated and subsequently showed, in vitro,

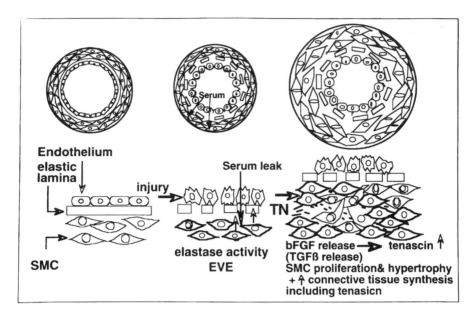

Fig. 10.6 Schema describing relationship of elastase to pulmonary vascular disease.

that serum factors or endothelial factors that might gain access to the subendothelium when the barrier is lost induce release of a serine elastase from pulmonary vascular smooth muscle cells.[36] This elastase can liberate biologically active smooth muscle cell mitogens, such as basic fibroblast growth factor, from extracellular matrix stores.[37]

The resulting smooth muscle cell hyperplasia contributes to the hypertrophy of the arterial wall. Release of other growth factors, such as transforming growth factor β which can induce increased synthesis of elastin and collagen, might also add to the thickening. We have further shown that there is also induction of the matrix glycoprotein tenascin, which co-operatively interacts with growth factors, such as epidermal growth factor and basic fibroblast growth factor, in inducing the proliferative response in the vessel wall.[38]

We have shown that hyperoxia-induced lung abnormalities and pulmonary hypertension in newborn rats can be largely alleviated by elastase inhibitors[39] and this has led to a clinical trial with promising results in preventing and reducing the severity of pulmonary hypertension.[40]

KEY POINTS FOR CLINICAL PRACTICE

1. It is important to think of etiologies of persistent pulmonary hypertension of the newborn in three categories: underdevelopment, maldevelopment, and maladaptation, as each may have differences in the medical or

surgical approach to treatment and in the expected response of vasodilators.

2. There are experimental and supportive clinical data to suggest that the vasoconstrictor, endothelin, is responsible for pulmonary vasoconstriction observed in utero and that nitric oxide and repression of K^+ channels are responsible for postnatal dilatation.

3. Treatment of persistent pulmonary hypertension of the newborn with inhaled nitric oxide (in doses ranging from as low as 6 ppm to 80 ppm) has been a major breakthrough, obviating the need for ECMO in many cases. However, in some refractory patients, the use of phosphodiesterase inhibitors and the future use of endothelin receptor blockade may also prove highly effective.

4. The refractoriness of the patient with pulmonary hypoplasia, e.g. severe congenital diaphragmatic hernia, to vasodilator therapy alone may necessitate new strategies to stimulate growth of peripheral arteries and alveoli. Heparin therapy may be useful in this regard, at least based upon experimental data.

5. The etiology of pulmonary maldevelopment may be related to an in utero insult resulting from severe hypoxia, hyperoxia, increased flow and or pressure, toxins, or inflammation.

6. New insights into the pathophysiology of the structural changes in the pulmonary circulation that occur in response to these injurious stimuli might lead to innovative therapies. We have shown that increased activity of an elastase has proven to be pivotal in orchestrating pulmonary vascular changes. The experimental use of elastase inhibitors has been shown to prevent or retard progression of pulmonary hypertension.

REFERENCES

1. Rabinovitch M. Pathophysiology of pulmonary hypertension. In: Emmanouilides GC, Allen HD, Riemenschneider TA, Gutgesell HP., eds. Moss and Adams Heart Disease in Infants, Children, and Adolescents. Including the Fetus and Young Adult. 5th edn. Baltimore: Williams and Wilkins, 1995; 1659–1695
2. Allen KM, Wharton J, Polak JM, Haworth SG. A study of nerves containing peptides in the pulmonary vasculature of healthy infants and children and of those with pulmonary hypertension. Br Heart J 1989; 62: 353–360
3. Durmowicz AG, Parks WC, Hyde DM, Mecham RP, Stenmark KR. Persistence, re-expression, and induction of pulmonary arterial fibronectin, tropoelastin, and type I procollagen mRNA expression in neonatal hypoxic pulmonary hypertension. Am J Pathol 1994; 145: 1411–1420
4. Allen K, Haworth SG. Human postnatal pulmonary arterial remodeling: ultrastructural studies of smooth muscle cell and connective tissue maturation. Lab Invest 1988; 48: 702–709

5. Frid MG, Moiseeva EP, Stenmark KR. Multiple phenotypically distinct smooth muscle cell populations exist in the adult and developing bovine pulmonary arterial media in vivo. Circ Res 1994; 75: 669–681

6. Das M, Stenmark KR, Dempsey EC. Enhanced growth of fetal and neonatal pulmonary artery adventitial fibroblasts is dependent on protein kinase C. Am J Physiol 1995; 269: L660–L667

7. Ziegler JW, Ivy DD, Kinsella JP, Abman SH. The role of nitric oxide, endothelin, and prostaglandins in the transition of the pulmonary circulation [Review]. Clin Perinatol 1995; 22: 387–403

8. Wang Y, Coceani F. Isolated pulmonary resistance vessels from fetal lambs. Contractile behavior and responses to indomethacin and endothelin-1. Circ Res 1992; 71: 320–330

9. Perreault T, De Marte J. Endothelin-1 has a dilator effect on neonatal pit pulmonary vasculature. J Cardiovasc Pharmacol 1991; 18: 43–51

10. Ivy DD, Kinsella JP, Abman SH. Physiologic characterization of endothelin A and B receptor activity in the ovine fetal pulmonary circulation. J Clin Invest 1994; 93: 2141–2148

11. Kourembanas S, Marsden PA, McQuillan LP, Faller DV. Hypoxia induces endothelin gene expression and secretion in cultured humans endothelium. J Clin Invest 1991; 88: 1054–1057

12. Lock JE, Olley PM, Coceani F et al. Pulmonary and systemic responses to 60-keto PGE1 in the conscious lamb. Prostaglandins 1979; 18: 303–309

13. Kinsella JP, Ivy DD, Abman SH. Ontogeny of NO activity and response to inhaled NO in the developing ovine pulmonary circulation. Am J Physiol 1994; 267: H1955–H1961

14. Halbower AC, Tuder RM, Franklin WA, Pollock JS, Forstermann U, Abman SH. Maturation-related changes in endothelial nitric oxide synthase immunolocalization in developing ovine lung. Am J Physiol 1994; 267: L585–L591

15. Steinhorn RH, Russell JA, Morin III FC. Disruption of cGMP production in pulmonary arteries isolated from fetal lambs with pulmonary hypertension. Am J Physiol 1995; 268: H1483–H1489

16. Chang JK, Moore P, Fineman JR et al. K+ channel pulmonary vasodilation in fetal lambs: role of endothelium-derived nitric oxide. J Appl Physiol 1992; 73: 188–194

17. Cornfield DN, McQueston JA, McMurtry IF, Rodman DM, Abman SH. Role of ATP-sensitive potassium channels in ovine fetal pulmonary vascular tone. Am J Physiol 1992; 263: H1363–H1368

18. Belik J, Halayko A, Rao K, Stephens N. Pulmonary vascular smooth muscle: biochemical and mechanical changes. J Appl Physiol 1991; 71: 1129–1135

19. Hislop A, Fairweather DVI, Blackwell RJ, Howard S. The effect of amniocentesis and drainage of amniotic fluid on lung development in *Macaca fascicularis*. Br J Obstet Gynaecol 1984; 91: 835–841

20. Collins MH, Moessinger AC, Kleinerman J et al. Fetal lung hypoplasia associated with maternal smoking: a morphometric analysis. Pediatr Res 1989; 19: 408–412

21. Karamanoukian HL, Glick PL, Zayek M et al. Inhaled nitric oxide in congenital hypoplasia of the lungs due to diaphragmatic hernia or oligohydramnios. Pediatrics 1994; 94: 715–718

22. Bohn D, Tamura M, Perrin D, Barker G, Rabinovitch M. Ventilatory predictors of pulmonary hypoplasia in congenital diaphragmatic hernia confirmed by morphometric assessment. J Pediatr 1987; 111: 423–431

23. Schranz D, Huth R, Hichel-Behnke I, Wipperman CF. Norepinephrine, enoximone and nitric oxide for treatment of myocardial stunning and pulmonary hypertension in a newborn with diaphragmatic hernia. J Pediatr 1995; 111: 423–431

24. Cullinane C, Cox PN, Silver MM. Persistent pulmonary hypertension of the newborn due to alveolar capillary dysplasia. Pediatr Pathol 1992; 12: 499–514

25. Endo M, Baron O, Keeley FW et al. The effect of heparin on pulmonary vascular maturation in the neonatal lamb. Submitted

26. Kinsella JP, Abman SH. Recent developments in the pathophysiology and treatment of persistent pulmonary hypertension of the newborn. J Pediatr 1995; 126: 853–864

27. Cornfield DN, Chatfield BA, McQueston JA, McMurtry IF, Abman SH. Effects of birth-related stimuli on L-arginine-dependent pulmonary vasodilation in ovine fetus. Am J Physiol 1992; 262: H1474–H1481

28. Thusu KG, Morin III FC, Russell JA, Steinhorn RH. The cGMP phosphodiesterase

inhibitor zaprinast enhances the effect of nitric oxide. Am J Respir Crit Care Med 1995; 152: 1605–1610

29. Steinhorn RH, Millard SL, Morin III FC. Persistent pulmonary hypertension of the newborn. Role of nitric oxide and endothelin in pathophysiology and treatment [Review]. Clin Perinatol 1995; 22: 405–428

30. Rosenberg AA, Kennaugh J, Koppenhafer SL, Loomis M, Chatfield BA, Abman SH. Elevated immunoreactive endothelin-1 levels in newborn infants with persistent pulmonary hypertension [see comments]. J Pediatr 1993; 123: 109–114

31. Kirshbom PM, Tsui SSL, DiBernardo LR et al. Blockade of endothelin-converting enzyme reduces pulmonary hypertension after cardiopulmonary bypass and circulatory arrest. Surgery 1995; 118: 440–445

32. Murphy JD, Rabinovitch M, Goldstein JD et al. The structural basis of persistent pulmonary hypertension of the newborn infant. J Pediatr 1981; 98: 962–967

33. McQueston JA, Kinsella JP, Ivy DD, McMurtry IF, Abman SH. Chronic pulmonary hypertension in utero impairs endothelium-dependent vasodilation. Am J Physiol 1995; 268: H288–H294

34. Zayek M, Cleveland D, Morin III FC. Treatment of persistent pulmonary hypertension in the newborn lamb by inhaled nitric oxide. J Pediatr 1993; 122: 743–750

35. Steinhorn RH, Morin III FC, Russel JA. The adventitia may be a barrier specific to nitric oxide in rabbit pulmonary artery. J Clin Invest 1993; 94: 1883–1888

36. Kobayashi J, Wigle D, Childs T, Zhu L, Keeley FW, Rabinovitch M. Serum-induced vascular smooth muscle cell elastolytic activity through tyrosine kinase intracellular signalling. J Cell Physiol 1994; 160: 121–131

37. Thompson K, Rabinovitch M. Exogenous leukocyte and endogenous elastases can mediate mitogenic activity in pulmonary artery smooth muscle cells by release of extracellular matrix-bound basic fibroblast growth factor. J Cell Physiol 1995; 166: 495–505

38. Jones PL, Rabinovitch M. Induction of tenascin and endothelial cell apoptosis are features of monocrotaline-induced progressive pulmonary vascular disease. Circulation 1995; 92: I-374

39. Koppel R, Han RNN, Cox D, Tanswell AK, Rabinovitch M. Alpha 1-antitrypsin protects neonatal rats from pulmonary vascular and parenchymal effects of oxygen toxicity. Pediatr Res 1994; 36: 763–770

40. Stiskal J, Dunn M, O'Brien K et al. Alpha 1-proteinase inhibitor (A1P1) therapy for the prevention of bronchopulmonary dysplasia (BPD) in premature infants. Pediatr Res 1996; 39: 247a

11

Evaluating headache in children

M. B. O'Neill

EPIDEMIOLOGY

Until recently few epidemiological studies on headaches in children were available from which clinicians could draw accurate information with regard to incidence and prevalence of the various types of headaches occurring in childhood. In one prospective study a cohort of 5,356 children were followed from birth until 5 years of age.[1] The families were contacted 8 times during this period to evaluate the frequency of headache occurrence. Postal questionnaires, telephone contact and clinic visits were utilized. Completed data were available on 4,405 children (82.2%). Headache occurred in 861 (19.5%). It was highly frequent in 9 (0.2%), fairly frequent in 23 (.5%), less frequent in 190 (4.3%) and infrequent in 639 (14.5%). No diagnosis of headache etiology was made. The frequency of headaches was correlated with increased leisure activities and lower socio-economic status.

Several population based studies of migraine in childhood have been published. A study of 1,003 children in a British general practice between the ages of 3–11 years attempted to determine the prevalence of migraine.[2] A direct structured interview technique was utilized. Migraine incidence was 4.7% of males and 5% of females. Migraine without aura was twice as common as migraine with aura. The relative frequencies of migraine headaches varied enormously. In children between 3–7 years of age the mean frequency was 6.8 headaches per year and in those children between 8–11 years of age it was 11.3 headaches/year with a range of 1–50. Migraine in adolescence was evaluated in a cohort of 1,523 males between 12–17 years of age were evaluated through a telephone interview. The prevalence of migraine was estimated at 3.8%, a cohort of 635 females of a similar age had a prevalence of 6.6%.[3]

Large numbers of children and adolescents have headaches, but few seek medical attention, only 15.1% of children[2] and under 20% of adolescents.[3]. No accurate reasons can be obtained for this. Clearly, there is a need for increased awareness among physicians[4] to address the need of headache sufferers.

CLASSIFICATION OF HEADACHES

Given that there is no diagnostic test for many of the headache syndromes that are encountered in clinical practice, the physician is dependent on the history and physical examination to make a diagnosis and sometimes a diagnosis cannot be made with certainty. To help remedy this situation the International Headache Society (IHS) defined expressive criteria for the diagnosis of the various headache syndromes.[5] The benefits of such a system are to reduce intraobserver diagnostic variability and to allow clear classification of the patient's clinical symptoms. These clinical criteria were put together by expert panels and represent a consensus viewpoint.

The utilization of diagnostic criteria represents a balance between sensitivity and specificity and the effectiveness of such an approach can only be validated by clinical trials. The results of such trials can then be used to enhance the criteria themselves. To date few pediatric headache studies[6,7] have been performed to evaluate the IHS criteria; in one retrospective study,[6] the clinical diagnosis, made by a neurologist, was regarded as the gold standard and this was compared against the IHS criteria for diagnosis of childhood migraine. Of the total sample of 254 children, 136 were diagnosed by the physician as having migraine. Utilizing the IHS criteria, the sensitivity of the criteria was 30.1% and the specificity was 94%. Some criteria were present infrequently, for example, headache duration was greater than 4 h in only 57%. Aggravation by physical activity was present in 40%. The pulsation quality of the headache was noted in 66% and nausea was present in 59%. In a study of 719 children and adolescents,[7] 24.3% with migraine and 33.2% with tension headaches did not fulfil the IHS criteria. In a smaller study of 45 children and adolescents with migraine, the IHS criteria were not met in 47% of patients. These studies suggest deficiencies in the current IHS criteria in the diagnosis of childhood headache. Such studies are important to improve the sensitivity and specificity of the criteria. The IHS criteria should be utilized to diagnose headache syndrome, recognising that, with increased research and a better understanding of the various clinical syndromes, they will change.

CLINICAL EVALUATION

For the practising physician evaluating a patient with headaches, the array of diagnostic possibilities is daunting when the IHS classification is reviewed (Table 11.1). To simplify this in the clinical context, an alternate approach can be utilized where headaches are classified as being acute, acute recurrent, chronic nonprogressive, chronic progressive, or mixed pattern.[10] Acute headaches are relatively short and are common with viral illnesses. Certain unusual acute headache syndromes include exertional headaches. Acute recurrent headaches are typified by various migraine syndromes (Table 11.2). The hallmark of these conditions are discrete episodes of headache with intervening intervals of normality which may last from weeks to months. Recurring migraine headaches have the same pattern, but over time they may change. Chronic progressive headaches are usually caused by tumors, pseudo tumour cerebri, hydrocephalus or brain abscesses. The headache is progressive with pain increasing in severity and the patient becoming progressively

Table 11.1 Headache classification according to the International Headache Society

1.	Migraine
2.	Tension-type headache
3.	Cluster headache and chronic paroxysmal hemicrania
4.	Miscellaneous headaches not associated with structural lesion
5.	Headache associated with head trauma
6.	Headache associated with vascular disorders
7.	Headache associated with non vascular intracranial
8.	Headache associated with substances or their withdrawal
9.	Headache associated with noncephalic infection
10.	Headache associated with metabolic disorder
11.	Headache or facial pain associated with disorder of cranium, neck, eyes, ears, nose, sinuses, teeth, mouth, or other facial or cranial structures
12.	Cranial neuralgias, nerve trunk pain, and deafferentation pain
13.	Headache not classifiable

more disabled. The headaches lasts longer than the traditional 72 h which is ascribed to a migraine headache. Chronic nonprogressive headaches are typified by tension headaches which can occur on a daily basis for weeks or months at a time. The headache remains the same and are usually not disabling for the patient. Mixed pattern headaches most commonly represent a combination of acute recurrent and chronic nonprogressive headaches, that is, migraine and tension headaches. In mixed pattern headaches, migraine should be addressed first and, if successfully addressed, the other headaches abate. In evaluating the diagnostic possibilities the 20 questions in Table 11.3 are useful. The use of developmentally appropriate questions enhances the diagnostic accuracy of the history taking.[8]

Table 11.2 Revised classification of migraine

1.1	Migraine without aura	
1.2	Migraine with aura	
	1.2.1	Migraine with typical aura
	1.2.2	Migraine with prolonged aura
	1.2.3	Familial hemiplegic migraine
	1.2.4	Basilar migraine
	1.2.5	Migraine aura without headache
	1.2.6	Migraine with acute onset aura
1.3	Ophthalmoplegic migraine	
1.4	Retinal migraine	
1.5	Childhood periodic syndromes that may be precursors to or associated with migraine	
	1.5.1	Benign paroxysmal vertigo of childhood
	1.5.2	Alternating hemiplegia of childhood
1.6	Complications of migraine	
	1.6.1	Status migrainous
	1.6.2	Migranous infarction
1.7	Migrainous disorder not fulfilling above criteria	

Table 11.3 Evaluating headaches by history

1.	Do you have more than one type of headache?
2.	How did the headache begin? Trauma? Infection?
3.	How long has it been present?
4.	Are the symptoms worsening or staying the same?
5.	How often do they occur?
6.	How long do they last?
7.	Do they occur at any special time or under specific circumstances?
8.	Are they preceded by warning signs?
9.	Where does it hurt?
10.	What is the quality of the pain? Pounding? Sharp?
11.	Do you have associated symptoms during the headache? Abdominal pain? Nausea, vomiting?
12.	Do you stop what you are doing during the headache?
13.	Do you have any other medical problems?
14.	Are you taking any medications regularly?
15.	Are there any activities that make the headache worse?
16.	Does any particular medication make the headache better?
17.	Does anyone else in your family have headaches?
18.	What do you think is causing your headaches?
19.	Can you tell when your child has a headache?
20.	Does your child cry with the pain?

From the history the pain severity must be assessed. Utilizing a 6 point scoring system is often useful. A score of 0 indicates no pain. A score of 1 indicates pain, but the child is only aware of it when he pays attention to it. A score of 2 indicates pain that can be ignored at times. A score of 3 indicates pain that can't be ignored, but allows for usual activities to be performed. A pain score of 4 indicates difficulty in concentration, but allows for easy activities to be performed and a score of 5 indicates pain that does not allow the child to do any activities. The pain severity must be correlated with the disability encountered as it pertains to school loss, recreational activity reduction and parental anxiety. Utilizing headache diaries where children over 7 years of age rate their headaches on a 0–5 scale, 4 times per day, one can obtain this information in a satisfactory fashion.[9]

Assessing pain and disability in adults is more complicated and for this the chronic pain index (CPI) has been developed. This incorporates a scoring system which evaluates the elements of pain and disability. It allows the patient to be assigned a score to indicate disability.

ACUTE RECURRENT HEADACHE

Migraine

The etiology of migraine is uncertain. Its elucidation is further hampered by the absence of an animal model. Several pathogenic mechanisms have been proposed which include: (i) the vascular theory of migraine; (ii) the theory of 5-hydroxytryptamine receptors' activation; and (iii) the theory of central neuronal hyperexcitability. None of these theories alone are persuasive as they all fail to account for the quality of the symptoms, their complexity and their relatively slow development. Migraine is a clinical condition which evolves over a period of time. Often there are characteristic prodromal features which may be followed by an aura. Subsequent to this phase there is an intense headache which occurs with resolution and recovery over a period of hours to days.

The old classification of migraine has been replaced by a newer one (Table 11.2). Familiarity with the newer definitions is important to enable clinical diagnosis given the absence of diagnostic tests. The new diagnostic criteria

Table 11.4 Diagnostic criteria of migraine with aura

MIGRAINE WITH AURA

Previously used terms: classic migraine; classical migraine; ophthalmic, hemiparesthetic, hemiplegic,or aphasic migraine

Diagnostic criteria

A.   At least two attacks fulfilling B

B.   At least three of the following four characteristics:

    1.   One or more fully reversible aura symptoms indicating focal cerebral cortical and/or brainstem dysfunction

    2.   At least one aura symptom develops gradually over more than 4 min or two or more symptoms occur in succession

    3.   No aura symptom lasts more than 60 min; if more than one aura symptom is present, accepted duration is proportionally increased

    4.   Headache follows aura with a free interval of less than 60 min (it may also being before or simultaneously with the aura.)

C.   At least one of the following:

    1.   History, physical, and neurologic examinations do not suggest one of the disorders listed in groups 5–11 (see Table 11.1)

    2.   History and/or physical and/or neurologic examinations do suggest such disorder, but it is ruled out by appropriate investigations

    3.   Such disorder is present, but migraine attacks do not occur for the first time in close temporal relation to the disorder

MIGRAINE WITH TYPICAL AURA

Diagnostic criteria

A.   Fulfils criteria for migraine with aura including all four criteria under B

B.   One or more aura symptoms of the following types:

    1.   Homonymous visual disturbance

    2.   Unilateral paresthesias and/or numbness

    3.   Unilateral weakness

    4.   Aphasia or unclassifiable speech difficulty

Table 11.5 Diagnostic criteria of migraine without aura

Migraine without aura
Previously used terms: common migraine, hemicrania simplex
Diagnostic criteria
A.   At least five attacks fulfilling B through D
B.   Headache lasting 4–72 h (untreated or unsuccessfully treated)
C.   Headache has at least two of the following characteristics:
      1.   Unilateral location
      2.   Pulsating quality
      3.   Moderate or severe intensity (inhibits or prohibits daily activities)
      4.   Aggravation by walking stairs or similar routine physical activity
D.   During headache at least one of the following:
      1.   Nausea and/or vomiting
      2.   Photophobia and phonophobia
E.   At least one of the following:
      1.   History, physical, and neurologic examinations do not suggest one of the disorders listed in groups 5 through 11 (see Table 11.1)
      2.   History and/or physical and/or neurologic examinations do suggest such disorder, but it is ruled out by appropriate investigations
      3.   Such disorder is present, but migraine attacks do not occur for the first time in close temporal relation to the disorder

---

for migraine in patients without aura and with typical aura are outlined in Tables 11.4 and 11.5.

Migraine heterogenicity

Appreciating that migraine is a heterogenous condition is important when dealing with children and adolescents who suffer from this condition given that up to 40% of children followed over a 5 year period will outgrow the condition, but the remainder will continue to be affected by it.[10] Amongst adults who suffer from migraine, there is significant disability caused by this condition,[11] with 19% taking time off work, a further 50% discontinuing normal activity for variable periods of time, 31% cancelling family events and 30% cancelling social events. Amongst adolescents who suffer from headaches, 10.1% of males and 8.6% of females miss part of a day's schooling and 2.4% of males and 2.7% of females miss a full day's schooling as a result of the disability caused by the headaches.[3] Most of these headache sufferers have migraine and much of the morbidity of headaches can be attributed to migraine, given that the pain associated with it is more severe than tension headaches. In younger children with migraine, 26% miss 1–2 days a year, 58% miss 3–5 days and 11% miss in excess of 5 days.[12]

The duration of pain is variable. The IHS criteria require pain to be present for 4 h, but acknowledges that in children it may be 2 h. In one study of school aged children, 7% had headache less than 2 h.[12] In another,[10] 46% had headaches for less than 3 h and, in one adult study,[13] 25% of the headaches were less than 4 h.

Migraine triggers

The identifiable triggers in children and adolescents suffering from migraine are variable. Recognized triggers include stress, fasting,[14] extremes of activity, sleep deprivation and foods. The proportion of identifiable triggers is variable and dependent on the history taking skill of the physician, the belief system of the family and their previous experience. Presumed triggers do not always produce the headaches on re-exposure. In clinical practice it is useful to discuss the concept of one trigger lowering the threshold for a migraine headache and another trigger inducing it. Migraneurs often have one or more triggers, e.g. fasting, lowers the threshold and a food trigger (in a susceptible child), for example chocolate, induces the headache.

Prior to embarking on a treatment plan, having made the diagnosis of migraine, it is essential to obtain the parents' perspective on what they wish to obtain from the consultation and to clearly define the impact of migraine in the child's and family's life. Adequately defining these two objectives allows for a rational therapeutic plan. The following three strategies are useful in dealing with migraine: (i) dietary therapy; (ii) relaxation therapy; and (iii) pharmacological therapy.

Elimination diet

Dietary modification, as a treatment modality in migraine, is controversial. Amongst 429 adult patients with migraine, 16.5% believed that their headaches were precipitated by cheese or chocolate and a further 18.4% reported sensitivity to alcoholic drinks.[15] Physician viewpoints, with regard to the effectiveness of dietary therapy, are variable. In a questionnaire study[16] of 327 physicians who were either members of the American Association for the Study of Headache, or British physicians, who had a known interest in migraine, the results were variable. 74% of the physicians felt diet was important in under 20% of patients, for 16% it was in 20–40%, for 3% it was 40-60% and for 2% it was 60–80%. Five percent of physicians were unable to estimate the impact of diet in migraine.

Many foods have been implicated as potential triggers for migraine and these include cheese, chocolates, soft drinks (aspartame), mushrooms, nuts, figs, banana, plums, smoked meats, meat extracts and hotdogs. The mechanism of migraine induction is uncertain and many of the studies do not evaluate the placebo effect of dietary therapy.

In clinical practice, I evaluate the potential impact of diet on migraine induction, recognizing the data limitation, because my philosophy is to prevent migraine attacks where possible, rather than attempt rescue once the migraine headache has occurred.

Pharmacological treatment

When migraine occurs infrequently, treatment with analgesics, e.g. paracetomol (acetaminophen), administered early in the prodromal phases is effective. Rest in a quiet room is often sought by the child or adolescent migraineur. Sumatriptan, a selective agonist of 5-hydroxytryptamine receptors, is effective in adults with migraine. There is limited experience with the use of subcutaneous sumatriptan in childhood. In one recent study[17] of 17 patients between the ages of 6–16 years, 15 of whom received 6 mg sumatriptan subcutaneously, 6 were better with an hour, 5 were better within 2 h, but 4 had no effect. In two younger children, both of whom received 3 mg each, both were well within 2 h. The failure rate of sumatriptan is 25% and side effects are transient, often being related to sensations of heaviness, neck pressure and flushing. Currently, an oral form of sumatriptan is being developed which will obviate the need for injection.

Prophylactic therapy

The use of medications to prevent the onset of migraine headaches is a joint decision between paediatrician, family and child, if old enough. A recent review[18] of prophylactic migraine medications indicated that none had good scientific evidence for their effectiveness. Despite this, medications that are used include propranolol and pizotifen. This latter medication causes drowsiness and weight gain in approximately 40% of patients and may take several weeks to be effective.[19]

Non pharmacological methods are effective in the treatment of migraine. These include relaxation therapy, plus or minus biofeedback, and self hypnosis. These modalities of treatment reduce the frequency of migraine headaches by 50%, but do not reduce their intensity. They however offer the sufferer an empowerment tool (see chronic nonprogressive headaches).

CHRONIC NONPROGRESSIVE HEADACHES

Within this group, tension headaches both episodic and chronic predominate. The diagnostic criteria utilized in the IHS classification are outlined in Table 11.6. This classification incorporates pericranial muscle tenderness which is not frequently seen or utilized in children or adolescents given the absence of structural criteria for its assessment. Recently, attempts have been made to provide objective criteria, but these are not in current usage.[20]

Prior to implementing a treatment strategy for headache treatment, potential triggers need to be evaluated, such as: (i) school problems either related to learning difficulties or bullies on the schoolyard; (ii) excessive after school activities which may be encouraged by the parent and complied with by the child against their will; and (iii) difficulties within the home which include marital conflict, unemployment and a recent stressful event, for example, death or relocation.

Table 11.6 The diagnostic criteria utilized in the International Headache Society classification for both episodic and chronic tension headaches

---

EPISODIC TENSION-TYPE HEADACHE

Previously used terms: tension headache, muscle contraction headache, psychomyogenic headache, stress headache, ordinary headache, essential headache, idiopathic headache,and pschogenic headache.

Diagnostic criteria

A.   At least 10 previous headache episodes fulfilling criteria B through D listed below; number of days with such headache 180/year (< 15/month)

B.   Headache lasting from 30 min to 7 days

C.   At least two of the following pain characteristics:
   1.   Pressing/tightening (nonpulsating) quality
   2.   Mild or moderate intensity (may inhibit, but does not prohibit activities)
   3.   Bilateral location
   4.   No aggravation by walking stairs or similar routine physical activity

D.   Both of the following:
   1.   No nausea or vomiting (anorexia may occur)
   2.   Photophobia and phonophobia are absent, or one but not the other is present

CHRONIC TENSION-TYPE HEADACHE

Previously used terms; chronic daily headache.

Diagnostic criteria

A.   Average headache frequency 15 days/month (180 days/year) for 6 months fulfilling criteria B through D

B.   At least two of the following pain characteristics:
   1.   Pressing/tightening quality
   2.   Mild or moderate severity (may inhibit but does not prohibit activities)
   3.   Bilateral location
   4.   No aggravation by walking stairs or similar routine physical activity

C.   Both of the following:
   1.   No vomiting
   2.   No more than one of the following: nausea, photophobia, or phonophobia

D.   At least one of the following:
   1.   History, physical, and neurologic examinations do not suggest one of the disorders listed in groups 5 through 11.
   2.   History and/or physical and/or neurologic examinations do suggest such disorder, but it is ruled out by appropriate investigations
   3.   Such disorder is present, but tension-type headache does not occur for the first time in close relation temporal

Chronic tension-type headache associated with disorder of pericranial muscles

Chronic tension-type headache not associated with disorder of pericranial muscles

---

Generally, children are unaware of the etiology of the headaches and asking them about them is unproductive. Should no trigger be evident, then obtaining the Minnesota multiphasic personality inventory is useful. It may indicate evidence of depression or hypochondriasis,[21] especially in adolescent patients.

The following is suggested strategy for children and adolescents with tension headaches:

1. Look for and correct the cause of the stress if possible.

2. Avoid giving the patient paracetamol (acetaminophen), or other analgesics unless the patient benefits from them.

3. Encourage normal activity (headaches may undermine the child's sense of well-being).

4. Discourage the parents assuming responsibility for the headaches (many parents become more concerned about their child's headaches than the child actually is. When this occurs, the child successfully transfers responsibility of the headaches to the parents which may result in secondary gain occurring).

5. Ensure the child performs their household chores and schoolwork. Missing school is to be discouraged as it leads to further stress when the child has to make up for lost time.

6. Explain to the child and adolescent that the headaches are not serious, nor do they indicate brain tumours or sinister diseases.

Children and adolescents with chronic daily headache are likely to blame others and use wishful thinking as coping mechanisms.[22] The use of biofeedback with or without relaxation training and self hypnosis have proved useful in the treatment of these headaches. Seven controlled relaxation studies without biofeedback have recently been evaluated.[23] Each study demonstrated a beneficial effect during therapy and follow-up. The frequency of the headaches was reduced by 50% with higher success rates being noted in children than in adults. The intensity of the headaches often remained unchanged.[24]

In a select population of adolescents with chronic tension headaches should the above manoeuvres prove unsuccessful then amitriptylline[25] should be tried. It may take 4 weeks for a therapeutic effect to be evident. Should the physician be unsuccessful in having a major impact in the elimination of chronic tension headaches, an alternate etiology should be sought, especially if the headache characteristics change in intensity or increased disability results.

CHRONIC PROGRESSIVE HEADACHE

Brain tumours

Physicians and parents alike worry about the potential presence of a brain tumour in any child who presents with headaches. Brain tumours are relatively infrequent occurrences in childhood, with an incidence of 3 per

100,000 population. Recently, the epidemiological aspects of headaches and brain tumours have been critically evaluated.[26] The study group were 3,291 children with brain tumours from 10 hospitals in the USA and Canada who were seen between the years 1930–1979. The review was performed between 1979–1984. Results indicated that 62% of children with brain tumours had chronic headaches caused by: (i) raised intracranial pressure; (ii) pressure on dural nerve ending; and (iii) stretching of intracranial vessels. In the headache group, 58% had supratentorial tumours, 70% had an infratentorial tumours and 34% presented with a spinal canal tumour and 34% had a spinal canal tumour. Headache as the only symptom of a brain tumour occurred in under 1% of patients, under 3% of patients had a normal neurological examination and in 55% of patients there were more than five abnormal neurological findings.

This study has given important clinical information to the practising physician with regard to symptoms and signs in children with brain tumours. Symptoms and signs associated with headache, but independent of tumour location are nausea, vomiting, papilloedema and hypoactive tendon reflexes. In contrast, children without headache who have tumours are more likely to have upper extremity weakness, irritability, optic atrophy and hypertonia. Supratentorial tumours which present with headache are associated with diplopia, an abnormality of personality, academic performance or speech, and are associated with the following signs: coma, stiff neck, pupillary abnormalities, anaesthesia or hyperesthesia of some portion of their body. Infratentorial tumours associated with headache have no specific symptom or neurological sign.

Interestingly, a large number of symptoms and signs are associated with the absence of headache in children with infratentorial tumours. These include, difficulty in walking, confusion, stupor, hyperactive reflexes, Babinski's sign, gait abnormalities, head tilt and oculomotor, abducens, facial and hypoglossal nerve paresis.

Children with brain tumours will invariably have multiple symptoms and signs which can be detected from history and physical assessment. This is reassuring for the physician, but implies the need for a careful history and physical assessment which needs to be repeated at the follow-up visit, especially if the headaches are not significantly improved, or if the pattern has changed. Concern that this is not happening has recently been raised.[27]

Benign intracranial hypertension

The diagnostic criteria for benign intracranial hypertension include the following:[5]

1. Increased intracranial pressure (greater than 200 mm water) measured by epidural, or intraventricular pressure monitoring, or by lumbar puncture.

2.   Normal neurological examination, except for papilloedema and possibly 6th nerve palsy.

3.   No mass lesion and no ventricular enlargement on neuro imaging.

4.   Normal, or low protein concentration and normal white cell count on the CSF.

5.   No clinical or neuro imaging suspicious of venous sinus thrombosis.

6.   The headache intensity and frequency related to variations of intracranial pressure with a time lag of less than 24 h.

The incidence of benign intracranial hypertension is approximately 0.3 per 100,000.[28] There are several aspects of this condition which are puzzling and despite recent postmortem studies the etiology is still unclear.[29] No theory explains why the ventricles do not dilate in response to the increased intracranial pressure.

The dominant clinical feature is headache which is usually pancephalic or frontal in location and is usually severe enough to interfere with daily routines. These high pressure headaches are accentuated by the Valsalva's manoeuvre which is useful to perform during the clinical evaluation. The patient may note that the headaches increase in intensity with bending over and that they are often frequent in the morning.[30]

Recently, an adolescent and adult study on benign intracranial hypertension has reenforced the association with obesity and recent weight.[31] It highlighted the findings of transient visual abnormalities which occurred in 68% and intracranial noises in 58% of patients. These findings often occurred on a daily basis.

While the clinical definition of benign intracranial hypertension requires the presence of papilloedema, this is not a uniform finding in childhood.[30] In some children, headaches become progressive over a short period of time, necessitating detailed neurological evaluation. This evaluation can lead to the diagnosis of benign intracranial hypertension without papilloedema. The frequency of this occurrence is uncertain. While the term benign is used to describe this condition visual failure can occur in up to 25% of patients, therefore long-term follow-up is essential.

Hydrocephalus

The development of headaches in a child with known hydrocephalus who has a shunt produces a diagnostic dilemma for the physician. If the symptoms are associated with vomiting, and altered consciousness, then shunt malfunction needs to be considered. In some cases, this may result in revision of the shunt if symptoms persist. If, however, the child presents with the recurring episodes of headaches the diagnosis of migraine needs to be entertained. Two recent case series (from the same institution) have indicated that when this diagnosis is made, and appropriate therapy instituted, symptoms resolve.[32,33] The authors suggest that in children with hydrocephalus with headache who have normal ventricular systems on CAT scanning, adequate shunt function, a positive family history of migraine, that migraine be considered in the differential diagnosis.

INVESTIGATION OF HEADACHES

In the past decade, computerized axial tomography (CT) scan and magnetic residence imaging (MRI) have become the techniques of choice in investigating children with headaches. The choice of modality is dependent upon the availability of the technology. For the practising physician there is a need to balance the expense of the procedure versus the benefit to the patient and the cost to the health care system.

Within the pediatric literature there are few studies to help physicians make appropriate choices. Few studies have evaluated the use of CT scan, or MRI, in children with headaches. In one Canadian study[34] of 157 children with headaches, seven CT scans were performed. The reasons were: (i) three due to parental anxiety: (ii) one because of atypical headaches; (iii) one because of focal neurological signs due to a tumour; (iv) one because of fever plus headache; and (v) one because of an abnormal skull x-ray performed by the referring physician. Only the patient with the brain tumour had an abnormal CT scan.

Two US studies have reported the use of CT scans and MRI in children with headaches. One study was of 104 children under 7 years of age, of whom 23 had CT scans and 7 had MRI.[35] None of these tests contributed significantly to either diagnosis or treatment. In a second study of 133 children, 78 had neuro imaging studies, 27 had CT scans, 45 had MRI and 6 had both.[36] The indications for CT scan included headache onset at a young age (under 5), atypical headache pattern, increased severity of frequency of headaches, abnormalities on ocular or neurological examination, headaches provoked by changing head position, focal symptoms and signs due to headaches, systemic symptoms for example fatigue and weight loss, and parental or physician concern about a cerebral mass. Parental or physician concern accounted for 30% of the indications. In one study from Israel of 312 children, 110 had CT scans of which only one had an abnormality, that is a brain tumour.[37]

MRI alone has also been used to evaluate headaches. In the largest study in children, of 1,375 patients presenting with headaches, 301 had MRIs.[38] Of these, 292 were reviewed retrospectively and 22 were abnormal. Of the abnormalities detected, only 6 were regarded as serious and these includes four tumours, one abscess and one with Moya-Moya disease.

It is obvious that dependent upon the location of the practising physician the technology available will be variable. In some countries, for example, the

US, MRI appears to be the predominant test utilized by neurologists for investigating children with headaches as opposed to CT scanning. For the practising physician there is a need to offer specific guidelines to enhance this decision making process, especially if access to technology is limited. In one study, 202 children, who had MRIs, were evaluated retrospectively over a 4 year period to determine the clinical predictors for significant MRI findings.[39] In this group, 7 patients had abnormal findings. These included 4 posterior fossa tumours, 2 cavernous hemangiomas, and 1 with a temporal lobe astrocytoma. The clinical history and examinations were correlated with the final diagnosis using logistic regression. The study indicated that there were four predictors of an abnormal MRI and these included: (i) headaches with an acute onset for less than one month; (ii) night-time headache; (iii) abnormal neurological exams; and (iv) abnormal neurological gait. Five of the seven children had abnormal findings on neurological examination and the two remaining had night-time headaches or acute onset of headache.

In a previously normal child with headache, the following criteria for performing CT scans are suggested:[34,40] (i) an accompanying change in personality; (ii) most of the headaches occur at night or during the early morning, or a marked change in headache characteristics; (iii) the headaches do not fit a recognized pattern, for example, stress induced or migraine; (iv) complicated migraine; (v) vomiting that is persisting, or increasing in frequency or (vi) neurological abnormalities on examination inclusive of visual abnormalities.

The importance of performing an investigation for parental reassurance has not been addressed by these studies and, as can be seen from others, accounts for 30% of the reason investigations are performed. It is essential for the practising physician to present the parent with the recognized indications for investigation and to warn them that, from anecdotal experience, early investigation can actually miss significant clinical lesions, for example, brain tumours.

Electroencephalogram (EEG)

The EEG has largely been replaced by CT scanning and thus is not indicated in children who present with headaches. From a research perspective, certain EEG abnormalities may be useful in evaluating those children who have migraine with aura.

Visual evoked responses (VER)

Given the absence of a diagnostic test for migraine, the clinician is dependent on the history and physical assessment to make the diagnosis. One paper has suggested that visual evoked responses in children with migraine can be utilized as a diagnostic test.[41] In a study of 44 children with migraine, with and without aura, and 8 children with the periodic syndrome, results were compared against 50 aged matched controls. The results indicated that fast wave amplitudes over 2 microvolts were able to distinguish migraine from non migraine sufferers. This had a specificity of 96%. More studies are required to verify these findings prior to the recognition of this test as being a specific diagnostic tool for migraine.

CONCLUSION

The evaluation of a child with headache is complex given that the differential diagnosis is extensive. A careful history and physical examination with judicious investigations will give correct diagnosis. Once made, an appropriate therapeutic plan should be instituted to ameliorate the suffering induced on the child and often the family by the headaches.

KEY POINTS FOR CLINICAL PRACTICE

1. Patients forget about their headache symptoms within two weeks of the headache occurring.

2. Utilizing a headache diary to log the symptoms severity and disability associated with the headaches is key in a chronic headache sufferer.

3. Never dispute the presence of pain in a headache sufferer.

4. In migraine use preventive strategies, rather than abortive ones.

5. Discuss with the parents the possibility of a brain tumour as an etiology of the headache in each consultation.

6. Migraine headache pattern can change over years, but not weeks; if the latter happens seek an alternative cause.

7. Investigate with neuroimaging if the patient meets the suggested criteria.

8. Discern if the reason or consultation, from the family physician and the parent, are the same (often it is not).

9. Ask a child to draw an aura, rather than describe it.

10. Use developmentally appropriate questions when obtaining a history from the younger child.

REFERENCES

1. Sillanpaa M, Piekkala P, Kero P. Prevalence of headache preschool age in a non selected child population. Cephalalgia 1991; 11: 239–242
2. Mortimer MJ, Kay J, Jaron A. Childhood migraine in general practice: clinical features and

characteristics. Cephalalgia 1992; 12: 238–242
3. Linet MS, Stewart WF, Celentano DD, Ziegler D, Sprecher M. An epidemiological study of headache amongst adolescents and young adults. JAMA 1989; 261: 2211–2216
4. Stewart WF, Lipton RB, Celentano DD, Reed ML. Prevalence of migraine headache in the United States. JAMA 1992; 267: 64–69
5. Olesen J. Headache Classification Committee of the International Headache Society. Classification and diagnostic criteria for headaches disorders, cranial neuralgia, and facial pain. Cephalgia 1988; 8 (Suppl. 7): 1–96
6. Maytal J, Lipton R, Young M, Shecter A. International Headache Society criteria and childhood migraines. Ann Neurol 1995; 38: 529(A)
7. Gallai V, Sarchielli P, Carboni F, Benedetti P, Mastropaolo C, Puca F. Applicability of the 1988 IHS criteria to headache patients under the age of 18 years attending twenty-one Italian headache clinics (The Juvenile Headache Collaborative Study Group). Headache 1995; 35: 146–153
8. Marcon RA, Labbe EE. Assessment and treatment of children's headaches from a developmental perspective. Headache 1990; 9: 586–592
9. McGrath PJ, Unruh AM. Pain in Children and Adolescents. New York: Elsevier, 1987
10. Bille B. Migraine in schoolchildren. Acta Paediatr Scand 1962; 51 (Suppl. 136): 13–151
11. Pryse-Phillips W, Findlay H, Tugswell, Edmads J, Murray TJ. The Canadian populations serving clinical epidemiological and societal impact of migraine and tension headache, Part 2. Can J Neurol Sci 1992; 19: 333–339
12. Sparks JP. The incidence of migraine in schoolchildren. Practitioner 1978; 221: 407–411
13. Henry P, Michel P, Brochet B, Dartigues JF, Tison S, Salamon R. A nation wide survey of migraine in France: prevalence and clinical features in adults. Cephalgia 1992; 12: 229–237
14. Dalton K, Dalton ME. Food intake before migraine attacks in children. J R Coll Gen Pract 1979; 29: 662–665
15. Peatfield RC. Relationships between food, wine and beer – precipitated migrainous headaches. Headache 1995; 35: 355–357
16. Blau JN, Diamond S. Dietary factors in migraine precipitation: physicians view. Headache 1985; 25: 184–187
17. MacDonald JT. Treatment of juvenile migraine with subcutaneous sumatriptan. Headache 1994; 24: 581–582
18. Igarashi M, May WN, Golden GS. Pharmacological treatment of childhood migraine. J Pediatr 1992; 120: 653–656
19. Symon DN, Russel G. Double blind placebo controlled trial of pizotifen syrup in the treatment of abdominal migraine. Arch Dis Child 1995; 72: 48–50
20. Sakai F, Ebihara S, Akiyama M, Horikawa M. Pericranial muscle hardness in tension type headaches. A non invasive measurement method and its clinical applications. Brain 1995; 188: 523–531
21. Ziegler DK, Paolo AM. Headache symptoms and psychological profile of headache prone individuals. Arch Neurol 1995; 52: 602–606
22. Holden EW, Gladstein J, Trulsen E, Wall B. Chronic daily headache in children and adolescents. Headache 1994; 34: 508–514
23. Duckro PM, Cantwell-Simons E. A review of studies evaluating biofeedback and relaxation training in the management of pediatric headache. Headache 1989; 29: 428–433
24. Bogaards MC, Kuile MM. Treatment of recurrent tension headache: analytic review. Clin J Pain 1994; 10: 174–190
25. Gobal H, Hamouz V, Hansen C et al. Chronic tension headache: amitriptylline reduces clinical headache duration and experimental pain sensitivity but does not alter pericranial muscle activity readings. Pain 1994; 59: 241–249
26. The Childhood Brain Tumor Consortium. The epidemiology of headache among children with brain tumour. J Neurooncol 1991; 10: 31–46
27. Edgeworth J, Bullock P, Baillie A, Gallagher A, Crouchman M. Why are brain tumors still being missed? Arch Dis Child 1996; 74: 148–151
28. Durcan FJ, Corbett JJ, Wall M. The incidence of pseudotumor cerebri. Arch Neurol 1994; 45: 875–877
29. Wall M, Dollar JM, Sadun AA, Kardon R. Idiopathic intracranial hypertension, lack of histologic evidence of cerebral edema. Arch Neurol 1995; 52: 141–145
30. Amacher AL, Spence JD. Spectrum of benign intracranial hypertension in children and

adolescents. Childs Nerv Syst 1985; 1: 81–86

31. Giuseffi V, Wall M, Siegel PZ, Rojas PB. Symptoms and disease associations with idiopathic intracranial hypertension (pseudotumor cerebri): a case control study. Neurology 1991; 41: 239–244

32. Nowak TP, James HE. Migraine headaches in hydrocephalic children: a diagnostic dilemma. Childs Nerv Syst 1989; 5: 310–314

33. James HE, Nowak TP. Clinical course and diagnosis of migraine headaches in hydrocephalic children. Pediatr Neurosurg 1991; 17: 310–316

34. Dooley JM, Camfield PR, O'Neill M, Vohra A. The value of CT scans for children with headache. Can J Neurol Sci 1990; 17: 309–310

35. Chu ML, Shinnar S. Headaches in children younger than seven years of age. Arch Neurol 1992; 49: 79–82

36. Maytal J, Bienkowski RS, Patel M, Eviatar L. The value of brain imaging in children with headaches. Pediatrics 1995; 96: 413–416

37. Nevo Y, Kramer U, Rieder-Groswasser I, Harel S. Clinical categorization of 312 children with chronic headache. Brain Dev 1994; 16: 441–444

38. Bass NE, Ruggieri PM, Cohen BH, Rothner AD, Zepp R, Patel N. Clinical usefulness of magnetic resonance imaging in pediatric headache. Ann Neurol 1995; 38: 527

39. Pinter JD, Medina LS, Davis RG, Zurakowski D, Barnes PD. Clinical predictors of brain lesions and utility of neuro imaging in children with headache. Ann Neurol 1995; 38: 524

40. Honig PJ, Charney EB. Children with brain tumors. Am J Dis Child 1982; 136: 121–124

41. Mortimer MJ, Good PA, Marsters JV, Addy DP. Visual evoked responses in children with migraine: a diagnostic test. Lancet 1990; 335: 75–77

12

Sleep problems and disorders

P. Hill

Sleep problems in childhood are common. Although this is well documented in preschool children and adolescents, sleep problems in primary school age children are also widespread. In a Belgian community study,[1] 43% had sleep difficulties, particularly delays getting off to sleep and parasomnias. One child in 25 was on regular sedatives.

Not all problems involving children's sleep are actually disorders of sleep itself. Difficulties settling to sleep and so-called night waking are not usually disorders of sleep process but nearly always arise out of a child's inability or reluctance to comply with parental expectations.

NORMAL SLEEP AND ITS VARIATIONS IN EARLY CHILDHOOD

The adult pattern of sleep cycles, each approximately 90 min long, progressing in depth through stages 1–4 and followed by a period of rapid eye movement (REM) sleep, is established early in childhood, usually by the age of 12 months. As is the case in adults, deep or slow-wave sleep consisting of stages 3 and 4 is relatively predominant in the first half of sleep and REM duration is longer during the last half. The major maturational changes during childhood are to do with the establishment of a single phase of sleep as the child progresses from a circadian (or technically an ultradian) rhythm based on a 4 h cycle in the neonatal period to one based on approximately 16 h of wakefulness and 8 h sleep by the early teens. It is thought that the 4 h cycle is dependent upon an endogenous pacemaker, probably located in the central hypothalamus, while the adolescent pattern is a function of compromise with environmental stimuli. The neonatal 4 h cycle does not, incidentally, depend upon feeding schedules since it can be found in infants fed intravenously and continuously.

Settling to sleep

Throughout the preschool years there is progressive organisation of the sleep-wake cycle into three main periods: morning awake, afternoon nap, afternoon awake and nocturnal sleep. This development is not purely endogenous and is supported or even driven by parental pressures. Most evident among these is the common requirement among Northern European and American societies that the young child settle to sleep early in the evening. This is quite often resisted by a child who experiences normal separation anxiety and ordinary fears of the dark so that the child demands the parent's presence while waiting to fall asleep. Such behaviour may be intensified by particularly high levels of general anxiety, 'difficult' temperament, or the practices of indulgent parents who accede to the child's demands. Alternatively the child may not be tired because of sleeping late in the morning: a delayed sleep-wake cycle. A common trap is for the parent to provide comfort by remaining near the child until asleep. This sidesteps the child's protest but does not provide the opportunity required for the child to learn how to settle to sleep alone, an acquired skill. Acquisition of the skill can be promoted by teaching parents to put their baby down to settle in the cot when drowsy but not asleep: an educational intervention which reduces the rate of settling troubles in the middle of the night.[2]

The management of such a problem is well described in various texts[3] and relies essentially on allowing the child progressively longer intervals between parental visits to the bedside to give reassurance, always leaving the room before the child falls asleep. This is parallelled by calm, firm supportive handling and limit setting over calls for drinks or coming out of the bedroom. Sometimes, one or two stairgates need to be placed in the bedroom doorway. Other effective techniques include promptly and firmly returning the child to bed when he or she leaves it or letting the child cry itself to sleep. These are often hard for parents to implement and, as they do not appear to result in more rapid resolution of the problem, there seems little to recommend them as initial manoeuvres.

A few children with neurological problems associated with visual impairment or with attention deficit hyperactivity disorder seem to have no phasic rhythm inducing sleep onset. Initial trials of melatonin given in supraphysiological doses each evening are favourable but relapse on discontinuation occurs.[4]

Night waking

About half of all night waking problems in preschool children are associated with evening settling difficulties. Most very young children wake a few times each night,[5] but usually settle themselves back to sleep without fuss. Some cannot or do not and it is these children who cry in the night and are regarded as night wakers, though the key problem is likely to be that they lack self-soothing strategies and cannot settle themselves to sleep when alone. This lack may be masked by a parent nursing them or staying with them until they fall asleep; something which may be a reflection of insecure maternal attachment.[6] The first clinical move is, therefore, to ensure that any lack of ability to settle oneself to sleep alone is dealt with in the evening before tackling the night waking problem.

If the child is able to settle in the evening but not get back to sleep during the night, it may be because the environmental stimuli are different in the middle of the night. The parents may be putting the child down or allowing the child to fall asleep in a room other than his bedroom, or the house is well lit and the TV on at bedtime but not in the night. Trying to match evening and night-time environment may help: settling the child in his or her own bedroom, turning down lights in the evening or allowing a nightlight during the night.

Generally speaking, the creation of the problem of night waking results from a complex interplay of factors including those intrinsic to the child (pain, itch, cough etc.) and unintentional perpetuation of the problem by parental attention to the disturbance.[7] Some children who wake during the night are overhydrated by too much milk or juice given to pacify them in the evening or at night wakings. They may also have their circadian rhythm disrupted by feeding which can stimulate digestion and inhibit the nocturnal lowering of body temperature. Wet nappies provide the clue.

There seem to be no grounds for thinking that pre-term infants are neurologically predisposed to night waking; if they do wake more frequently, this can be attributed to different parental handling practices.[8] Breast fed babies wake more frequently than bottle fed but the reasons for this are not necessarily chemical. Cows' milk allergy can cause crying in babies and, thereby, interfere with sleep. Avoiding cows' milk protein and switching to a hydrolysate formula will relieve the problem.[9]

Those children who are able to settle themselves in the evening but cannot do so when they wake during the night can be taught self-settling by a similar programme of graded intervals to that employed in the evening; it is just harder work for the parents to manage such a programme in the middle of the night. They may need advice to share the burden between them on a rota basis or given sanction to take the child into bed with them until the parents feel able to tackle the problem directly. Sharing a bed with a small child is a common practice but whether it is safe is much debated. Data from New Zealand[10] suggest that the rate of SIDS is slightly raised among infants who share a bed with another person but McKenna et al.[11] point out the phylogenic antecedents and stress the essential normality of the practice, disputing the increased risk. For toddlers and older children, the SIDS argument is probably irrelevant yet there is evidence that, if sharing a bed with a parent is a regular practice, the child has a higher rate of emotional and behaviour problems though the cause is obscure.[12]

An alternative approach with a child who has a predictable time of waking is for the parents to wake the child some 30 min beforehand and then settle the child back to sleep. The parent then cuts down the number of active wakings over a period of several weeks.[13] Providing the child with a wrist-worn actigraph which can be downloaded into a computer is an innovative and experimental technique that will allow more precise timing of wakening episodes.[14] Which approach to choose does not matter very much: specific methods have not been shown to be superior over concerned support, written advice or the passage of time.

Duration of sleep

There are obvious variations between children as to the amount of sleep they need. Exactly how much sleep is required at each age is hard to determine with any accuracy because of inherent individual variation and habit. It may be a misplaced concern since sleep deprivation has little objective adverse impact apart from tiredness, irritability and reduced concentration. It has been suggested that growth hormone secretion during slow-wave sleep is probably to limit catabolism secondary to starvation during sleep rather than to promote growth[15].

Just like adults, children can be described as 'morning' or 'evening' persons most active on waking or in the evening accordingly. Indeed, a markedly 'evening' disposition has been thought to explain night settling difficulties though it seems more plausible that it merely contributes to them. Young children who wake early and do not return to sleep can be a major burden to parents who are themselves evening persons. Little can be done except provide play materials in the bedroom and ensure the child's safety by, for instance, putting in a stairgate or locking the kitchen door. Resourceful families with otherwise compliant children can rig up a signalling system using a time switch on a bedside light to indicate when it is appropriate to go into the parents, wake siblings or go downstairs.

Settling and waking problems are common but taxing on parents, especially if they have no way of distancing themselves from the child because of living in a small flat or bed and breakfast accommodation. The understandable reluctance to prescribe hypnotics for small children need not become an ideological rod with which to beat exhausted parents. By sedating their child for two or three nights, the parents can obtain some respite and sleep themselves which may enable them to tackle the problem more actively and consistently. I prefer trimeprazine or dichloralphenazone, but promethazine is an alternative. Benzodiazepines can produce a state of irritable unhappiness and are best avoided. Parents need to be advised to give a sufficiently large dose at least 1 h before it is intended to work; they often expect instant results and, therefore, wait until the last moment when the child is upset and aroused.

Dreaming

Dreams are a universal experience and frightening dreams are very common in childhood. Nightmares are distinguished clinically from sleep terrors (see below) by the fact that the child can remember them. This may mean that the child becomes reluctant to go to bed or settle to sleep for a few nights. Nightmares are common and need only arouse medical interest if they are excessively frequent (for instance more than once a week over a period) or repetitive in content. A traumatic experience such as a road traffic accident can be followed by dreams with a stereotypic content for 2 or 3 years, even if there are no other clinical signs. In my experience the content need not be an accurate recollection of the accident and in young children there can be a fixed repetitive content which would require symbolic interpretation and may even defy that. An example of this is provided below:

A four-year old boy survived unhurt a motorway accident in which his brother was killed and he was admitted overnight to hospital. For three years he experienced a dream in which he saw a man with a stick standing by a road and facing away from him. This recurred three or four nights a week and would wake him in a state of overwhelming fear. He did not know who the man was, nor what he was doing. In the dream he would try to see the man's face or speak to him but never succeeded in either. The dream would consistently occur following any visit to a hospital.

Various strategies can assist the resolution of recurrent nightmares. Simple discussion of past traumata or present stresses is sensible. Encouraging the child to tell the story of the dream at bedtime and then impose a happy ending on it can be carried out by a parent while settling the child. It is possible to suppress REM sleep with imipramine or most other tricyclics (not trimipramine) and in the case of children with the full syndrome of post-traumatic stress disorder this may be a humane way of providing settled sleep for a few weeks. It may break a cycle and result in permanent abolition of a post-traumatic nightmare.

PARASOMNIAS

The term parasomnia is imprecise and has been used to describe any episodic behaviour in sleep. More recently there has been a tendency to use it more selectively to refer to disturbances of the architecture of sleep, particularly the arousal disorders: sleep walking and sleep terrors.

Most small children show a transitional and partial waking towards the end of the first sleep cycle when deep (stage 4) slow-wave sleep stops and there is a rapid transition to light sleep. They sigh, rub their eyes with the back of their hand, may open them briefly but then roll over and return to sleep. The process is unremarkable but is at the benign end of a continuum of behaviours which are, in their severer forms, often associated with emotional arousal.[16] All are effectively produced by an overshoot from a phase of slow-wave sleep with well-organised, symmetrical, regular delta rhythm into confused consciousness as there is an eruption from deep to very shallow sleep or even electrophysiological wakefulness, sometimes called the 'four to zero shift'.

Sleepwalking

Quiet sleepwalking can be observed in about 15% of children aged 5–12 years.[17] Following a rather brief first slow-wave sleep stage, the child sits up in bed (and may be found so doing) before walking purposelessly and sedately with open eyes and an unsteady, even ataxic gait. He may head for a wardrobe and urinate in it in the confused belief that it is the lavatory. The EEG shows a partial awakening with a mixture of non-REM and paroxysmal sleep patterns or may be indistinguishable from wakefulness. Clinically the child is in lowered, dissociated consciousness. Ordinary children can be induced to walk during sleep by getting them upright and setting them on their feet.

Agitated sleepwalking is less common though seems physiologically similar. The child rushes from his bed and may plunge from a window or escape through a house door. He is likely to mumble or speak briefly but inappropriately. Contrary to folklore, some such children injure themselves, occasionally severely, in falls from windows and it is crucial to ensure that windows and doors are locked. A comparable phenomenon is the confusional arousal in which the child stays in bed but thrashes around and appears fearful of something although it is impossible to discover what. The parents say that although the child's eyes are open they cannot communicate and the child pushes them away when they try questioning or reassurance.

Sleep terrors

A sleep terror (previously known as a night terror) is a dramatic occurrence with a familiar picture. It is most likely to occur in children aged between 3–11 years though its precise prevalence is unknown since most parents refer to sleep terrors as nightmares. About an hour and a half after falling asleep, the child abruptly sits up and screams. The parents find the child sitting in or standing by the bed, obviously frightened, with a wide-eyed stare and dilated pupils. The child is breathing rapidly, sweating and has a very high pulse rate; the normal dampening of vegetative and emotional functions typical of slow-wave sleep has been abruptly removed. The child may shout incoherently or speak a few short phrases. Many children will be evidently hallucinated and attempt to push an imaginary object or person away. The parents' attempts to soothe are typically rejected; they cannot console the child, who does not acknowledge their presence or accept their offer of a cuddle unless the child wakes completely. After a period varying from a few seconds to as long as half an hour the child lies back down in bed and falls asleep.

Parasomnias generally

All the above share common characteristics. They occur in a state of confused consciousness and cannot be recalled subsequently. There is a rapid shift from deep to shallow sleep at the end of the first sleep cycle. A family history is common, probably reflecting a dominant inheritance, at least if there is persistence beyond childhood.[18] They can be precipitated by stress or intercurrent physical illness but can also arise spontaneously. It does not matter if parents wake a child experiencing a parasomnia but it is difficult to do so.

The natural history of parasomnias is benign in most instances. Although quite common in childhood they are rare in adult life. Many children will only sleepwalk or experience a sleep terror a few times. Accordingly, the appropriate thing to do in many instances is reassure. For more persistent problems, anticipatory waking is worth trying. The most likely time for the parasomnia is established by the parents keeping a diary. Once the time can be predicted, the child is woken gently by the parents 15 min before the parasomnia is due. This is repeated every night for a week. Lask[19] reports good and lasting results but anecdotal reports from others (self included) indicate that it is often difficult to predict a time. In some, mainly older, children the outcome may be that the parasomnia appears later in the night. It is possible to block deep slow-wave sleep with a variety of agents, mainly benzodiazepines, and so stop a parasomnia occurring. My practice is to reserve this for severe cases where anticipatory waking is impossible because of infrequent but severe episodes or where it has failed. Diazepam, 2–8 mg or clonazepam 0.5 mg at bedtime is given regularly for a month and then tailed off to be reinstated if there is recurrence. Only very occasional cases have needed more than 1 month and in such circumstances it is wise to consider the possibility of nocturnal complex seizures.

Other episodic behaviours in sleep which do not necessarily show the close association with abrupt emergence from slow-wave sleep include head rolling, sleep talking and toothgrinding (bruxism). These tend to occur in light sleep and not in REM sleep as is often thought. It is rarely necessary to treat them though severe bruxism can present dental problems in which case, anecdotal reports suggest the effectiveness of a tricyclic such as dothiepin taken shortly before bedtime. Plastic mouthguards worn at night and relaxation training also have their advocates.

NOCTURNAL COMPLEX SEIZURES

Although not a disorder of sleep, these can give rise to odd behaviour during sleep and can mimic a parasomnia, particularly when the focus is in the frontal lobe. Seizures can then take the form of rhythmic automatisms, rocking or thrashing, quite often with accompanying vocalisations which can include shouts and screams. They may be followed by complex motor actions: partial dressing, running out of the bedroom or even, in one of my cases, doing the washing up. This is sometimes termed episodic nocturnal wandering and is usually seen in older teenagers. EEG recording during this phase does not reveal seizure activity and it may well be a form of post-ictal automatism.

Routine inter-ictal EEG will not necessarily be abnormal in nocturnal seizures and monitoring during sleep is essential, if possible with a domestic recorder over several nights. If this is not possible, observation in hospital with simultaneous recording using a low-light video or security camera in parallel with an EEG is an alternative. The electrodes need placing low on the forehead, even below the eyebrows in the orbit, in order to pick up seizure activity from the inferior frontal cortex.

In the clinical differentiation from parasomnias, it may be helpful to note the fact that seizures may occur at any stage of the night and sometimes several times a night. Their onset and cessation are typically abrupt and the seizure activity itself is brief except in the case of post-ictal automatisms. The assessment and differential diagnosis is difficult and reference to Stores' review[20] is essential.

It now seems likely that episodic posturing in sleep, commonly termed hypnogenic paroxysmal dystonia, is itself epileptic and frequently responds to carbamazepine.[21]

HEAD BANGING AND ROLLING

Rhythmic rolling of the head from side to side or banging it against the sides of the cot as a prelude to sleep is not uncommon among babies and toddlers. It may recur during the night, curiously unassociated with calling for parents even though the picture is of a child who has woken and is trying to get back to sleep. Determined bangers hammer their heads against a pillow or cotside rocking forward and backward in an all-fours position. It seems to instil a dreamy, abstracted state of mind and child practitioners are insistent on carrying it out in order to get to sleep. How much is intentional, how much is automatic and possibly arising in light sleep is unclear. The children do not harm themselves beyond some mild bruising. Most cases grow out of it, so the management is essentially one of containment: tethering the cot, padding its sides, ignoring it as far as is possible. Various management strategies have been tried for children who persist with the habit: setting a loud metronome to beat synchronously and then slowing it incrementally each subsequent night, sedation with antihistamines, prohibiting parental intervention to avoid covert reinforcement, fitting movement- or noise- sensitive alarms. None of these can be guaranteed to work and some experimentation is inevitable. The occasional case proves to be very difficult to treat successfully.

REM SLEEP BEHAVIOUR DISORDER

In normal REM sleep, striated muscle tone is inhibited and there is a virtual paralysis of voluntary movement. Some adults and children do not seem to have this as part of their REM sleep, so that they retain the ability to act out their dreams and may injure themselves or others in so doing.[22] Typically, there is jerking of the limbs and shouting, punching and kicking. Most cases described in children have had brain stem lesions[20] and respond to REM blockade using tricyclics or clonazepam.[23]

NARCOLEPSY

Although the diagnosis of narcolepsy is usually made in young adults, the condition has frequently been present in partial form for years beforehand.

One can expect about half of all cases to present one of the four elements of the narcoleptic tetrad (attacks of irresistible sleep, cataplexy, sleep paralysis, hypnagogic hallucinations) before the age of 15 and it is exceptional for the full tetrad to present before puberty.[24] The most common picture in middle childhood is that of lengthy sleep at night (10 h or more) and a reluctance to give up the practice of naps during the day.[25] Affected children are quite commonly obese.[24]

The daytime sleep attacks are ultimately irresistible though can be fought off for a while. They may occur at any time and last from a few minutes to hours. For diagnostic purposes it is important to clarify that they are not a consequence of insufficient or poor quality nocturnal sleep. In childhood and early adolescence lengthy night sleep is a common symptom and may be followed by substantial difficulty rousing in the morning when irritability or even confusion are evident.

Cataplexy presents as droopiness or falls when muscle tone is lost secondary to strong emotion: surprise, laughter, or anger. It is effectively REM sleep atonia in the waking state and can be misdiagnosed as clumsiness, conversion hysteria or attention-seeking behaviour, especially if only a few muscle groups are affected. Usually there is no loss of consciousness though occasionally a cataplectic attack can progress into sleep. Children tend to describe it as 'dizziness'.

Sleep paralysis, the subjective experience of muscular atonia, and auditory, visual or tactile hypnogogic hallucinations at the point of falling asleep are the result of entering REM sleep straightaway at sleep onset, a sign which can be confirmed by polysomnography. Both experiences are frightening and can result in the child's refusal to settle to sleep alone, even for daytime naps when they can occur. The child's report of hallucinations can give rise to suspicions of schizophrenia. Sleep paralysis can also occur as an isolated symptom, especially when a child wakes out of a nightmare but is still affected by REM motor inhibition.

Clearly it is necessary to keep the possibility of narcolepsy in mind when confronted by a sleepy child. Questioning about the clinical features of the tetrad can be extended by asking about microsleeps in which the child pauses in activity for about 5–10 s, eyes open but poorly responsive to external stimuli. This can easily be mistaken for an absence seizure though lasts a little longer. It can adversely affect academic progress at school.

A sleep EEG shows that the child enters REM sleep immediately when falling asleep with fragmentation and disruption of subsequent REM episodes. In virtually all affected cases the HLA-DR2 antigen can be demonstrated,[26,27] though its frequency in the general population is 30–35%. The multiple sleep latency test is a quick screen which can be carried out at home. The child is allowed to have five naps, 2 h apart, during the day and the time taken for the child to fall asleep is discreetly measured. If the mean time taken to fall asleep is less than 7 min, pathological sleepiness (not necessarily secondary to narcolepsy) is present.

Management of narcolepsy is best undertaken in an expert centre. This allows mutual support from other sufferers. Information for child and parents about the condition allows parents to understand the cataplectic falls or the fear of falling asleep secondary to hypnagogic hallucinations and sleep paralysis. Arrangements with the child's school should be made to allow a nap in late morning and early afternoon since there is often a refractory period of 2 h or so which can then be capitalised upon.

Most cases will require medication. Various stimulants – mazindol, methylphenidate, pemoline, amphetamine or even coffee– can provide relief and each has its advantages and disadvantages. Height, weight and blood pressure need regular monitoring. Cataplexy may be unaffected by stimulants and require clomipramine or viloxazine in a single daily dose for its control

KLEINE LEVIN SYNDROME

This rare condition presents in teenage boys with episodes lasting several days in which there is drowsy, confused behaviour with irritability, social withdrawal and overeating. In such a phase, the young person may be sexually disinhibited and experience dream-like experiences, often horrifying. Episodes recur every few weeks or months but without a precise cycle. Before an episode there may be a day or two of depersonalisation, altered time perception and a feeling or disengagement from surrounding events. Weight gain following the overeating can be dramatic with the appearance of livid stretch marks on abdomen and thighs. Between episodes, the boy is entirely normal and has only a hazy, embarrassed memory of the disturbed behaviour and experiences. An illustrative case is as follows:

> *A 15-year old boy, head of house at his school and an outstanding sportsman, began to develop patches of behaviour in which he would retire to bed and refuse to get dressed. At the same time he would raid the fridge and steal food from other peoples' plates at meals. He masturbated openly in front of his sister, making suggestive remarks. He appeared drowsy and was uncooperative, resisting attempts to get him to moderate his behaviour. He complained of `visions' of dogs running into a barbed wire fence, severing their own heads.*

Routine EEG and hypnograms (a processed EEG identifying stages of sleep) are normal as is cerebral imaging so the diagnosis is made clinically. It is unlikely to be missed though can be mistaken for depression or bulimia if a mental state examination is not undertaken. The cause is quite unknown.

It will be a long time before anyone collects enough cases for a controlled trial but the anecdotal evidence from several case reports is that lithium taken prophylactically is very effective at preventing relapse. In the above case it provided total protection but relapse followed within days if it was stopped. Carbamazepine is either ineffective or weak as a prophylactic. Appetite suppressants such as D-fenfluramine and stimulants such as methylphenidate may limit the overeating but have little major effect. The natural history is for the condition usually to burn out in early adult life.

MISCELLANEOUS HYPERSOMNIAS

Some adolescents and adults sleep more, and more readily, than others. Drowsiness in the afternoon is unusual in middle childhood but becomes common after puberty. Frequent, long naps during the day associated with rapid falling asleep at night and difficulty waking in the morning may be simply normal variation but can also be seen after viral infections when it seems to be a response to chronic tiredness rather than sleepiness. A further group may have daytime sleepiness associated with hypotension and Raynaud's phenomenon.[28] These conditions are sometimes collectively termed idiopathic CNS hypersomnia.

Some authorities identify a separate syndrome of sleep drunkenness in which there is no excessive daytime sleepiness but the adolescent finds it almost impossible to wake spontaneously in the morning. Attempts by others to wake him are met by irritability and are often unsuccessful. Clearly this blends into normal behaviour but in a few individuals is sufficient of a problem to be regarded as a disorder. In some it is associated with partial waking and complex automatic behaviour at the ordinary time of rousing. Severe cases need waking early and a single dose of methylphenidate or amphetamine given orally so that waking an hour later is easier.

A periodic monthly hypersomnia lasting several days and ending when menstruation begins has been described in a small series from Stanford.[29] This starts within two years of menarche and burns itself out in early adult life.

Obstructive sleep apnoea syndrome

Brief apnoeic spells lasting a few seconds are quite common among babies in their first few months of life and a well-recognised problem in low-birth-weight babies. Most of these are central in origin but there are various conditions which produce an obstructive apnoea in infancy and childhood. These include hypertrophied tonsils and adenoids, obesity, Pierre-Robin and Down syndromes, cerebral palsy and muscular dystrophy. These factors can coexist and interact to yield an end result of upper airway partial obstruction and loud snoring. Characteristically, the child adopts an unusual sleeping position and sweats copiously during the night. Sleep is unsettled and there is frequent waking. In consequence, the child is drowsy and inattentive during the day so that school progress is affected. A number of affected children also show daytime behavioural problems, such as hyperactivity, irritability, rebelliousness and aggressive behaviour at home.[30]

Investigation requires simple examination of upper airways followed by polysomnography and overnight oximetry though the latter is insufficiently discriminating if it is the only test.[31]

Where the cause is adenotonsillar hypertrophy, then tonsillectomy, adenoidectomy or both are effective.[32].

INSOMNIA AT SLEEP ONSET

Toddlers may be reluctant to settle to sleep for the reasons given above. Adolescents typically find reasons to stay up late and may establish a sleep rhythm for themselves which is out of phase with their parents but the total sleep time they enjoy is normal. Occasionally their parents label this pattern as insomnia but if left to their own devices the adolescents show a short sleep latency and most are almost certainly chronically sleep deprived. Nevertheless, there are grounds for thinking that some of the reluctance of adolescents to go to bed may be grounded in biology and a delayed sleep phase may be something which ordinarily develops at puberty.[33] It has long been established that afternoon drowsiness is a phenomenon which appears at puberty and occurs independently of heavy or alcoholic lunches.[34]

Teenagers who adopt late bedtimes can go to extremes and find themselves seriously out of synchrony with the rest of the world. The conventional approach to this is to persuade them to go to bed progressively 2 h **later** each night, thus walking them around the clock until a more sensible bedtime is arrived at. Recently, however, there has been interest in vitamin B_{12} and a couple of cases have been reported in which a short course of methylcobalamin, 3 mg daily orally, has been dramatically effective in restoring normal sleep cycle synchrony.[35] It may also be useful in cases of hypernychthemeral syndrome in which blind people adopt a sleep-wake cycle of longer than 24 h so move in and out of synchrony with everyone else.

True insomnia in the sense of difficulties in falling asleep, staying asleep or obtaining enough sleep to be refreshed, is most likely to result from anxiety,[36] though licit or illicit self-medication and excessive caffeine intake should also be considered.

SLEEP PROBLEMS IN CHILDREN WITH GENERAL LEARNING DISABILITY

In a thorough review of this topic, Stores[37] makes the point that this is an area of considerable concern to a number of parents yet is very poorly studied. Immature and disordered sleep physiology is an understandable feature of generally delayed development and problems typical of normal preschool children: settling difficulties, nocturnal waking and short sleep time, are all common among mentally handicapped children of school-age. They may be more difficult to deal with because the child is simply larger than a toddler or because of associated communication problems.

Some conditions show particular associations: daytime hypersomnia is characteristic of Prader-Willi syndrome and obstructive sleep apnoea likely in

Down's syndrome and the mucopolysaccharidoses. There seems to be a general association between the degree of intellectual retardation and sleep problems but disentangling the causal mechanisms is difficult. Various factors such as obesity and sleep architecture abnormalities can coexist[38] and an approach to formulating the problem in terms of the individual child's characteristics is more fruitful than assuming the primary developmental condition predicts the sleep problem.

SLEEP PROBLEMS ASSOCIATED WITH OTHER CLINICAL CONDITIONS

Chronic physical disorder can adversely affect sleep quality. Pain, cough or itching are obvious instances but difficulties in turning over at night can be overlooked yet cause substantial discomfort and disrupt sleep. Enuresis is not definitely a disorder of sleep but can be difficult to treat in a heavy sleeper. Head injury, epilepsy, and chronic fatigue syndromes can disrupt sleep by means of a number of mechanisms.

The toxic effects of medication on sleep are usually underestimated but bronchodilators can stimulate the CNS and cause almost as much disruption of sleep as can wheezing or coughing. A number of illicit drugs can, of course, affect sleep and a confidential history of both licit and illicit drug taking needs to be taken from any adolescent who has an abnormal sleep pattern.

Severe depressive disorder in adolescence is associated with the same sorts of sleep disruption as in adults: difficulties getting off to sleep and frequent waking during the night as well as a shortened time to the first episode of REM sleep.[39] Rather similar adverse effects on the quality of sleep can be seen in anorexia nervosa which suggests that starvation is the fundamental cause. Much less consistent findings have emerged when hyperkinetic disorder has been studied and the simplest thing to say is that in this condition there is no pattern of disturbed sleep which has been established and indeed no definite evidence that sleep is affected.

CONCLUSION

Sleep problems and disorders are common among children and teenagers. They can adversely affect the quality of life of parents, disrupt family life and compromise the academic progress of children. Asking about disturbances during the night and sleepiness during the day is a reasonable addition to routine history taking. It may lead to an intervention with resultant health gain for child and family. Treatment of sleep disorders is rewarding both in terms of resolving the lead clinical problem and in improving daytime behaviour and relationships with parents.[40]

KEY POINTS FOR CLINICAL PRACTICE

1. It is helpful to conceptualise failure to settle to sleep in the evening as an inability to settle to sleep alone and unaided; a lack of a skill which can be learned.

2. So-called night waking is quite likely to be fundamentally the child's inability to settle himself back to sleep unaided.

3. Anticipatory waking may be effective for both night waking and parasomnias.

4. Nightmares following a traumatic experience can be blocked with tricyclics.

5. Sleep walking, especially in its agitated form, is potentially dangerous.

6. Sleep terrors are not remembered by the child in the morning.

7. Nocturnal complex seizures can mimic parasomnias.

8. The waking EEG may be normal in the case of nocturnal seizures.

9. Narcolepsy in children presents with a partial picture, and especially with prolonged night-time sleep.

10. Cataplexy can be restricted to a few muscle groups. It is often subjectively described as 'dizziness'.

11. Microsleeps in narcolepsy can mimic absence seizures.

12. Children who snore may have obstructive sleep apnoea.

13. An adolescent who complains of insomnia is most likely to be anxious.

14. Treatment of sleep disorders can improve daytime behaviour and school performance.

REFERENCES

1. Kahn A, Van de Merckt C, Rebuffat E et al. Sleep problems in healthy preadolescents. Pediatrics 1989; 84: 542–546
2. Adair R, Zuckerman B, Bauchner H, Philipp B, Levenson S. Reducing night waking in infancy: a primary care intervention. Pediatrics 1992; 89: 585–588
3. Hall D, Hill P, Elliman D. The Child Surveillance Handbook, 2nd Edn. Oxford: Radcliffe Medical Press, 1994

4. Jan JE, Espezel H, Appleton RE. The treatment of sleep disorders with melatonin. Dev Med Child Neurol 1994; 36: 97–107
5. Minde K, Popiel K, Leos N, Falkner S, Parker K, Handley-Derry M. The evaluation and treatment of sleep disturbances in young children. J Child Psychol Psychiatry 1993; 34: 521–533
6. Benoit D, Zeanah C, Boucher C, Minde K. Sleep disorders in early childhood: association with insecure maternal attachment. J Am Acad Child Adolesc Psychiatry 1992; 31: 86–93
7. Messer D, Richards MPM. The development of sleeping difficulties. In: St James Roberts I, Harris G, Messer D, eds. Infant Crying, Feeding and Sleeping: Problems and Treatments. London: Harvester Wheatsheaf, 1993
8. Wolke D, Meyer R, Ohrt B, Riegel K. The incidence of sleeping problems in preterm and fullterm infants discharged from neonatal special care units: an epidemiological study. J Child Psychol Psychiatry 1995; 36: 203–223
9. Kahn A, Mozin MJ, Rebuffat E., Sottiaux M, Muller MF. Milk intolerance in children with persistent sleeplessness: a prospective double-blind crossover evaluation. Pediatrics 1989; 84: 595–603
10. Mitchell EA, Scragg R. Are infants sharing a bed with another person at increased risk of sudden infant death syndrome? Sleep 1993; 16: 387–389
11. McKenna JJ, Thoman EB, Anders TF, Sadeh A, Schechtman VL, Glotzbach SF. Infant-parent co-sleeping in an evolutionary perspective: implications for understanding infant sleep development and the sudden infant death syndrome. Sleep 1993; 16: 263–282
12. Madansky D, Edelbrock C. Cosleeping in a community sample of 2- and 3-year-old children. Pediatrics 1990; 86: 197–203
13. Rickert VI, Johnson CM. Reducing nocturnal awakening and crying episodes in infants and young children: a comparison between scheduled awakenings and systematic ignoring. Pediatrics 1988; 81: 203–212
14. Sadeh A, Larie P, Scher A, Tirosh E, Epstein R. Actigraphic home-monitoring sleep disturbed and control infants and young children: a new method for pediatric assessment of sleep-wake patterns. Pediatrics 1991; 87: 494–499
15. Horne J. Why we Sleep: the Functions of Sleep in Humans and Other Mammals. Oxford: Oxford University Press, 1988
16. Hill P. Sleep disorders in childhood and adolescence. In: Horne J. ed. Sleep Disorders: Current Approaches. Southampton, Duphar Medical Relations, 1989
17. Klackenberg G. Somnambulism in childhood – prevalence, course and behavioral correlates. Acta Psychiatr Scand 1982; 71: 495–499
18. Hallstrom R. Night terrors in adults through three generations. Acta Psychiatr Scand 1972; 48: 350–352
19. Lask B. Novel and non-toxic treatment for night terrors. BMJ 1988; 297: 592
20. Stores G. Confusions concerning sleep disorders and the epilepsies in children and adolescents. Br J Psychiatry 1991; 158: 1–7
21. Hirsch E. Abnormal paroxysmal postures and movements during sleep: partial epilepsy or paroxysmal hypnogenic dystonia? In: Horne J. ed. Sleep '90. Bochum: Pontenagel Press, 1990
22. Mahowald MW, Schenck CH. REM sleep behaviour disorder. In: Kryger MH, Roth T, Dement WC. eds. Principles and Practice of Sleep Medicine. Philadelphia: Saunders, 1992
23. Horne J. Sleep and its disorders in children. J Child Psychol Psychiatry 1992; 33: 473–487
24. Dahl RE, Holttum J, Trubruck L. A clinical picture of child and adolescent narcolepsy. J Am Acad Child Adolesc Psychiatry 1994; 33: 834–841
25. Guilleminault C. Narcolepsy and its differential diagnosis. In: Guilleminault C. ed.Sleep and Its Disorders in Children. New York: Raven Press, 1987
26. Honda Y, Asaka A, Tanaka Y, Juji T. Discrimination of narcolepsy by using genetic markers and HLA. Sleep Res 1983; 12 :254
27. Langdon N, Welsh KI, Van Dam M, Vaughan RW, Parkes JD. Genetic markers in narcolepsy. Lancet 1984; ii: 1178–1180
28. Guilleminault, C. Disorders of excessive sleepiness. Ann Clin Res 1986; 17: 209–219
29. Billiard M, Guilleminault C, Dement WC. A menstruation-linked periodic hypersomnia, Kleine-Levin syndrome or a new clinical entity? Neurology 1975; 25: 436–443
30. Ali NJ, Pitson DJ, Stradling JR. Snoring, sleep disturbance and behaviour in 4-5 year olds. Arch Dis Child 1993; 68; 360–366

31. Douglas NJ, Thomas S, Jan MA. Clinical value of polysomnography. Lancet 1992; 339: 347–350
32. Stradling J, Thomas G, Warley ARH, Williams P, Freeland A. Effect of adenotonsillectomy on nocturnal hypoxaemia, sleep disturbance and symptoms in snoring children. Lancet 1990; 335: 249–253
33. Carskadon MA, Vieira C, Acebo C. Association between puberty and delayed phase preference. Sleep 1993; 16: 258–262
34. Carskadon MA, Harvey K, Duke P, Anders TF, Litt IF, Dement WC. Pubertal changes in daytime sleepiness. Sleep 1980; 2: 453–460
35. Ohta T, Ando K, Iwata T et al. Treatment of persistent sleep-wake schedule disorders in adolescents with methylcobalamin (vitamin B_{12}). Sleep 1991; 14: 414–418
36. Hill P. Adolescent Psychiatry. Edinburgh: Churchill Livingstone, 1989: 239–240
37. Stores G. Sleep studies in children with a mental handicap. J Child Psychol Psychiatry 1992; 33: 1303–1317
38. Hertz G, Cataletto M, Feinsilver SH, Angulo M. Sleep and breathing patterns in patients with Prader Willi syndrome (PWS): effects of age and gender. Sleep 1993; 16: 366–371
39. Hill P. Sleep disorders in depression and anxiety: issues in childhood and adolescence. J Psychosom Res 1994; 38(Suppl. 1): 61–67
40. Minde K, Faucon A, Falkner S. Sleep problems in toddlers: effects of treatment on their daytime behaviour. J Am Acad Child Adolesc Psychiatry 1994; 33: 1114–1121

Paediatric literature review – 1995

T. J. David

ALLERGY & IMMUNOLOGY

Allergy

Colloff MJ, Taylor C, Merrett TG. The use of domestic steam cleaning for the control of house dust mites. Clin Exp Allergy 1995; 25: 1061–1066. *Steam cleaning kills dust mites and reduces concentrations of dust mite antigen.*

Kwittken PL, Sweinberg SK, Campbell DE et al. Latex hypersensitivity in children: clinical presentation and detection of latex-specific immunoglobulin E. Pediatrics 1995; 95: 693–699. *Children with spina bifida and bladder exstrophy have an increased risk.*

Patel L, Radivan FS, David TJ. Management of anaphylactic reactions to food. Arch Dis Child 1995; 71: 370–375. *Review.*

Roesler TA, Bock SA, Leung DYM. Management of the child presenting with allergy to multiple foods. Clin Pediatr 1995; 34: 608–612. *Belief in multiple food allergies is much more common than true hypersensitivity to multiple foods.*

Shaheen SO. Changing patterns of childhood infection and the rise in allergic disease. Clin Exp Allergy 1995; 25: 1034–1037. *Review.*

Immunology

Rosen FS, Cooper MD, Wedgwood RJP. The primary immunodeficiencies. N Engl J Med 1995; 333: 431–440. *Review.*

CARDIOVASCULAR

Cameron JW, Rosenthal A, Olson DA. Malnutrition in hospitalized children with congenital heart disease. Arch Pediatr Adolesc Med 1995; 149: 1098–1102. *Acute and chronic malnutrition occurred in 33% and 64% of the patients, respectively.*

De Giovanni JV. Treatment of arrhythmias by radiofrequency ablation. Arch Dis Child 1995; 73: 385–391. *Review.*

Friedland IR, du Plessis J, Cilliers A. Cardiac complications in children with *Staphylococcus aureus* bacteremia. J Pediatr 1995; 127: 746–748. *Clinically silent endocarditis was detected in 4 (11%) of 36 hospitalized children with staphylococcal bacteremia.*

Meijboom F, Szatmari A, Deckers JW et al. Cardiac status and health-related quality of life in the long term after surgical repair of tetralogy of Fallot in infancy and childhood. J Thoracic Cardiovasc Surg 1995; 95: 883–891. *Encouraging data on late quality of life, physical status and intelligence. See also pp. 786–792.*

Morley R, Leeson Payne C, Lister G et al. Maternal smoking and blood pressure in 7.5 to 8 year old offspring. Arch Dis Child 1995; 72: 120–124. *Maternal smoking may have long term consequences for blood pressure in children.*

COMMUNITY

Blum NJ, Williams GE, Friman PC et al. Disciplining young children: the role of verbal instructions and reasoning. Pediatrics 1995; 96: 336–341. *Review.*

Committee on Children with Disabilities. Guidelines for home care of infants, children, and adolescents with chronic disease. Pediatrics 1995; 96: 161–164. *Review.*

Committee on Community Health Services. Health care for children of farmworker families. Pediatrics 1995; 95: 952–953. *Review and recommendations.*

Cox JE, Bithoney WG. Fathers of children born to adolescent mothers. Predictors of contact with their children at 2 years. Arch Pediatr Adolesc Med 1995; 149: 962–966. *Studies indicate that paternal involvement results in more effective maternal parenting. For review about stepfathers see Arch Dis Child 1995; 73: 487–489.*

Dieckmann RA, Vardis R. High-dose epinephrine in pediatric out-of-hospital cardiopulmonary arrest. Pediatrics 1995; 95: 901–913. *Does not seem to be useful.*

Foulds J, Godfrey C. Counting the costs of children's smoking. BMJ 1995; 311: 1152–1154. *In 1994, 12% of English schoolchildren aged 11–15 were regular smokers.*

Hourihane JO, Rolles CJ. Morbidity from excessive intake of high energy fluids: the `squash drinking syndrome'. Arch Dis Child 1995; 72: 141–143. *Report of 8 children in whom a range of symptoms (e.g. poor appetite) improved when the intake of energy rich fluids was reduced.*

James JA, Laing GJ, Logan S. Changing patterns of iron deficiency anaemia in the second year of life. BMJ 1995; 311: 230. *In an inner-city general practice one quarter of 14 month and 2 year old children were anaemic.*

Kaltenthaler EC, Elsworth AM, Schweiger MS et al. Faecal contamination on children's hands and environmental surfaces in primary schools in Leeds. Epidemiol Infect 1995; 115: 527–534. *Those schools with high hand counts were more likely to have had a reported outbreak of gastroenteritis.*

Patterson JM. Promoting resilience in families experiencing stress. Pediatr Clin North Am 1995; 42: 47–63. *Review.*

Rautava P, Lehtonen L, Helenius H et al. Infantile colic: child and family three years later. Pediatrics 1995; 96: 43–47. *The children in the colic group had more sleeping problems and more frequent temper tantrums (at 3 years of age) than the control group. See also Arch Pediatr Adolesc Med 1995; 149:533-536.*

Taylor EH, Edwards RL. When community resources fail. Assisting the frightened or angry parent. Pediatr Clin North Am 1995; 42: 209–216. *Review.*

Williams CL, Dwyer J, Agostoni C et al. A summary of conference recommendations on dietary fibre in childhood. Pediatrics 1995; 96: 1023–1028. *Minimal dietary fibre intake for children 3 years of age should be equivalent to at least age plus 5 g/day. See other papers on fibre in supplement.*

Accidents

Bijur PE, Trumble A, Harel Y et al. Sports and recreation injuries in US children and adolescents. Arch Pediatr Adolesc Med 1995; 149: 1009–1016. *Sports account for 36% of injuries from all causes. For equestrian injuries see Pediatrics 1995; 95:487–489.*

Brogan TV, Bratton SL, Dowd MD et al. Severe dog bites in children. Pediatrics 1995; 96: 947–950. *Large dogs that are familiar to the child are usually involved. For genital dog bites see Clin Pediatr 1995; 34: 331–333.*

Kemp A, Sibert J. Preventing scalds to children. BMJ 1995; 311: 643–644. *Review.*

Koskiniemi M, Kyykka T, Nybo T et al. Long-term outcome after severe brain injury in preschoolers is worse than expected. Arch Pediatr Adolesc Med 1995; 149: 249–254. *Follow-up data into adult life in 39 children.*

Murray TM, Livingston LA. Hockey helmets, face masks, and injurious behaviour. Pediatrics 1995; 95: 419–421. *Head and face protection elimates occular facial and dental injuries but is linked with an increase in catastrophic spinal injuries because players adopt a false sense of security when using head and face protection.*

Nixon JW, Kemp AM, Levene S et al. Suffocation, choking, and strangulation in childhood in England and Wales: epidemiology and prevention. Arch Dis Child 1995; 72: 6–10. *Of the 21 choking deaths, 11 occurred while eating and 10 resulted from foreign bodies (only 1 was a toy).*

Pless IB, Taylor HG, Arsenault L. The relationship between vigilance deficits and traffic injuries involving children. Pediatrics 1995; 95: 219–224. *Objective evidence of deficits in vigilance and attention when children are involved with traffic injuries were compared with controls.*

Rimell FL, Thome A, Stool S et al. Characteristics of objects that cause choking in children. JAMA 1995; 274: 1763–1766. *Balloons caused 29% of deaths.*

Roberts I. Injuries to child pedestrians. BMJ 1995; 310: 413–414. *The key to prevention is a change in transport policy. For injury prevention counseling by pediatricians see Pediatrics 1995; 96: 1–4.*

Roberts I. Deaths of children in house fires. BMJ 1995; 311: 1381–1382. *Review.*

Roberts I, Norton R, Jackson R et al. Effect of environmental factors on risk of injury of child pedestrians by motor vehicles: a case-control study. BMJ 1995; 310: 91–94. *Reducing traffic volume and restricting curb parking may help. For driveway injuries see Pediatrics 1995; 95: 405–408.*

Roberts I, Pless B. Social policy as a cause of childhood accidents: the children of lone mothers. BMJ 1995; 311: 925–928. *Children of lone mothers have injury rates that are twice those of children in two parent families.*

Smith GA, Dietrich AM, Garcia CT et al. Epidemiology of shopping cart-related injuries to children. An analysis of national data for 1990 to 1992. Arch Pediatr Adolesc Med 1995; 149: 1207–1210. *Injuries related to shopping trolleys are an important cause of pediatric morbidity. For playground accidents see Acta Paediatr 1995; 84: 573–576, and for infant walkers see Pediatrics 1995; 95: 778–780.*

Child abuse

Bond GR, Dowd MD, Landsman I et al. Unintentional perineal injury in prepubescent girls: a multicenter, prospective report of 56 girls. Pediatrics 1995; 95: 628–631. *The injuries were most commonly to the labia minora. In only 1 was the hymen involved. Hymenal injury suggests sexual abuse.*

Bonnier C, Nassogne MC, Evrard P. Outcome and prognosis of whiplash shaken infant syndrome; late consequences after a symptom-free interval. Dev Med Child Neurol 1995; 37: 943–956. *Full clinical appearance of neurological deficits takes 4 months for the interruption of brain growth, 6–12 months for lesions of the central nervous system long pathways, up to 2 years for epilepsy, and 3–6 years for behavioural and neurospychological signs.*

Carty H, Ratcliffe J. The shaken infant syndrome. BMJ 1995; 310: 344–345. *Review.*

De San Lazaro C. Making paediatric assessment in suspected sexual abuse a therapeutic experience. Arch Dis Child 1995; 73: 174–176. *Review.*

Llewellyn A. The abuse of children with physical disabilities in mainstream schooling. Dev Med Child Neurol 1995; 37: 740–743. *Review.*

Skau K, Mouridsen SE. Munchausen sydrome by proxy: a review. Acta Paediatr 1995; 84: 977–982. *Review.*

Smith R. Osteogenesis imperfecta, non-accidental injury, and temporary brittle bone disease. Arch Dis Child 1995; 72: 169–171. *Controversial review. For other opinions see pp. 171–176.*

Enuresis

Wille S, Anveden I. Social and behavioural perspectives in enuretics, former enuretics and non-enuretic controls. Acta Paediatr 1995; 84: 37–40. *Children with primary nocturnal enuresis were well adjusted individuals and displayed similar social and behavioural traits as their peers.*

Handicap

Armitage IM, Burke JP, Buffin JT. Visual impairment in severe and profound sensorineural deafness. Arch Dis Child 1995; 73: 53–56. *Of 87 children with profound deafness, 29 (35%) had visual impairment.*

Bandini LG, Puelzl-Quinn H, Morelli JA et al. Estimation of energy requirements in persons with severe central nervous system impairment. J Pediatr 1995; 126: 828–832. *Standardized equations overestimate energy needs of individuals with severe CNS impairment. For malnutrition and cerebral palsy see J Pediatr; 1995: 126: 833–839.*

Coleby M. The school-aged siblings of children with disabilities. Dev Med Child Neurol 1995; 37: 415–426. *Siblings demonstrated restricted contact with friends, behaviour difficulties, and increased anxiety.*

Committee on Sports Medicine and Fitness. Atlantoaxial instability in Down's syndrome: subject review. Pediatrics 1995; 96: 151–154. *Review. See also Arch Dis Child 1995; 72: 115–119.*

Crichton JU, Mackinnon M, White CP. The life-expectancy of persons with cerebral palsy. Dev Med Child Neurol 1995; 37: 567–576. *The 30 year survival was 87%.*

Hutchinson T. The classification of disability. Arch Dis Child 1995; 73: 91–99. *Review.*

Larnert G, Ekberg O. Positioning improves the oral and pharyngeal swallowing function in children with cerebral palsy. Acta 1995; 84: 689–692. *In the reclined position with the neck flexed, aspiration decreased in all five children, oral leak diminished in two children and retention improved in one child.*

Morton RE, Khan MA, Murray-Leslie C et al. Atlantoaxial instability in Down's syndrome: a five year follow up study. Arch Dis Child 1995; 72: 115–119. *Radiographs can reliably detect children with chronic instability who may be at risk of gradually developing symptoms.*

Newton RW, Wraith JE. Investigation of developmental delay. Arch Dis Child 1995; 72: 460–465. *Review. See also J Pediatr 1995; 127: 193–199.*

Powls A, Botting N, Cooke RWI et al. Motor impairment in children 12 to 13 years old with a birthweight of less than 1250 g. Arch Dis Child 1995; 72: F62–F66. *Many very low birthweight children have impaired motor skills which persist into adolescence.*

Rosenbloom L. Diagnosis and management of cerebral palsy. Arch Dis Child 1995; 72: 350–354. *Review.*

Sala DA, Grant AD. Prognosis for ambulation in cerebral palsy. Dev Med Child Neurol 1995; 37: 1020–1026. *Review. See also pp. 997–1005.*

Slaney SF, Wilkie AOM, Hirst MC et al. DNA testing for fragile X syndrome in schools for learning difficulties. Arch Dis Child 1995; 72: 33–37. *There are still unrecognised cases of fragile X syndrome.*

Immunisation

Barnett ED, Chen R. Children and international travel: immunizations. Pediatr Infect Dis J 1995; 14: 982–992. *Review.*

Dagan R, Slater PE, Duvdevani P et al. Decay of maternally derived measles antibody in a highly vaccinated population in southern Israel. Pediatr Infect Dis J 1995; 14: 965–969. *Infants older than 6 months of age in a well-immunized population may be poorly protected against measles.*

De Serres G, Boulianne N, Meyer F et al. Measles vaccine efficacy during an outbreak in a highly vaccinated population: incremental increase in protection with age at vaccination up to 18 months. Epidemiol Infect 1995; 115: 315–323. *Vaccine efficacy rose from 85% in children vaccinated at 12 months of age to ≥ 94% in those vaccinated at 15 months and older.*

Evans MR. Children who miss immunisation: implications for eliminating measles. BMJ 1995; 310: 1367–1368. *At current immunisation coverage, 6.8% of children would remain completely unimmunised with a two dose measles schedule incorporating a preschool booster.*

Farrington P, Pugh S, Colville A et al. A new method for active surveillance of adverse events from diphtheria/tetanus/pertussis and measles/mumps/

rubella vaccines. Lancet 1995; 345: 567–569. *Completion of vaccination by 4 months instead of 10 months after the change in the UK to an accelerated immunisation schedule may have resulted in a 4-fold decrease in febrile convulsions attributable to DTP vaccine.*

Grosheide PM, Klokman-Houweling JM, Conyn-van Spaendonck MAE. Programme for preventing perinatal hepatitis B infection through screening of pregnant women and immunisation of infants of infected mothers in the Netherlands, 1989–92. BMJ 1995; 311: 1200–1202. *Prevention for perinatal hepatitis B in an area of low prevalence, when incorporated into existing health care, is feasible and achieves satisfactory coverage rates.*

Hall CB. The recommended childhood immunisation schedule of the United States. Pediatrics 1995; 95: 135–137. *Review.*

Halsey NA, Hall CB. Workshop on conflicting guidelines for the use of vaccines. Pediatrics 1995; 95: 938–941. *Review.*

Hsu CY, Huang LM, Lee CY et al. Local massage after vaccination enhances the immunogenicity of diphtheria- tetanus-pertussis vaccine. Pediatr Infect Dis J 1995; 14: 567–572. *But mild fever and pain were common after massage.*

James JM, Wesley Burks A, Roberson PK et al. Safe administration of the measles vaccine to children allergic to eggs. N Engl J Med 1995; 332: 1262–1266. *The MMR vaccine can be safely administered in a single dose to children with allergy to eggs even those with severe hypersensitivity.*

Krause PR, Klinman DM. Efficacy, immunogenicity, safety, and use of live attenuated chickenpox vaccine. J Pediatr 1995; 127: 518–525. *Review. See also Pediatrics 1995; 95: 791–796.*

Miller E. Acellular pertussis vaccines. Arch Dis Child 1995; 73: 390–391. *Review.*

Nussinovitch M, Harel L, Varsano I. Arthritis after mumps and measles vaccination. Arch Dis Child 1995; 72: 348–349. *The mumps component is the cause. For gait disturbance after MMR see Lancet 1995; 345: 316.*

Ramsay ME, Miller E, Ashworth LAE et al. Adverse events and antibody response to accelerated immunisation in term and preterm infants. Arch Dis Child 1995; 72: 230–232. *These findings support the current recommendations that preterm children are vaccinated at chronological age according to the national schedule.*

Rylance G, Bowen C, Rylance J. Measles and rubella immunisation: information and consent in children. BMJ 1995; 311: 923–924. *Appropriate and necessary involvement of today's socially aware older children may have secondary benefit in influencing the opinions and actions of tomorrow's parents.*

Simpson N, Lenton S, Randall R. Parental refusal to have children immunised: extent and reasons. BMJ 1995; 310: 227 *Homeopathy was given as the reason in 21%, and religion in 16%.*

Strebel PM, Ion-Nedelcu N, Baughman MPH et al. Intramuscular injections within 30 days of immunization with oral poliovirus vaccine – a risk factor for vaccine-associated paralytic poliomyelitis. N Engl J Med 1995; 332: 500–506. *Provocation paralysis, may rarely occur in a child who receives multiple intramuscular injections shortly after exposure to oral poliovirus vaccine. See also pp. 529–530 and Pediatr Infect Dis J 1995; 14: 840–846.*

Infant feeding

Barros FC, Victora CG, Semer TC et al. Use of pacifiers is associated with decreased breast-feeding duration. Pediatrics 1995; 95: 497–499. *Pacifier use is strongly associated with early weaning and should not be recommended for breast fed infants.*

Birch LL, Fisher JA. Appetite and eating behaviour in children. Pediatr Clin North Am 1995; 42: 931–953. *Review.*

Black MM, Dubowitz H, Hutcheson J et al. A randomized clinical trial of home intervention for children with failure to thrive. Pediatrics 1995; 95: 807–814. *Weekly home visits for one year by lay home visitors, supervised by a community health nurse. May have some beneficial impact on child development.*

Committee on Pediatric AIDS. Human milk, breastfeeding, and transmission of human immunodeficiency virus in the United States. Pediatrics 1995; 96: 977–979. *Review.*

Cooper WO, Atherton HD, Kahana M et al. Increased incidence of severe breastfeeding malnutrition and hypernatremia in a metropolitan area. Pediatrics 1995; 96: 957–960. *Breast fed infants under 6 weeks of age can develop severe hypernatraemia in the face of inadequate milk supply.*

Goldfarb J. Extended breastfeeding in the United States. Clin Pediatr 1995; 34: 648–649. *Review. See also pp. 642–647.*

Hodes M. Feeding disorders. Prescribers J 1995; 35: 192–198. *Review.*

Maggioni A, Lifshitz F. Nutritional management of failure to thrive. Pediatr Clin North Am 1995; 42: 791-810. *Review.*

Petter LPM, Hourihane JO, Rolles CJ. Is water out of vogue? A survey of the drinking habits of 2–7 year olds. Arch Dis Child 1995; 72: 137–140. *Young children consume large quantities of squash which constitutes a substantial energy supply.*

Sanders TAB. Vegetarian diets and children. Pediatr Clin North Am 1995; 42: 955–965. *Review.*

Scott FW. AAP recommendations on cow milk, soy, and early infant feeding. Pediatrics 1995; 96: 515–517. *Review.*

SIDS

Byard RW, Burnell RH. Apparent life threatening events and infant holding practices. Arch Dis Child 1995; 73: 502–504. *Certain infants may not respond normally to airway occlusion while being held or nursed.*

Gilman EA, Cheng KK, Winter HR et al. Trends in rates and seasonal distribution of sudden infant deaths in England and Wales, 1988–92. BMJ 1995; 310: 631–632. *The rates fell dramatically in 1992.*

Klonoff-Cohen H, Edelstein SL. Bed sharing and the sudden infant death syndrome. BMJ 1995; 311: 1269–1272. *No significant relation between routine bed sharing and SIDS.*

Mitchell EA, Stewart AW, Clements M et al. Immunisation and the sudden infant death syndrome. Arch Dis Child 1995; 73: 498–501. *There was a reduced chance of SIDS in the 4 days immediately following immunisation.*

Taylor JA, Sanderson M. A reexamination of the risk factors for the sudden infant death syndrome. J Pediatr 1995; 126: 887–891. *If women refrained from smoking while pregnant, up to 30% of SIDS might be prevented. For nicotine effects see Arch Dis Child 1995; 73: 549–551 and for bottle feeding and SIDS see BMJ 1995; 310: 88–90.*

Tonkin SL, Davis SL, Gunn TR. Nasal route for infant resuscitation by mothers. Lancet 1995; 345: 1353–1354. *Recommends the nasal route of air entry be taught to parents for resuscitation of babies.*

Warnock DW, Delves HT, Campell CK et al. Toxic gas generation from plastic mattresses and sudden infant death syndrome. Lancet 1995; 346: 1516–1520. *Does not support the hypothesis that toxic gases from antimony, arsenic or phosphorus are a cause of SIDS. See also pp. 1503–1504, 1557–1558, 345: 386–387, 720 & 1044–1046, and BMJ 1995; 310: 1216–1217.*

Surveillance/screening

Hall DMB, Michel JM. Screening in infancy. Arch Dis Child 1995; 72: 93–96. *Review.*

Phelan PD. Neonatal screening for cystic fibrosis. Thorax 1995; 50: 705–706. *Review. For evidence of benefit of early diagnosis by screening see pp. 712–718.*

Richardson MP, Williamson TJ, Lenton SW et al. Otoacoustic emissions as a screening test for hearing impairment in children. Arch Dis Child 1995; 72: 294–297. *A feasible screening test. For screening in Europe, see Int J Pediatr Otorhinolaryngol 1995; 31: 175–182.*

Robertson C, Aldridge S, Jarman F et al. Late diagnosis of congenital sensorineural hearing impairment: why are detection methods failing. Arch Dis

Child 1995; 72: 11–15. *Poor screen test efficacy, incomplete population coverage, and parental and professional denial.*

DERMATOLOGY

Denning DW, Evans EGV, Kibbler CC et al. Fungal nail disease: a guide to good practice. BMJ 1995; 311: 1277–1281. *Review.*

Van der Stichele RH, Dezeure EM, Bogaert MG. Systematic review of clinical efficacy of topical treatments for head lice. BMJ 1995; 311: 604–608. *Only for permethrin has sufficient evidence been published to show efficacy.*

ENDOCRINOLOGY

Service FJ. Hypoglycemic disorders. N Engl J Med 1995; 332: 1144–1150. *Review.*

Diabetes

Clarke CM, Lee DA. Prevention and treatment of the complications of diabetes mellitus. N Engl J Med 1995; 332: 1210-1217. *Review.*

von Muhlendahl KE, Herkenhoff H. Long-term course of neonatal diabetes. N Engl J Med 1995; 333: 704–708. *Some patients have permanent diabetes, but others have transient or lasting remissions.*

Growth

Castillo-Duran C, Rodriguez A, Venegas G et al. Zinc supplementation and growth of infants born small for gestational age. J Pediatr 1995; 127: 206–211. *Chilean infants born small for gestational age have better weight and linear growth during the first 6 months of life if they receive zinc supplementation.*

Cole TJ, Freeman JV, Preece MA. Body mass index reference curves for the UK, 1990. Arch Dis Child 1995; 73: 25–29. *Centile curves for British children are presented. See also 72: 38–41.*

Cole TJ. Conditional reference charts to assess weight gain in British infants. Arch Dis Child 1995; 73: 8–16. *Compares an infant's current weight with that predicted from their previous weight, allowing for the fact that on average, light infants tend to grow faster than heavier infants.*

Conter V, Cortinovis I, Rogari P et al. Weight growth in infants born to mothers who smoked during pregnancy. BMJ 1995; 310: 768–771. *The deficits of weight at birth in children born to mothers who smoked during pregnancy are overcome by 6 months of age.*

Crowley S, Hindmarsh PC, Matthews DR et al. Growth and the growth hormone axis in prepubertal children with asthma. J Pediatr 1995; 126: 297–303. *Inhaled steroids retard linear growth velocity in children with asthma.*

Freeman JV, Cole TJ, Chinn S et al. Cross sectional stature and weight reference curves for the UK, 1990. Arch Dis Child 1995; 73: 17–24. *New reference curves have been estimated from birth to 20 years for children in 1990. See also Drug Ther Bull 1995; 33: 94.*

Greco L, Power C, Peckham C. Adult outcome of normal children who are short or underweight at age 7 years. BMJ 1995; 310: 696–700. *One in three normal children who was short or underweight at age 7 became a short or underweight adult.*

Hindmarsh PC, Swift PGF. An assessment of growth hormone provocation tests. Arch Dis Child 1995; 72: 362–368. *Review.*

Williams SP, Durbin GM, Morgan MEI et al. Catch up growth and pancreatic function in growth retarded neonates. Arch Dis Child 1995; 73: F158–F161. *Impaired pancreatic exocrine function at birth is associated with severe intrauterine malnutrition and with impaired catch up growth during the first 6 months of life.*

Wollmann HA, Kirchner T, Enders H et al. Growth and symptoms in Silver-Russell syndrome: review on the basis of 386 patients. Eur J Pediatr 1995; 154: 958–968. *Normative data.*

ENT

Prescott CAJ. Nasal obstruction in infancy. Arch Dis Child 1995; 72: 287–289. *Review.*

Otitis media

Barnett ED, Klein JO. The problem of resistant bacteria for the management of acute otitis media. Pediatr Clin North Am 1995; 42: 509–517. *Review. For review of antibiotic resistant pneumococci, see pp. 519–537 and for antibiotic resistance in Group A streptococci see pp. 539–551.*

Berman S. Otitis media in children. N Engl J Med 1995; 332: 1560–1565. *Review.*

Clements DA, Langdon L, Bland C et al. Influenza A vaccine decreases the incidence of otitis media in 6 to 30-month-old children in day care. Arch Pediatr Adolesc Med 1995; 149: 1113–1117. *Influenza is a preventable cause of otitis media. For respiratory syncitial virus as a cause see Pediatrics 1995; 84: 419–423.*

Ey JL, Holberg CJ, Aldous MB et al. Passive smoke exposure and otitis media in the first year of life. Pediatrics 1995; 95: 670–677. *Is a significant risk factor.*

Heikkinen T, Ruuskanen O. Signs and symptoms predicting acute otitis media. Arch Pediatr Adolesc Med 1995; 149: 26–29. *The absence of earache does not preclude acute otitis media.*

Heikkinen T, Ruuskanen O, Ziegler T et al. Short-term use of amoxicillin-clavulanate during upper respiratory tract infection for prevention of acute otitis media. J Pediatr 1995; 126: 313–316. *Otitis media developed in 18% of children receiving amoxicillin clavulanate and 22% of children receiving placebo. For treatment failure with these antibiotics see 126: 799–806.*

Mandel EM, Casselbrant ML, Rockette HE et al. Efficacy of 20-versus 10-day antimicrobial treatment for acute otitis media. Pediatrics 1995; 96: 5–13. *More children were effusion free by the day 20 visit if given antimicrobial treatment for 20 days rather than for 10 days, but recurrence of otitis media during the study period was not prevented by the additional 10 days of treatment.*

Niemela M, Uhari M, Mottonen M. A pacifier increases the risk of recurrent acute otitis media in children in day care centres. Pediatrics 1995; 96: 884–888. *A pacifier is a significant risk factor for recurrent acute otitis media.*

Pichichero ME, Pichichero CL. Persistent acute otitis media: I. Causative pathogens. Pediatr Infect Dis J 1995; 14: 178–183. *The most common pathogens were Pneumococcae (24%), Haemophilus influenzae (7%), Branhamella catarrhalis (7%), Beta haemolytic streptococci (6%) and Staphylococcus aureus (5%). For treatment failure see 14: 183–188.*

Pichichero ME, Pichichero CL. Persistent acute otitis media: II. Antimicrobial treatment. Pediatr Infect Dis J 1995; 14: 183–188. *Treatment failure occurs even when no pathogen is isolated and despite demonstrated in vitro activity against culture proven pathogens.*

Glue ear

Couriel JM. Glue ear: prescribe, operate, or wait. Lancet 1995; 345: 3–4. *Review.*

GASTROENTEROLOGY

Andrew M, Marzinotto V, Pencharz P et al. A cross-sectional study of catheter-related thrombosis in children receiving total parenteral nutrition at home. J Pediatr 1995; 126: 358–363. *A high risk of catheter related deep vein thrombosis. See also Arch Pediatr Adolesc Med 1995; 149: 288–291 and Arch Dis Child 1995; 73: 147–150.*

Barbe T, Losay J, Grimon G et al. Pulmonary arteriovenous shunting in children with liver disease. J Pediatr 1995; 126: 571–579. *The risk is highest in biliary atresia and the polysplenia syndrome.*

Challacombe DN. Screening tests for coeliac disease. Arch Dis Child 1995; 73: 3–7. *Review.*

Davies AEM, Sandhu BK. Diagnosis and treatment of gastro-oesophageal reflux. Arch Dis Child 1995; 73: 82–86. *Review. For reflux and irritability see pp. 121–125.*

Macarthur C, Saunders N, Feldman W. *Helicobacter pylori*, gastroduodenal disease, and recurrent abdominal pain in children. JAMA 1995; 273: 729–734. *Review. See also Pediatrics 1995; 96: 211–215.*

Mowat AP, Davidson LL, Dick MC. Earlier identification of biliary atresia and hepatobiliary disease: selective screening in the third week of life. Arch Dis Child 1995; 72: 90–92. *Review.*

Papadopoulou A, Rawashdeh MO, Brown GA et al. Remission following an elemental diet or prednisolone in Crohn's disease. Acta Paediatr 1995; 84: 79–83. *An elemental diet was better than prednisolone in proximal disease.*

Rubaltelli FF, Dario C, Zancan L. Congenital nonobstructive, nonhemolytic jaundice: effect of tin-mesoporphyrin. Pediatrics 1995; 95: 942–944. *It inhibits heme catabolism and thus the production of bilirubin.*

Stringer MD, Puntis JWL. Short bowel syndrome. Arch Dis Child 1995; 73: 170–173. *Review.*

Sturman JA, Chesney RW. Taurine in pediatric nutrition. Pediatr Clin North Am 1995; 42: 879–897. *Review.*

Terrault N, Wright T. Interferon and hepatitis C. N Engl J Med 1995; 332: 1509–1511. *Review.*

Thompson NP, Montgomery SM, Pounder RE et al. Is measles vaccination a risk factor for inflammatory bowel disease? Lancet 1995; 345: 1071–1074. *It may be. See also pp. 1062–1063.*

Cystic fibrosis

Borowitz DS, Grand RJ, Durie PR. Use of pancreatic enzyme supplements for patients with cystic fibrosis in the context of fibrosing colonopathy. J Pediatr 1995; 127: 681–684. *Review. For gut inflammation and pancreatic enzymes see Lancet 1995; 346: 1265–1266. For radiological features see Lancet 1995; 346: 1496–1497.*

Green MR, Buchanan E, Weaver LT. Nutritional management of the infant with cystic fibrosis. Arch Dis Child 1995; 72: 452–456. *Review. For head growth see pp. 150–152.*

Homnick DN, Spillers CR, Cox SR et al. Single-and multiple-dose-response relationships of beta-carotene in cystic fibrosis. J Pediatr 1995; 127: 491–494. *Dose-proportional increase in β-carotene concentrations were found, although clearance was independent of dose.*

Schwarzenberg SJ, Wielinski CL, Shamieh I et al. Cystic fibrosis-associated colitis and fibrosing colonopathy. J Pediatr 1995; 127: 565–570. *Affected persons have taken larger doses of pancreatic enzymes. See also Lancet 1995; 345: 752–756 and 346: 499–500, 1106–1107, 1247–1251 & 1265–1266.*

GENETICS & MALFORMATIONS

Genetics

Blau HM, Springer ML. Gene therapy – a novel form of drug delivery. N Engl J Med 1995; 333: 1204–1207. *Review. For gene therapy of cystic fibrosis see pp. 823–831 & 871–872.*

Evans K, Gregory CY, Fryer A et al. The role of molecular genetics in the prenatal diagnosis of retinal dystrophies. Eye 1995; 9: 24–28. *Around half the blindness in children in the developed world is genetically determined.*

Fryer A. Genetic testing of children. Arch Dis Child 1995; 73: 97–99. *Review.*

Krontiris TG. Oncogenes. N Engl J Med 1995; 333: 303–306. *Review.*

Postma DS, Bleecker ER, Amelung PJ et al. Genetic susceptibility to asthma – bronchial hyperresponsiveness coinherited with a major gene for atopy. N Engl J Med 1995; 333: 894–900. *A trait for elevated serum total IgE is coinherited with a trait for bronchial hyperresponsiveness. See also BMJ 1995; 311: 776–779 and Lancet 1995; 346: 1262–1265 & 1243.*

Turk J. Fragile X syndrome. Arch Dis Child 1995; 72: 3–5. *Review.*

Malformations

Britz-Cunningham SH, Shah MM, Zuppan CW et al. Mutations of the connexin43 gap-junction gene in patients with heart malformations and defects of laterality. N Engl J Med 1995; 332: 1323–1329. *These mutations are associated with visceroatrial heterotaxia.*

Drolet BA, Clowry L, McTigue MK et al. The hair collar sign: marker for cranial dysraphism. Pediatrics 1995; 96: 309–313. *Consists of a ring of long, dark, coarse hair surrounding a midline scalp nodule.*

Roberts HE, Moore CA, Cragan JD et al. Pediatrics 1995; 96: 880–883. *The widespread use of prenatal diagnostic techniques does not entirely explain the decreasing prevalence of neural tube defects.*

Rothman KJ, Moore LL, Singer MR et al. Teratogenicity of high vitamin A intake. N Engl J Med 1995; 333: 1369–1373. *Among babies born to women receiving a high intake of vitamin A, about 1 infant in 57 had a malformation attributable to the supplement. See also pp. 1414–1415.*

Weng EY, Mortier GR, Graham JM. Beckwith-Wiedemann syndrome. Clin Pediatr 1995; 34: 317–326. *Review.*

Young ID. Diagnosing Prader-Willi syndrome. Lancet 1995; 345: 1590. *Review.*

HAEMATOLOGY

Nuss R, Manco-Johnson M. Hemostasis in Ehlers-Danlos syndrome. Patient report and literature review. Clin Pediatr 1995; 34: 552–555. *Subdural haematuria misdiagnosed as child abuse.*

Ratip S, Skuse D, Porter J et al. Psychosocial and clinical burden of thalassaemia intermedia and its implications for prenatal diagnosis. Arch Dis Child 1995; 72: 408–412. *Over half of the patients had problems with sexual maturation and functioning.*

Reid MM. Chronic idiopathic thrombocytopenic purpura: incidence, treatment, and outcome. Arch Dis Child 1995; 72: 125–128. *A high spontaneous recovery rate is notable.*

Shannon KM, Keith JF, Mentzer WC et al. Recombinant human crythropoietin stimulates erythropoiesis and reduces erythrocyte transfusions in very low birth weight preterm infants. Pediatrics 1995; 95: 1–8. *A weekly dose of 500 U/kg is safe and effective. See also pp. 9–10.*

Shearer MJ. Vitamin K. Lancet 1995; 345: 229–234. *Review.*

Warwick R, Modi N. Guidelines for the administration of blood products. Arch Dis Child 1995; 72: 379–381. *Review.*

Webb DKH. Irradiation in the prevention of transfusion associated graft-versus-host disease. Arch Dis Child 1995; 73: 388–389. *Review.*

Sickle cell disease

Charache S, Terrin ML, Moore RD et al. Effect of hydroxyurea on the frequency of painful crises in sickle cell anemia. N Engl J Med 1995; 332: 1317–1322. *Reduced the rate of painful crises in adults. See also pp. 1372–1374.*

Falletta JM, Woods GM, Verter JI et al. Discontinuing penicillin prophylaxis in children with sickle cell anaemia. J Pediatr 1995; 127: 685–690. *Children with sickle cell anaemia who have not had a prior severe pneumococcal infection or a splenectomy and are receiving comprehensive care may safely stop prophylactic penicillin therapy at 5 years of age.*

Singhal A, Thomas P, Kearney T et al. Acceleration in linear growth after splenectomy for hypersplenism in homozygous sickle cell disease. Arch Dis Child 1995; 72: 227–229. *Accelerated linear growth after the reduction in erythropoietic stress may implicate a specific nutrient deficiency in hypersplenic children with SS.*

Vichinsky EP, Haberkern CM, Neumayr L et al. A comparison of conservative and aggressive transfusion regimens in the perioperative management of sickle cell disease. N Engl J Med 1995; 333: 206–213. *A conservative transfusion regimen was as effective as an aggressive regimen in preventing perioperative complications.*

INFECTIOUS DISEASE

Abramson O, Dagan R, Tal A et al. Severe complications of measles requiring intensive care in infants and young children. Arch Pediatr Adolesc Med 1995; 149: 1237–1240. *Adult respiratory distress syndrome and air leaks were the most severe complications.*

Anonymous. Diagnosis and treatment of streptococcal sore throat. Drug Ther Bull 1995; 33: 9–12. *Review.*

Begg N, Balraj V. Diphtheria: are we ready for it. Arch Dis Child 1995; 73: 568–572. *Review.*

Bhatti N, Law MR, Morris JK et al. Increasing incidence of tuberculosis in England and Wales: a study of the likely causes. BMJ 1995; 310: 967–969. *Major role for socioeconomic factors. See also pp. 963–966.*

Brogan TV, Nizet V, Waldhausen JHT et al. Group A streptococcal necrotizing fasciitis complicating primary varicella: a series of fourteen patients. Pediatr Infect Dis J 1995; 14: 588–594. *An unusual but important association.*

Cohen B. Parvovirus B19: an expanding spectrum of disease. BMJ 1995; 311: 1549–1552. *Review.*

Hussain SM, Luedtke GS, Baker CJ et al. Invasive group B streptococcal disease in children beyond early infancy. Pediatr Infect Dis J 1995; 14: 278–281. *Review of 143 cases.*

Jenkinson D. Natural course of 500 consecutive cases of whooping cough: a general practice population study. BMJ 1995; 310: 299–302. *Most cases of whooping cough are relatively mild. Adults also get whooping cough, especially from their children, and get the same symptoms as children. For erythromycin prophylaxis see Pediatr Infect Dis J 1995; 14: 969–975.*

McCracken GH. Emergence of resistant *Streptococcus pneumoniae*: a problem in pediatrics. Pediatr Infect Dis J 1995; 14: 424–428. *Review. See also pp. 420–423.*

McKendrick MW. Acyclovir for childhood chickenpox. Cost is unjustified. BMJ 1995; 310: 108–109. *Review.*

Mulholland EK, Falade AG, Corrah PT et al. A randomized trial of chloramphenicol vs. trimethoprim-sulfamethoxazole for the treatment of malnourished children with community-acquired pneumonia. Pediatr Infect Dis J 1995; 14: 959–965. *Equally effective.*

Ryan M, Hall SM, Barrett NJ et al. Toxoplasmosis in England and Wales 1981 to 1992. Commun Dis Rep CDR Wkly 1995; 5: R13–R21. *Review. See also pp.R21-R27. For neurological/developmental outcome see Pediatrics 1995; 95: 11–20.*

Schlesinger Y, Buller RS, Brunstrom JE et al. Expanded spectrum of herpes simplex encephalitis in childhood. J Pediatr 1995; 126: 234–241. *Review. See also Pediatr Infect Dis J 1995; 14: 827–832 & 832–835.*

Tracey KJ. TNF and Mae West or: death from too much of a good thing. Lancet 1995; 345: 75 76. *Review.*

AIDS

Bryson YJ, Pang S, Wel LS et al. Clearance of HIV infection in a perinatally infected infant. N Engl J Med 1995; 332: 832–838. *Report of an infant perinatally infected in whom the infection subsequently cleared. See also pp. 883–884.*

Clumeck N. Primary prophylaxis against opportunistic infections in patients with AIDS. N Engl J Med 1995; 332: 739–740. *Review. See also pp. 693–705.*

Danner SA, Carr A, Leonard JM et al. A short-term study of the safety, pharmacokinetics, and efficacy of ritonavir, an inhibitor of HIV-1 protease. N Engl J Med 1995; 333: 1528–1532. *Well tolerated but clinical benefit remains to be established. See also pp. 1534–1539.*

Peckham C, Gibb D. Mother-to-child transmission of the human immunodeficiency virus. N Engl J Med 1995; 333: 298–302. *Review. For immunologic characterization of children vertically infected with HIV, see J Pediatr 1995; 126: 368–374.*

Simonds RJ, Lindegren L, Thomas P et al. Prophylaxis against *Pneumocystis carinii* pneumonia among children with perinatally acquired human immunodeficiency virus infection in the United States. N Engl J Med 1995; 332: 786–790. *If pneumocystis is to be prevented, prophylaxis must be offered to more children than the guidelines currently recommend.*

Gastroenteritis

Ho L, Bradford BJ. Hypernatremic dehydration and rotavirus enteritis. Clin Pediatr 1995; 34: 440–441. *Report of 5 cases.*

Phillips CA. Bird attacks on milk bottles and campylobacter infection. Lancet 1995; 346: 386. *Drinking milk from bottles attacked by birds is unsafe.*

Meningitis

Begg NT, Cartwright KAV, Corbel MJ et al. Control of meningococcal disease: guidance for consultants in communicable disease control. Commun Dis Rep CDR Wkly 1995; 5: R189–R195. *Review. See also pp. R196–R199.*

Britto J, Nadel S, Habibi P et al. Gastrointestinal perforation complicating meningococcal disease. Pediatr Infect Dis J 1995; 14: 393–394. *Report of two cases.*

Grimwood K, Anderson VA, Bond L et al. Adverse outcomes of bacterial meningitis in school-age survivors. Pediatrics 1995; 95: 646–656. *One in four school-age meningitis survivors has either serious and disabling sequelae or a functionally important behaviour disorder, neuropsychologic or auditory dysfunction adversely affecting academic performance.*

Jones DM, Kaczmarski EB. Meningococcal infections in England and Wales: 1994. Commun Dis Rep CDR Wkly 1995; 5: R125–R130. *Review. For meningococcal vaccines see pp. R130–R135, and for early management see pp. R135–R137.*

Kanra GY, Ozen H, Secmeer G et al. Beneficial effects of dexamethasone in children with pneumococcal meningitis. Pediatr Infect Dis J 1995; 14: 490–494. *Incidence of hearing impairment was significantly less than in the placebo group, 3.7% vs 23%.*

Wald ER, Kaplan SL, Mason EO et al. Dexamethasone therapy for children with bacterial meningitis. Pediatrics 1995; 95: 21–28. *Dexamethasone did not significantly improve audiologic, neurologic, or developmental outcome in children with bacterial meningitis. See also pp.29–31 and J Neurol Neurosurg Psychiatry 1995; 59: 31–37.*

Kilpi T, Peltola H, Jauhiainen T et al. Oral glycerol and intravenous dexamethasone in preventing neurologic and audiologic sequelae of childhood bacterial meningitis. Pediatr Infect Dis J 1995; 14: 270–278. *Oral glycerol prevented neurologic sequelae in infants and children with bacterial meningitis more effectively than intravenous dexamethasone.*

Riedo FX, Plikaytis BD, Broome CV. Epidemiology and prevention of meningococcal disease. Pediatr Infect Dis J 1995; 14: 643–657. *Review.*

Shields MD, Adams D, Beresford P et al. Managing meningitis in children: audit of notifications, rifampicin chemoprophylaxis, and audiological referrals. Quality Health Care 1995; 4: 269–272. *Steps often overlooked included notification, chemophrophylaxis of contacts and assessment of hearing at follow up.*

Singhi SC, Singhi PD, Srinivas B et al. Fluid restriction does not improve the outcome of acute meningitis. Pediatr Infect Dis J 1995; 14: 495–503. *In the population studied fluid restriction did not improve outcome and indeed appeared to increase the likelihood of adverse outcome. For therapy with protein C concentrate see J Pediatr 1995; 126: 646–652.*

Tunkel AR, Scheld WM. Acute bacterial meningitis. Lancet 1995; 346: 1675–1680. *Review.*

MEDICINE IN THE TROPICS

Bennett J, Azhar N, Rahim F et al. Further observations on ghee as a risk factor for neonatal tetanus. Int J Epidemiol 1995; 24: 643–647. *Reduction in umbilical ghee use, hand washing and tetanus immunization of mothers would all be helpful.*

Bern C, Nathanail L. Is mid-upper-arm circumference a useful tool for screening in emergency settings. Lancet 1995; 345: 631–633. *It is not a useful substitute for low weight for height.*

Isenberg SJ, Leonard APT, Wood M. A controlled trial of povidone-iodine as prophylaxis against ophthalmia neonatorum. N Engl J Med 1995; 332: 562–566. *More effective than silver nitrate or erythromycin, less toxic and costs less. See also pp.600–601.*

Moosa AA, Quortum HA, Ibrahim MD. Rapid diagnosis of bacterial meningitis with reagent strips. Lancet 1995; 345: 1290–1291. *Reagent strips can distinguish normal from infected CSF and are of value in the diagnosis of meningitis.*

Osborne CM. The challenge of diagnosing childhood tuberculosis in a developing country. Arch Dis Child 1995; 72: 369–374. *Review.*

Gastroenteritis

Bhan MK, Woo EC, Fontaine O et al. Multicentre evaluation of reduced-osmolarity oral rehydration salts solution. Lancet 1995; 345: 282–285. *Has beneficial effects in acute non-cholera diarrhoea.*

Bhattacharya SK, Bhattacharya MK, Manna B et al. Risk factors for development of dehydration in young children with acute watery diarrhoea: a case-control study. Acta Paediatr 1995; 84: 160–164. *Significant risk factors were withdrawal of breastfeeding during diarrhoea and not giving oral rehydration solution during diarrhoea.*

Lebenthal E, Khin-Maung U, Rolston DDK et al. Thermophilic amylase-digested rice-electrolyte solution in the treatment of acute diarrhea in children. Pediatrics 1995; 95: 198–202. *This is an effective form of rehydration.*

Molina S, Vettorazzi C, Peerson JM et al. Clinical trial of glucose-oral rehydration solution (ORS), rice dextrin-ORS, and rice flour-ORS for the management of children with acute diarrhea and mild or moderate dehydration. Pediatrics 1995; 95: 191–197. *The three solutions had similar efficacy for children with acute watery diarrhoea and mild or moderate dehydration.*

Sazawal S, Black RE, Bhan MK et al. Zinc supplementation in young children with acute diarrhea in India. N Engl J Med 1995; 333: 839–844. *Supplementation results in reduction in the duration and severity of diarrhea.*

Immunisation

Coster TS, Killeen KP, Waldor MK et al. Safety, immunogenicity, and efficacy of live attenuated *Vibrio cholerae* 0139 vaccine prototype. Lancet 1995; 345: 949–952. *A safe live attenuated vaccine candidate for cholera caused by the 0139 serogroup.*

Mulholland K. Measles and pertussis in developing countries with good vaccine coverage. Lancet 1995; 345: 305–307. *Review. See also pp. 272–273 and pp. 858–859.*

Whittle HC, Maine N, Pilkington J et al. Long-term efficacy of continuing hepatitis B vaccination in infancy in two Gambian villages. Lancet 1995; 345: 1089–1092. *Vaccination progressively decreased HBV transmission by chronic carriers. See also pp. 1065–1066.*

Infant feeding

Prasad B, de Costello AM. Impact and sustainability of a 'baby friendly' health education intervention at a district hospital in Bihar, India. BMJ 1995; 310: 621–633. *Training doctors and midwives improves feeding practices but refresher training is needed to sustain the improvement.*

Malaria

Aidoo M, Lalvani A, Allsopp CEM et al. Identification of conserved antigenic components for a cytotoxic T lymphocyte-inducing vaccine against malaria. Lancet 1995; 345: 1003–1007. *Provides a basis for the rational design of malaria vaccines. For failure of SPf66 vaccine see Lancet 1995; 346: 462–467 & 1554–1556.*

D'Alessandro U, Olaleye BO, McGuire W et al. Mortality and morbidity from malaria in Gambian children after introduction of an impregnated bednet programme. Lancet 1995; 345: 479–483. *Impregnated nets worked, but at a cost the country could not afford. See also pp. 1056–1057.*

Defo BK. Epidemiology and control of infant and early childhood malaria: a competing risks analysis. Int J Epidemiol 1995; 24: 204–217. *Antenatal care attendance, improved housing conditions and childhood immunization practices are potentially cost-effective strategies for malaria control.*

Marsh K, Forster D, Waruiru C et al. Indicators of life-threatening malaria in African children. N Engl J Med 1995; 332: 1399–1404. *The presence of impaired consciousness or respiratory distress identified those at high risk for death.*

Sadiq ST, Glasgow KW, Drakeley CJ et al. Effects of azithromycin on malariometric indices in The Gambia. Lancet 1995; 346: 881–882. *Despite clearing pre-existing parasitaemia, azithromycin did not significantly prevent new parasitaemia.*

Steele RW, Baffoe-Bonnie B. Cerebral malaria in children. Pediatr Infect Dis J 1995; 14: 281–285. *Review of 187 cases in Ghana.*

Vitamin A

Baqui AH, de Francisco A, Arifeen SE et al. Bulging fontanelle after supplementation with 25000 IU of vitamin A in infancy using immunization contacts. Acta Paediatr 1995; 84: 863–866. *Nine infants (10.5%) supplemented with vitamin A had episodes of bulging of the fontanelle compared with two infants (2.5%) in the placebo group (p < 0.05).*

Bates CJ. Vitamin A. Lancet 1995; 345: 31–35. *Review. See also Arch Dis Child 1995; 72: 106–109.*

Rahi JS, Sripathi S, Gilbert CE et al. Childhood blindness in India: causes in 1318 blind school students in nine states. Eye 1995; 9: 545–550. *The major causes were: (i) corneal staphyloma, scar and phthisis bulbi (mainly attributable to vitamin A deficiency); (ii) microphthalmos, anophthalmos and coloboma; (iii) retinal dystrophies and albinism; and (iv) cataract, uncorrected aphakia and amblyopia.*

Semba RD, Munasir Z, Beeler J et al. Reduced seroconversion to measles in infants given vitamin A with measles vaccination. Lancet 1995; 345: 1330–1332. *Simultaneous high dose vitamin A may interfere with seroconversion to live measles vaccine in infants with maternal antibody. See pp. 1317 and 346: 503–504.*

METABOLIC

Chan GM, Hoffman K, McMurry M. Effects of dairy products on bone and body composition in pubertal girls. J Pediatr 1995; 126: 551–556. *Young girls whose dietary calcium intake was provided primarily by dairy products at or above the recommended dietary allowances had an increased rate of bone mineralization.*

Jones TW, Borg WP, Boulware SD et al. Enhanced adrenomedullary response and increased susceptibility to neuroglycopenia: mechanisms underlying the adverse effects of sugar ingestion in healthy children. J Pediatr 1995; 126: 171–177. *Contributing factor to adverse behavioural and cognitive effects after sugar ingestion.*

Mazariegos-Ramos E, Guerrero-Romero F, Rodriguez-Moran M et al. Consumption of soft drinks with phosphoric acid as a risk factor for the development of hypocalcemia in children: a case-control study. J Pediatr 1995; 126: 940–942. *The intake of > 1.5 l/week of soft drinks containing phosphoric acid is a risk factor for the development of hypocalcemia.*

Poulton J, Brown GK. Investigation of mitochondrial disease. Arch Dis Child 1995; 73: 94–96. *Review.*

Walter JH. Late effects of phenylketonuria. Arch Dis Child 1995; 73: 485–486. *Review.*

Wraith JE. The mucopolysaccharidoses: a clinical review and guide to management. Arch Dis Child 1995; 72: 263–267. *Review.*

Rickets

Pivnick EK, Kerr NC, Kaufman RA et al. Rickets secondary to phosphate depletion. Clin Pediatr 1995; 34: 73–78. *Prolonged treatment with antacids containing aluminium or magnesium may lead to phosphate depletion.*

Train JJA, Yates RW, Sury MRJ. Hypocalcaemic stridor and infantile nutritional rickets. BMJ 1995; 310: 48–49. *Stridor may be a presenting feature.*

MISCELLANEOUS

Abu-Arafeh I, Russell G. Prevalence and clinical features of abdominal migraine compared with those of migraine headache. Arch Dis Child 1995; 72: 413–417. *The similarities between the two conditions are so close as to suggest that they have a common pathogenesis. For pizotifen to treat migraine see pp. 48–50.*

Fraser DR. Vitamin D. Lancet 1995; 345: 104–107. *Review.*

Meydani M. Vitamin E. Lancet 1995; 345: 170–175. *Review.*

Miller ML, Szer I, Yogev R et al. Fever of unknown origin. Pediatr Clin North Am 1995; 42: 999–1015. *Review.*

Morland B. Lymphadenopathy. Arch Dis Child 1995; 73: 476–479. *Review.*

Oakley A, Bendelow G, Barnes J et al. Health and cancer prevention: knowledge and beliefs of children and young people. BMJ 1995; 310: 1029–1033. *Children and young people possess considerable knowledge about cancer.*

Platt MJ, Pharoah POD. Child health statistical review, 1995. Arch Dis Child 1995; 73: 541–548. *Review.*

Royal College of Physicians. Alcohol and the young. Summary of a report of a joint working party of the Royal College of Physicians and the British Paediatric Association. J R Coll Phys Lond 1995; 29: 470–474. *Review.*

Yanagawa H, Yashiro M, Nakamura Y et al. Epidemiologic pictures of Kawasaki disease in Japan: from the nationwide incidence survey in 1991 and 1992. Pediatrics 1995; 95: 475–479. *The incidence rates of Kawasaki disease in Japan are 10 times higher than in the west.*

Yaron M, Lowenstein SR, Koziol-McLain J. Measuring the accuracy of the infrared tympanic thermometer: correlation does not signify agreement. J Emerg Med 1995; 13: 617–621. *Tympanic thermometry may miss children with significant fever.*

NEONATOLOGY

Albert D. Management of suspected tracheobronchial stenosis in ventilated neonates. Arch Dis Child 1995; 72: F1–F2. *Review. See also pp. F3–F7*

Ballin A, Arbel E, Kenet G et al. Autologous umbilical cord blood transfusion. Arch Dis Child 1995; 73: F181–F183. *Safe, provided that bacteriological testing has been done.*

Barker DP, Simpson J, Pawula M et al. Randomised, double blind trial of two loading dose regimens of diamorphine in ventilated newborn infants. Arch Dis Child 1995; 73: F22–F26. *A 50 mcg/kg loading dose is safe and effective; a higher dose is not beneficial.*

Barton JS, Tripp JH, McNinch AW. Neonatal vitamin K prophylaxis in the British Isles: current practice and trends. BMJ 1995; 310: 632–633. *Continuing confusion regarding dose and frequency of administration.*

Bass JL, Mehta KA. Oxygen desaturation of selected term infants in car seats. Pediatrics 1995; 96: 288–290. *Premature and term infants can be at risk of oxygen desaturation in car seats.*

Chetcuti PAJ, Ball RJ. Surfactant apoprotein B deficiency. Arch Dis Child 1995; 73: F125–F127. *Review.*

Chiriboga CA, Vibbert M, Malouf R et al. Neurological correlates of fetal cocaine exposure: transient hypertonia of infancy and early childhood. Pediatrics 1995; 96: 1070–1077. *Cocaine-induced effects are usually symmetri-*

cal, transient, and the majority of exposed children outgrow hypertonia by 24 months of life. See also pp. 259–264.

Coulthard MG, Vernon B. Managing acute renal failure in very low birthweight infants. Arch Dis Child 1995; 73: F187–F192. *Review.*

Fardy CH, Silverman M. Antioxidants in neonatal lung disease. Arch Dis Child 1995; 73: F112–F117. *Review.*

Fishman MA. Validity of brain death criteria in infants. Pediatrics 1995; 96: 513–515. *Review. See also pp. 518–520.*

Forsyth JS, Crighton A. Low birthweight infants and total parenteral nutrition immediately after birth. I. Energy expenditure and respiratory quotient of ventilated and non-ventilated infants. Arch Dis Child 1995; 73: F4–F7. *A mix of carbohydrate and fat from day 1 may not only meet energy needs but may also reduce respiratory quotient. See also pp. F8–F16.*

Haouari N, Wood C, Griffiths G et al. The analgesic effect of sucrose in full term infants: a randomised controlled trial. BMJ 1995; 310: 1498–1500. *Reduces crying and the autonomic effects of a painful procedure.*

Kaplan P, Levinson M, Kaplan BS. Cerebral artery stenoses in Williams syndrome cause strokes in childhood. J Pediatr 1995; 126: 943–945. *Extensive narrowing of lumens of many cerebral arteries caused strokes with brain damage and chronic hemipareses in two children with Williams syndrome. See also pp. 945–948.*

Kinsella JP, Abman SH. Recent developments in the pathophysiology and treatment of persistent pulmonary hypertension of the newborn. J Pediatr 1995; 126: 853–864. *Review.*

Lebenthal E. Gastrointestinal maturation and motility patterns as indicators for feeding the premature infant. Pediatrics 1995; 95: 207–209. *Review.*

Lopriore E, Vandenbussche FPHA, Tiersma ESM et al. Twin-to-twin transfusion syndrome: new perspectives. J Pediatr 1995; 127: 675–680. *Review.*

Neuzil J, Darlow BA, Inder TE et al. Oxidation of parenteral lipid emulsion by ambient and phototherapy lights: potential toxicity of routine parenteral feeding. J Pediatr 1995; 126: 785–790. *Intralipid is highly susceptible to oxidation and elevated levels of oxidized lipids can be formed during its clinical use, especially when combined with phototherapy. See also pp. 747–748.*

Perlman JM, Risser R. Cardiopulmonary resuscitation in the delivery room. Arch Pediatr Adolesc Med 1995; 149: 20–25. *Check the airway one more time before compressing the chest.*

Rehan VK, Menticoglou SM. Mechanisms of visceral damage in fetofetal transfusion syndrome. Arch Dis Child 1995; 73: F48–F50. *Review.*

Richards C, Holmes SJK. Intestinal dilatation in the fetus. Arch Dis Child 1995; 72: F135–F138. *Review.*

Russell GAB, Cooke RWI. Randomised controlled trial of allopurinol prophylaxis in very preterm infants. Arch Dis Child 1995; 73: F27–F31. *There was no difference in the primary endpoint periventricular leucomalacia between the treated and control groups.*

Sanderson C, Hall DMB. The outcomes of neonatal intensive care. BMJ 1995; 310: 681–682. *Review.*

Wiswell TE, Baumgart S, Gannon CM et al. No lumbar puncture in the evaluation for early neonatal sepsis: will meningitis be missed? Pediatrics 1995; 95: 803–806. *If lumbar puncture is omitted as part of the early evaluation, the diagnosis of bacterial meningitis occasionally will be delayed or missed completely.*

Cerebral palsy

Adamson SJ, Alessandri LM, Badawi N et al. Predictors of neonatal encephalopathy in full term infants. BMJ 1995; 311: 598–602. *Intrapartum hypoxia was not the cause of neonatal encephalopathy in most cases in this population.*

Eken P, Toet MC, Groenendaal F et al. Predictive value of early neuroimaging, pulsed Doppler and neurophysiology in full term infants with hypoxic-ischaemic encephalopathy. Arch Dis Child 1995; 73: F75–F80. *The cerebral function monitor and somatosensory evoked potentials provided the most useful information.*

Martin E, Barkovich AJ. Magnetic resonance imaging in perinatal asphyxia. Arch Dis Child 1995; 72: F62–F70. *Review.*

Murphy DJ, Sellers S, MacKenzie IZ et al. Case-control study of antenatal and intrapartum risk factors for cerebral palsy in very preterm singleton babies. Lancet 1995; 346: 1449–1454. *Factors associated with an increased risk of cerebral palsy were chorioamnionitis, prolonged rupture of membranes, and maternal infection.*

Nelson KB, Grether JK. Can magnesium sulfate reduce the risk of cerebral palsy in very low birthweight infants? Pediatrics 1995; 95: 263–269. *Suggests a protective effect.*

Chronic lung disease/bronchopulmonary dysplasia

Gray PH, Burns YR, Mohay HA et al. Neurodevelopmental outcome of preterm infants with bronchopulmonary dysplasia. Arch Dis Child 1995; 73:

F128–F134. *Bronchopulmonary dysplasia is not independently associated with adverse neurodevelopmental outcome.*

Groneck P, Speer CP. Inflammatory mediators and bronchopulmonary dysplasia. Arch Dis Child 1995; 73: F1–F3. *Review.*

Harris MA, Sullivan CE. Sleep pattern and supplementary oxygen requirements in infants with chronic neonatal lung disease. Lancet 1995; 345: 831–832. *In infants with chronic neonatal lung disease, arousal mechanisms minimise oxygen desaturation but induce sleep disruption.*

Jones R, Wincott E, Elbourne D et al. Controlled trial of dexamethasone in neonatal chronic lung disease: a 3-year follow-up. Pediatrics 1995; 96: 897–906. *Despite early benefits, there were no clear effects at 3 years.*

Linder N, Kuint J, German B et al. Hypertrophy of the tongue associated with inhaled corticosteroid therapy in premature infants. J Pediatr 1995; 127: 651–653. *Report of three infants in whom hypertrophy of the tongue developed during beclomethasone inhalation therapy.*

CRIB and other risk scoring systems

de Courcy-Wheeler RHB, Wolfe CDA, Fitzgerald A et al. Use of the CRIB (clinical risk index for babies) score in prediction of neonatal mortality and morbidity. Arch Dis Child 1995; 73: F32–F36. *CRIB adjusted mortality did not demonstrate better performance in units providing the highest level of care.*

Hope P. CRIB, son of Apgar, brother to APACHE. Arch Dis Child 1995; 72: F81–F83. *Review. See also Lancet 1995; 345: 1020–1022.*

Infant feeding

Nissen E, Lilja G, Mattiesen AS et al. Effects of maternal pethidine on infants' developing breast feeding behaviour. Acta Paediatr 1995; 84: 140–145. *Infants exposed to pethidine had delayed and depressed sucking and rooting behaviour.*

Jaundice

Fok TF, Wong W, Cheng AFB. Use of eyepatches in phototherapy: effects on conjunctival bacterial pathogens and conjunctivitis. Pediatr Infect Dis J 1995; 14: 1091–1094. *Significantly more infants in the eyepatches group had purulent eye discharge and clinical conjunctivitis than the controls.*

Garg AK, Prasad RS, Al Hifzi I. A controlled trial of high-intensity double-surface phototherapy on a fluid bed versus conventional phototherapy in neonatal jaundice. Pediatrics 1995; 95: 914–916. *Significantly more effective in reducing bilirubin than conventional phototherapy.*

Kappas A, Drummond GS, Henschke C et al. Direct comparison of Sn-Mesoporphyrin, an inhibitor of bilirubin production, and phototherapy in controlling hyperbilirubinemia in term and near-term newborns. Pediatrics 1995; 95: 468–574. *A single dose of SnMP entirely supplanted the need for phototherapy in jaundiced term and near-term newborns.*

NEPHROLOGY

Woolf AS, Winyard PJD. Unravelling the pathogenesis of cystic kidney diseases. Arch Dis Child 1995; 72: 103–105. *Review.*

Zilleruelo G, Strauss J. HIV nephropathy in children. Pediatr Clin North Am 1995; 42: 1469–1485. *Review.*

Haemolytic uraemic syndrome

Boyce TG, Swerdlow DL, Griffin PM. *Escherichia coli* 0157: H7 and the hemolytic-uremic syndrome. N Engl J Med 1995; 333: 364–368. *Review.*

Nephrotic syndrome

Mendoza SA, Tune BM. Management of the difficult nephrotic patient. Pediatr Clin North Am 1995; 42: 1459–1468. *Review.*

Polito C, La Manna A, Todisco N et al. Bone mineral content in nephrotic children on long-term, alternate-day prednisone therapy. Clin Pediatr 1995; 34: 234–236. *Bone mineral content. See also pp. 237–240.*

Urinary tract infection

Blethyn AJ, Jenkins HR, Roberts R et al. Radiological evidence of constipation in urinary tract infection. Arch Dis Child 1995; 73: 534–535. *Confirms an association between recurrent urinary tract infection and faecal loading. See also Arch Pediatr Adolesc Med 1995; 149: 623–627. For radiological assessment of constipation, see pp. 532–533.*

Gordon I. Vesico-ureteric reflux, urinary-tract infection, and renal damage in children. Lancet 1995; 346: 489–488. *Review.*

Hellerstein S. Urinary tract infections. Old and new concepts. Pediatr Clin North Am 1995; 42: 1433–1457. *Review.*

Merrick MV, Notghi A, Chalmers N et al. Long term follow up to determine the prognostic value of imaging after urinary tract infections. Part I: reflux. Arch Dis Child 1995; 72: 388–392. *Reflux is important as a risk factor for progressive renal damage, but principally when associated with other risk factors, in particular further episodes of infection. For data on scarring see pp.393–396.*

Smellie JM, Rigden SPA, Prescod NP. Urinary tract infection: a comparison of four methods of investigation. Arch Dis Child 1995; 72: 247–250. *Ultrasonography is unreliable in detecting reflux renal scarring, or inflammatory change and, alone, is inadequate for investigating urinary tract infection in children. See also pp. 251–258.*

NEUROLOGY

Cole GF, Stuart CA. A long perspective on childhood multiple sclerosis. Dev Med Child Neurol 1995; 37: 661–666. *Report of 28 cases. See also pp. 667–672.*

North K, Joy P, Yuille D et al. Cognitive function and academic performance in children with neurofibromatosis type 1. Dev Med Child Neurol 1995; 37: 427–436. *Low incidence of intellectual disability but high incidence of specific learning disability.*

Tracey I, Scott RB, Thompson CH et al. Brain abnormalities in Duchenne muscular dystrophy: phosphorus-31 magnetic resonance spectroscopy and neuropsychological study. Lancet 1995; 345: 1260–1264. *The findings parallel those in dystrophic muscle.*

Epilepsy

Appleton RE. Epilepsy. Prescribers J 1995; 35: 182–191. *Review. For quality of life see Dev Med Child Neurol 1995; 37: 689–696.*

Barone SR, Kaplan MH, Krilov LR. Human herpesvirus-6 infection in children with first febrile seizures. J Pediatr 1995; 127: 95–97. *Acute HHV-6 infection is a frequent cause of febrile convulsions.*

Benbadis SR, Wolgamuth BR, Goren H et al. Value of tongue biting in the diagnosis of seizures. Arch Int Med 1995; 155: 2346–2349. *Particularly if it is lateral it is highly specific to generalized tonic-clonic seizures.*

Besag FMC, Wallace SJ, Dulac O et al. Lamotrigine for the treatment of epilepsy in childhood. J Pediatr 1995; 127: 991–997. *Lamotrigine is well tolerated and is effective especially for absence seizures and atonic seizures.*

Kieslich M, Jacobi G. Incidence and risk factors of post-traumatic epilepsy in childhood. Lancet 1995; 345: 187. *High incidence of seizures after subdural and subarachnoid haematoma.*

Kuhn BR, Allen KD, Shriver MD. Behavioural management of children's seizure activity. Intervention guidelines for primary-care providers. Clin Pediatr 1995; 34: 570–575. *Review.*

O'Donohoe NV. The EEG and neuroimaging in the management of the epilepsies. Arch Dis Child 1995; 73: 552–557. *Review. For further review see pp. 557–562.*

Rantala H, Uhari M, Hietala J. Factors triggering the first febrile seizure. Acta Paediatr 1995; 84: 407–410. *Those with seizures had a significantly higher temperature than matched controls before hospitalization.*

Schoenenberger RA, Tanasijevic MJ, Jha A et al. Appropriateness of antiepileptic drug level monitoring. J Am Med Ass 1995; 274: 1622–1626. *Only 27% of 10,000 examinations were appropriate.*

Stores G, Zaiwalla Z, Styles E et al. Non-convulsive status epilepticus. Arch Dis Child 1995; 73: 106–111. *Occurs in a variety of epilepsies, especially the Lennox-Gastaut syndrome. Clinical manifestations ranged from obvious mental deterioration to subtle changes.*

OPHTHALMOLOGY

Clark RSB, Orr RA, Atkinson CS et al. Retinal haemorrhages associated with spinal cord arteriovenous malformation. Clin Pediatr 1995; 34: 281–283. *Retinal haemorrhage followed rupture of a spinal cord arteriovenous malformation.*

Cunningham S, Fleck BW, Elton RA et al. Transcutaneous oxygen levels in retinopathy of prematurity. Lancet 1995; 346: 1464–1465. *Variability of transcutaneous oxygen levels in the first two weeks of life is a significant predictor of severe retinopathy.*

ORTHOPAEDICS

Casey ATH, O'Brien M, Kumar V et al. Don't twist my child's head off: iatrogenic cervical dislocation. BMJ 1995; 311: 1212–1213. *Wry neck in children may be due to atlantoaxial subluxation.*

Fink AM, Berman L, Edwards D et al. The irritable hip: immediate ultrasound guided aspiration and prevention of hospital admission. Arch Dis Child 1995; 72: 110–114. *Advocates early aspiration, but lacks follow up data or controls.*

Wong M, Isaacs D, Howman-Giles R et al. Clinical and diagnostic features of osteomyelitis occurring in the first three months of life. Pediatr Infect Dis J 1995; 14: 1047–1053. *Demonstrates the potential diagnostic reliability of radionuclide bone scans.*

Yagupsky P, Bar-Ziv Y, Howard CB et al. Epidemiology, etiology, and clinical features of septic arthritis in children younger than 24 months. Arch Pediatr Adolesc Med 1995; 149: 537–540. *The diagnosis in young children requires a high index of suspicion, and the disease cannot be excluded on the basis of lack of fever or normal results of laboratory tests.*

PSYCHIATRY

Anonymous. The management of hyperactive children. Drug Ther Bull 1995; 33: 57–64. *Review.*

Black D, Newman M. Television violence and children. BMJ 1995; 310: 273–274. *Review. See also Pediatrics 1995; 95: 949–951.*

Carter BD, Edwards JF, Kronenberger WG et al. Case control study of chronic fatigue in pediatric patients. Pediatrics 1995; 95: 179–186. *Some may have treatable psychological conditions.*

DeVile CJ, Sufraz R, Lask BD et al. Occult intracranial tumours masquerading as early onset anorexia nervosa. BMJ 1995; 311: 1359–1360. *Report of 3 cases.*

Hazell P, O'Connell D, Heathcote D et al. Efficacy of tricyclic drugs in treating child and adolescent depression: a meta-analysis. BMJ 1995; 310: 897–901. *No more effective than placebo.*

Kaplan CA, Thompson AE, Searson SM. Cognitive behaviour therapy in children and adolescents. Arch Dis Child 1995; 73: 472–475. *Review.*

Russell J. Treating anorexia nervosa. BMJ 1995; 311: 584 *Review.*

RESPIRATORY

Hakonarson H, Moskovitz J, Daigle KL et al. Pulmonary function abnormalities in Prader-Willi syndrome. J Pediatr 1995; 126: 565–570. *Restrictive ventilatory impairment occurs primarily as a result of respiratory muscle weakness.*

Hanning CD, Alexander-Williams JM. Pulse oximetry: a practical review. BMJ 1995; 311: 367–370. *Review.*

Menon K, Sutcliffe T, Klassen TP. A randomized trial comparing the efficacy of epinephrine with salbutamol in the treatment of acute bronchiolitis. J Pediatr 1995; 126: 1004–1007. *Epinephrine was more effective. See also Arch Pediatr Adolesc Med 1995; 149: 686–692.*

Ninan TK, Macdonald L, Russell G. Persistent nocturnal cough in childhood: a population based study. Arch Dis Child 1995; 73: 403–407. *In those aged 8–13, in the absence of symptoms of asthma, nocturnal cough is likely to be a manifestation of atypical in only a minority.*

Paulson TE, Spear RM, Peterson BM. New concepts in the treatment of children with acute respiratory distress syndrome. J Pediatr 1995; 127: 163–175. *Review.*

Rhodes SK, Shimoda KC, Wald LR et al. Neurocognitive deficits in morbidly obese children with obstructive sleep apnoea. J Pediatr 1995; 127: 741–744. *Affected children with obstructive sleep apnoea had deficits in learning, memory, and vocabulary.*

Rock MJ. The diagnostic utility of bronchoalveolar lavage in immunocompetent children with unexplained infiltrates on chest radiograph. Pediatrics 1995; 95: 373–377. *Bronchoalveolar lavage may yield a diagnosis in patients unresponsive to empiric antibiotic therapy.*

Wilson N, Sloper K, Silverman M. Effect of continuous treatment with topical corticosteroid on episodic viral wheeze in preschool children. Arch Dis Child 1995; 72: 317–320. *No effect on acute episodes of wheeze in this group of children.*

Asthma

Anto JM, Sunyer J. Nitrogen dioxide and allergic asthma: starting to clarify an obscure association. Lancet 1995; 345: 402–403. *Review.*

Barnes PJ. Inhaled glucocorticoids for asthma. N Engl J Med 1995; 332: 868–875. *Review. For single dose prednisone therapy see Pediatrics 1995; 96: 224–229.*

Bien JP, Bloom MD, Evans RL et al. Intravenous theophylline in pediatric status asthmaticus. A prospective, randomized, double-blind, placebo-controlled trial. Clin Pediatr 1995; 34: 475–481. *No benefit in adding theophylline to treatment with methylprednisolone and albuterol for status asthmaticus.*

Burr ML. Pollution: does it cause asthma. Arch Dis Child 1995; 72: 377–387. *Review. See also 73: 418–422.*

Butz AM, Malveaux FJ, Eggleston P et al. Social factors associated with behavioural problems in children with asthma. Clin Pediatr 1995; 34: 581–590. *There is a group of children at risk for behaviour problems, specifically in families that lack adequate social and financial resources. See also Arch Pediatr Adolesc Med 1995; 149: 565–572.*

Choong K, Zwaigenbaum L, Onyett H. Severe varicella after low dose inhaled corticosteroids. Pediatr Infect Dis J 1995; 14: 809–811. *Life threatening chickenpox in child who was on inhaled beclomethasone 5.8 mcg/kg/day. See also BMJ 1995; 310: 327.*

Chou KJ, Cunningham SJ, Crain EF. Metered-dose inhalers with spacers vs nebulizers for pediatric asthma. Arch Pediatr Adolesc Med 1995; 149:

201–205. *Inhalers with spacers may be an effective alternative to nebulizers for treatment of children with acute asthma. For subsensitivity to bronchodilator after salmeterol see Lancet 1995; 346: 201–206.*

Hughes CH, Baumer JH. Moving house: a risk factor for the development of childhood asthma? BMJ 1995; 311: 1069–1070. *A strong association between house moves in families with young children to previously inhabited, centrally heated dwellings and the subsequent development of asthma.*

Johnston SL, Pattemore PK, Sanderson G et al. Community study of role of viral infections in exacerbations of asthma in 9–11 year old children. BMJ 1995; 310: 1225–1229. *Upper respiratory viral infections are associated with 80 to 85% of asthma exacerbations in school age children. For chlamydia as a trigger see Arch Pediatr Adolesc Med 1995; 149: 341–342.*

Jones KP, Mullee MA, Middleton M et al. Peak flow based asthma self-management: a randomised controlled study in general practice. Thorax 1995; 50: 851–857. *Rigid adherence to long term daily peak flow measurement in the management of mild asthma in general practice does not appear to produce large changes in outcomes.*

Martinez FD, Wright AL, Taussig LM et al. Asthma and wheezing in the first six years of life. N Engl Med J 1995; 332: 134–138. *The majority of infants with wheezing have transient conditions and do not have increased risks of asthma. See also pp. 181–182.*

Powell CVE, Primhak RA. Asthma treatment, perceived respiratory disability, and morbidity. Arch Dis Child 1995; 72: 209–213. *Perceived symptoms and morbidity are high in children with diagnosed asthma.*

Robins AW, Lloyd BW. Most consultants deviate from asthma guidelines. BMJ 1995; 311: 508. *Only 21% of British paediatricians use cromoglycate as the first step. See also BMJ 1995; 311: 663–666.*

Svedmyr J, Nyberg E, Asbrink-Nilsson E et al. Intermittent treatment with inhaled steroids for deterioration of asthma due to upper respiratory tract infections. Acta Paediatr 1995; 84: 884–888. *Peak flow was significantly higher with budesonide than with placebo.*

Welliver RC. RSV and chronic asthma. Lancet 1995; 34: 789–790. *Review.*

Zoritch B. Nitric oxide and asthma. Arch Dis Child 1995; 72: 259–262. *Review.*

Cystic fibrosis

Barbero GJ. The undoing of a diagnosis. The effect of a misdiagnosis of a disease. Arch Paediatr Adolesc Med 1995; 149: 1341–1344. *Report of the management and outcome of 18 children in whom cystic fibrosis had been misdiagnosed.*

Eigen H, Rosenstein BJ, FitzSimmons S et al. A multicenter study of alternate-day prednisone therapy in patients with cystic fibrosis. J Pediatr 1995; 126: 515–523. *During the first 24 months the percentage of the predicted forced vital capacity was greater in the 1 mg/kg group and the 2 mg/kg group when each was compared with placebo.*

Konstan MW, Byard PJ, Hoppel CL et al. Effect of high-dose ibuprofen in patients with cystic fibrosis. N Engl J Med 1995; 332: 848–854. *High-dose ibuprofen significantly slows the progression of the lung disease. See also pp. 886–887. For failure of amiloride see Arch Dis Child 1995; 73: 427–430.*

Range SP, Knox AJ. rhDNase in cystic fibrosis. Thorax 1995; 50: 321–322. *Review.*

Croup

Cruz MN, Stewart G, Rosenberg N. Use of dexamethasone in the outpatient management of acute laryngotracheitis. Pediatrics 1995; 96: 220–223. *Reduction in severity of illness within 24 h after treatment.*

Doull I. Corticosteroids in the management of croup. BMJ 1995; 311: 1244. *Nebulised corticosteroids are the treatment of choice.*

RHEUMATOLOGY

Athreya BH. Vasculitis in children. Pediatr Clin North Am 1995; 42: 1239–1261. *Review.*

Cabral DA, Malleson PN, Petty RE. Spondyloarthropathies of childhood. Pediatr Clin North Am 1995; 42: 1051–1069. *Review.*

Cassidy JT, Langman CB, Allen SH et al. Bone mineral metabolism in children with juvenile rheumatoid arthritis. Pediatr Clin North Am 1995; 42: 1017–1033. *Review.*

Giannini EH, Cawkwell GD. Drug treatment in children with juvenile rheumatoid arthritis. Pediatr Clin North Am 1995; 42: 1099–1125. *Review.*

Lehman TJA. A practical guide to systemic lupus erythematosus. Pediatr Clin North Am 1995; 42: 1223–1237. *Review.*

Lloyd-Thomas AR, Lauder G. Reflex sympathetic dystrophy in children. BMJ 1995; 310: 1648–1649. *The features are neuropathic pain and autonomic dysfunction.*

Sansome A, Dubowitz V. Intravenous immunoglobulin in juvenile dermatomyositis – four year review of nine cases. Arch Dis Child 1995; 72: 25–28. *All showed clinical improvement.*

Uziel Y, Laxer RM, Blaser S et al. Cerebral vein thrombosis in childhood systemic lupus erythematosus. J Pediatr 1995; 126: 722–727. *Report of three cases.*

Uziel Y, Miller ML, Laxer RM. Scleroderma in children. Pediatr Clin North Am 1995; 42: 1171–1203. *Review.*

SURGERY

Britton JR, Britton HL. Gastric aspirate volume at birth as an indicator of congenital intestinal obstruction. Acta Paediatr 1995; 84: 945–946. *Neonates with intestinal obstruction have a 10 fold higher gastric aspirate volume at birth.*

Catto-Smith AG, Coffey CMM, Nolan TM et al. Fecal incontinence after the surgical treatment of Hirschsprung disease. J Pediatr 1995; 172: 954–957. *After surgical treatment 53% had significant fecal soiling and 27% less severe soiling.*

Christesen HBT. Prediction of complications following unintentional caustic ingestion in children. Is endoscopy always necessary? Acta Paediatr 1995; 84: 1177–1182. *Children who are non-symptomatic are not at risk of complications and do not need endoscopic examination.*

Hall PA, Payne JF, Stack CG et al. Parents in the recovery room: survey of parental and staff attitudes. BMJ 1995; 310: 163–164. *Most parents wanted to be there; their presence was judged to be helpful in 98% once the staff became used to the idea.*

Kelly DA, Buckels JAC. The future of small bowel transplantation. Arch Dis Child 1995; 72: 447–451. *Review.*

Najmaldin A. Minimal access surgery in paediatrics. Arch Dis Child 1995; 72: 106–109. *Review.*

Samuel M, Burge DM, Griffiths DM. Gastric volvulus and associated gastro-oesophageal reflux. Arch Dis Child 1995; 73: 462–464. *Common features at presentation were episodic colicky abdominal pain, non-bilious vomiting, upper abdominal distension, haematemesis, and failure to thrive.*

THERAPEUTICS

Anonymous. Managing acute pain in children. Drug Ther Bull 1995; 33: 41–44. *Review.*

Anonymous. Managing chronic pain in children. Drug Ther Bull 1995; 33: 52–55. *Review.*

Birkebaek NH, Esberg G, Andersen K et al. Bone and collagen turnover during treatment with inhaled dry powder budesonide and beclomethasone dipropionate. Arch Dis Child 1995; 73: 524–527. *The suppression of bone and collagen turnover seems to be more marked during treatment with beclomethasone dipropionate.*

Committee on Drugs. Treatment guidelines for lead exposure in children. Pediatrics 1995; 96: 155–160. *Review.*

Mackie IC. Children's dental health and medicines that contain sugar. BMJ 1995; 311: 141–142. *Review. For sugar free paracetomol see BMJ 1995; 311: 362.*

Tramer M, Moore A, McQuay H. Prevention of vomiting after paediatric strabismus surgery: a systematic review using the numbers-needed-to-treat method. Br J Anaesth 1995; 75: 556–561. *For droperidol, four children have to be given the drug to prevent one vomiting; the benefits of this and other agents is unproven.*

Index